Societies of Wolves and Free-ranging Dogs

Wolves are charismatic emblems of wilderness. Dogs, which descended from wolves, are models of urbanity. Do free-ranging dogs revert to pack living, or are their societies only reminiscent of a wolfish heritage?

Focusing on behavioral ecology, this is the first book to assess societies of both gray wolves and domestic dogs living as urban strays and in the feral state. It provides a comprehensive review of wolf genetics, particularly of New World wolves and their confusing admixture of wolf, coyote, and dog genomes. Spotte draws on the latest scientific findings across the specialized fields of genetics, sensory biology, reproductive physiology, space use, foraging ecology, and socialization. This interdisciplinary approach provides a solid foundation for a startling and original comparison of the social lives of wolves and free-ranging dogs.

Supplementary material, including a full glossary of terms, is available online at www.cambridge.org/9781107015197.

Stephen Spotte is a marine scientist with research and field experience ranging from the Arctic to the Amazon basin. He has been curator or director of three US public aquariums, was a research scientist at the Marine Sciences and Technology Center, University of Connecticut, and is presently Adjunct Scientist at Mote Marine Laboratory in Sarasota, Florida.

Societies of Wolves
and Free-ranging Dogs

STEPHEN SPOTTE

Mote Marine Laboratory
Sarasota, Florida

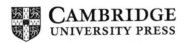
CAMBRIDGE
UNIVERSITY PRESS

CAMBRIDGE
UNIVERSITY PRESS

University Printing House, Cambridge CB2 8BS, United Kingdom

One Liberty Plaza, 20th Floor, New York, NY 10006, USA

477 Williamstown Road, Port Melbourne, VIC 3207, Australia

314-321, 3rd Floor, Plot 3, Splendor Forum, Jasola District Centre, New Delhi - 110025, India

79 Anson Road, #06-04/06, Singapore 079906

Cambridge University Press is part of the University of Cambridge.

It furthers the University's mission by disseminating knowledge in the pursuit of education, learning and research at the highest international levels of excellence.

www.cambridge.org
Information on this title: www.cambridge.org/9781107656086

© S. Spotte 2012

First published 2012

A catalogue record for this publication is available from the British Library

ISBN 978-1-107-01519-7 Hardback
ISBN 978-1-107-65608-6 Paperback

Additional resources for this publication at www.cambridge.org/9781107015197

For my grandsons
Nicholas, Jacob, Oscar, and Adler
May friendly barks accompany you

There are some authors who have thought that dogs and wolves are one kind: namely, that vulgar dogs are tame wolves and that ravening wolves are wild dogs.

Edward Topsell, *Historie of Four-footed Beastes* (1607)

Contents

Preface   *page* xi
Acknowledgments   xv
List of abbreviations   xvi

1   What makes a wolf   1

1.1   Wolves in the beginning   1
1.2   Modern wolves   2
1.3   Great Lakes wolf   4
1.4   Red wolf   8
1.5   Eastern coyote   12
1.6   The color of wolves   15

2   What makes a dog   19

2.1   Domestication   19
2.2   Early dogs   21
2.3   Coydogs and wolfdogs   26
2.4   Dingoes   30

3   Visual and tactile communication   33

3.1   Metaphors and semiotics   33
3.2   Signal and response   38
3.3   Agonistic behavior   40
3.4   The physiological stress response   42
3.5   Visual and tactile signaling   43

4   Olfactory and vocal communication   59

4.1   Odor and pheromone reception   59
4.2   Scent-marking   66
4.3   Vocalization   73
4.4   Wolf howls   83

5   Space   90

5.1   Use of space   90
5.2   Territorial disputes   95
5.3   Pack dynamics   96
5.4   Natural controls on wolf populations   99
5.5   Painting the social fence   105
5.6   Space use by free-ranging dogs   107

6   Foraging   119

6.1   Wolves as predators   119
6.2   Competitors of wolves   130
6.3   Wolves hunting and scavenging   131
6.4   Prey selection by wolves   137
6.5   The dilemma of cooperative hunting   141
6.6   Foraging by free-ranging dogs   142

7   Courtship and conception   150

7.1   The reproductive cycle – part 1   150
7.2   Courtship in owned dogs   158
7.3   Courtship in free-ranging dogs   163
7.4   Courtship in wolves   167

8   Reproduction and parenting   174

8.1   The reproductive cycle – part 2   174
8.2   Wolf dens and rendezvous sites   182
8.3   Dens and rendezvous sites of free-ranging dogs   186
8.4   Wolf litters   187
8.5   Free-ranging dog litters   190
8.6   Helping and the altruism dilemma   193

9   Socialization   205

9.1   The socialization sequence   205
9.2   Play and bonding   212
9.3   Confinement and social order in wolves   221
9.4   Dominance in free-ranging dogs   227
9.5   Leadership   229
9.6   Dingoes   234

Notes   239
References   312
Index   362

Preface

Behavior and ecology are "two sides of the same coin,"[1] a viewpoint I endorse and use in this brief essay on the social lives of wolves and free-ranging dogs. My goal has been to write a timely, simple, relevant book. Timely with current research findings, simple in minimizing technical information, and relevant by deepening our understanding of wolves and of dogs that run loose in a contentious world of shrinking spaces.

The wolves discussed include gray wolves (*Canis lupus*) and their admixtures: the Great Lakes wolf (including the Algonquin wolf) and the red wolf, more aptly named red coyote. When referring to first-generation wolf × domestic dog admixtures I use wolfdog; coydog is the term applied when the first-generation offspring are progeny of coyotes (*Canis latrans*) and domestic dogs. A free-ranging dog is any dog of domestic origin uncontrolled by humans and includes truly feral animals like dingoes, rural and urban strays, and wandering pets. Dingoes that have interbred with domestic dogs are known as wild canids or wild dogs in Australia, but to keep things consistent I refer to their first-generation offspring as dingo-dogs. Although not entirely logical (both are actually domestic dogs), the term has a pleasing sound when spoken aloud.

Why focus on free-ranging dogs and exclude those with owners? Because only dogs living in partial or complete independence from humans offer insight into how their societies function ecologically. With few exceptions these animals today exist at the peripheries of human societies, passing through almost unnoticed. The wolf literature, although vast and comprehensive, is a honeycomb of specialties. Wolves gave rise to domestic dogs and yet few studies have placed the two side by side and compared social aspects of their behavioral ecology. My objective is to do this, bringing to light some of the biology underlying societies of wolves and free-ranging dogs.

In the interest of scholarship I seldom cite unrefereed, or "gray," literature (e.g. federal and state government reports) and undocumented statements from books and websites. I also omit mention of popular books with certain exceptions, notably Adolph Murie's groundbreaking *The Wolves of Mount McKinley*, Lois Crisler's extraordinary memoir *Arctic Wild*, and the remarkable account of L. David Mech titled *The Arctic Wolf: Living with the Pack*. All offer rare insight into how wolves live in nature, information not available elsewhere.

These classics bear out a singular truth: that intense observation of wild animals shifts their social lives into clearer focus while paradoxically extending our distance from them.

What follows is more narrative than text, the chapter titles low barriers erected to intermittently disrupt and redirect the flow of information. Canid evolution, and that of domestic dogs in particular, has been remarkably messy, and this story of their heritage and societies as I tell it might seem similarly eclectic. There are no chapters labeled behavior, evolution, and so forth as if these categories were not congeries and could somehow teeter along in isolation. Attempting to establish arbitrary classifications at any level implies the capacity to pry apart and reassemble nature in convenient pieces. Like a dog's genes, what I have to say has been unavoidably mixed and integrated.

Wolf genetics is a turbulent sea of confusion. Nowhere except in a limited region of southeastern Canada and the contiguous United States have so many forms of the genus *Canis* coexisted in the recent past, and nowhere else is their collective heritage quite so muddled. Attempting to sort out how these different lineages and populations admixed and their behavior adapted to changing prey and landscapes can offer fascinating insights. The genetic composition of a wolf, coyote, or dog has bearing on how it looks and interacts with its own kind, others closely related to it, or with us, including whether or not we consider it worth protecting. In the absence of such knowledge we have only breeders' manuals, pedigree registries, and nature television, sources revealing what wolves and dogs have become but little about how they arrived. Before describing what an animal does, understanding what it is seems a useful prelude.

To keep matters clear I largely ignore the idea of subspecies except in historical usage. Consistent with this I treat dingoes as free-ranging dogs and the New Guinea singing dog as a dingo.[2] All are derived lineages of *Canis lupus* (domestic dogs and gray wolves share 99.8% of their mitochondrial DNA).[3] As one researcher wrote: "Dogs are gray wolves, despite their diversity in size and proportion."[4] Improbable as it seems, that includes the Pekingese mincing toward you with a bow on its head and wearing a form-fitted jacket.[5] I omit discussion of two wild dogs only distantly related to the wolf and its immediate descendants. The dhole (*Cuon alpinus*) split from the rest of the dogs about 7.6 million years ago[6] and is actually more closely related to the jackals. The African wild dog (*Lycaon pictus*) occupies an even more basal place in canid evolution.[7]

References have been relegated to endnotes along with parenthetical and explanatory information I felt interrupted the text. No doubt some readers will whine about this decision, even bark or howl. To help overcome the anxiety and exhaustive effort of paging back and forth I recommend a bookmark. References and notes constitute part of a book's structure, not its narrative, just as the image in a painting can be viewed and assessed satisfactorily without examining the brush strokes.

Terms that appear in italics are defined in the text, others in the endnotes, but definitions of all can be found in the online glossary (see back cover) with two exceptions: descriptions of visual and haptic agonistic behaviors are summarized in Table 3.1, acoustical characterizations of wolf vocalizations in Table 4.2. I felt a detailed glossary was necessary to assure readers that terms and concepts introduced are subsequently applied and discussed as defined, and because the subject matter straddles several specialties each with its own vocabulary. Overall, my intention was to make things easier for general readers or those who might be specialists in one field but not the others. I kept graphs and tables to a minimum and decided that color photographs were unnecessary. The world contains many beautiful pictures of canids, and their addition would not have enhanced what I have to say. As Sartre told us, "Images are fleeting, blurred, individual; they reflect our particularity. But words are social, they universalize."

The behavior of social animals such as wolves and dogs is largely about communication. Attempts at identifying and classifying their interactions often leads to questions posed by linguistics, which are suited only to humans. How does animal communication function in a social context (pragmatics), and what could communication actually "mean" to the animals themselves (semantics)? As I discuss, such links remain unconnected in every species except our own. Language *is* us, and in trying to determine what animals do we have lots of description available and limited enlightenment.

The insistence that behavior and biology are inseparable might seem frustrating to those who measure only behavior's visible aspects. However, mechanism underlies expression at every level, and behaviorists ignore this truth at their peril. So-called "cognitive" studies are misnamed when the variables are limited to cognition's outward displays; that is, when the observer describes a result and ignores the cause. Observation alone offers limited explanatory power if its goal is understanding how and why animals behave as they do. Exceptions arise in restricted contexts (e.g. ecology) where behavior becomes a dependent variable used to evaluate larger effects. I discuss some situations in which observation's cloudy lens has adequate resolving power (e.g. prey switching, habitat-biased dispersal), helping explain why if not how.

Progress in understanding the social behavior of wolves and dogs has been slow and hesitant, stymied in part by an inability to divorce our own probable responses from those of the subjects. Linking a dog's whine with *what seems to us* is frustration, yelp *with what surely must be* fear because a comparable signal would be fearful to us, is not a fruitful approach. Solid experimental designs should prevent conclusions from overreaching the data, but research has always been compromised by the difficulty of keeping our self-awareness suitably distant from the phenomenal consciousness of our subjects. The footprints of human bias contaminate the best experiments. We measure the howls of wolves and barks of dogs acoustically, count scent-marks, and try to determine context in a wolf's stare, but in the end any interpretations seldom pass beyond conjecture. These and similar phenomena present themselves as abducent ghosts not yet unanchored in biology and therefore unexplained or coherently explainable. Animals exist in realms we can barely penetrate as tourists, much less scientists. As N. Kathryn Hayles wrote, "If every species constructs for itself a different world, which is the world?"

Stephen Spotte
Mote Marine Laboratory
Sarasota, Florida

Acknowledgments

I thank Michael Spotte for advice and assistance with the graphics, Charles W. Radcliffe and Patrick W. Concannon for stimulating conversations about canids, and authors and editors who allowed me to reproduce illustrations from their published work. As always, thanks to the staff of the Marine Biological Laboratory-Woods Hole Institution of Oceanography Library, Woods Hole, Massachusetts.

Abbreviations

AOB	accessory olfactory bulb
AOS	accessory olfactory system
BISF	Beltrami Island State Forest
BMR	basal metabolic rate
DAP	dog-appeasing pheromone
ESS	evolutionarily stable strategy
FLU	flexed-leg urination
FSH	follicle-stimulating hormone
GnRH	gonadotropin-releasing hormone
LH	luteinizing hormone
MHC	major histocompatibility complex
MOB	main olfactory bulb
MOE	main olfactory epithelium
MOS	main olfactory system
mRNA	messenger RNA
mtDNA	mitochondrial DNA
ORs	odorant receptors
RLU	raised-leg urination
SNF	Superior National Forest
SNPs	single-nucleotide polymorphisms
SQA	squat-urination
STU	standing-urination
TAARs	trace amine-associated receptors
TRs	taste receptors
VNO	vomeronasal organ
VRs	vomeronasal receptors

1   What makes a wolf

The zoological order Carnivora includes the canids. When discussing its members the term *carnivoran* is preferable to carnivore because it excludes unrelated predators.[1] Modern canids appeared about 10 million years before the present (years BP) and diverged into two branches, the dogs and the foxes.[2] Depending on how you divide them, living canids number about 35 species.[3] They have 78 *chromosomes*, and all are known to *admix*.[4] The golden jackal (*Canis aureus*) and gray wolf (*Canis lupus*) have been considered the domestic dog's possible ancestors,[5] and although all evidence points to the gray wolf,[6] some raise other possibilities, such as an extinct and unknown wolf-like canid.[7] Two of these are the dingo and a hypothetical and now extinct wild dog similar to the dingo.[8] The next closest relatives of gray wolves and domestic dogs are the coyote and Ethiopian wolf (*Canis simensis*), less accurately called the Simien jackal.[9] As later chapters should help clarify, implications of these relationships reach out from the past, affecting the behavior and social lives of all members of the genus *Canis*, including the domestic dogs we keep as pets.

1.1   Wolves in the beginning

The family Canidae (*Canis* means dog in Latin) evolved in North America, first appearing in the late *Miocene* 6 million years BP.[10] When North America and Asia formed a high-latitude connection in the late *Cenozoic* (3 million years BP) some canids migrated across, where they continued to evolve, and one returned later as the gray wolf.[11] The record infers that North American wolves and the coyote separated about 1–2 million years BP,[12] although genetic findings point to the gray wolf's origin being only 250 000 years BP.[13] According to a slightly different hypothesis, the gray wolf might have evolved in Asia and migrated to North America about 300 000 years BP across the Bering land bridge when sea levels were lower than today.[14]

   At one time the gray wolf was the world's most widely distributed carnivoran,[15] ranging from Portugal to Siberia and throughout the Arctic, south into the Arabian peninsula and the rest of the Middle East, from the Himalayas to the Indian peninsular plains, and east into China.[16] Before Europeans arrived gray wolves could be found nearly everywhere in North America, from the Arctic deep into

Mexico. The exception was the southeastern US, thought by some to be occupied by an animal with relict descendants known today as the red wolf (*C. rufus*),[17] although this is doubtful (Section 1.4).

On the central plains modern ancestors of today's wolves preyed on American bison (*Bison bison*), toward the north and into Canada on moose (*Alces alces*), caribou (*Rangifer tarandus*), and elk (*Cervus canadensis*), and elsewhere on antelope, wild sheep and wild goats, and various species of deer. To European settlers wolves were vermin. Fur trappers, bounty hunters, farmers, government poisoning programs, and, it seems, any citizen with a gun, eventually killed them off,[18] sparing a few survivors in national parks and remote regions unsuited to human habitation or exploitation. The unfortunate experience of Old World wolves is similar and started much earlier.[19]

The opening of the North American landscape by European immigrants and their descendants altered ecosystems, making them better habitats for rodents, rabbits, and other small mammals, the principal prey of the coyote, which is indigenous to North America.[20] Before 1850 coyotes occupied an area west of the Mississippi River into the Sierra Nevada Mountains and California, south into Mexico, and north into Alberta.[21] Today their latitudinal range from Central America to northern Alaska exceeds that of any other terrestrial mammal.[22]

This rapid expansion began early in the twentieth century in conjunction with the sharp decline in wolf *populations* brought about by "predator control," clearing forests for timber and agriculture, and human competition for large game.[23] The coyote is smaller and less conspicuous than the wolf. It requires less space,[24] lives in flexible societies,[25] is comfortable near humans in urban and suburban areas,[26] scavenges efficiently,[27] and can exist on small prey[28] adapted to disturbed habitats.[29] Wolves often prefer forested areas, coyotes open spaces.[30] As the wolves and forests disappeared the coyotes moved in, and in the east they took up living in wooded areas too.[31]

Although fluid dispersal of a species is not a guarantee of rapid gene flow, mobility heightens the likelihood of genetic exchange.[32] The consequence can be surprisingly small genetic variations among broadly dispersed populations. Coyotes have a more diverse *genotype* than wolves[33] brought about by an astonishing capacity to disperse and high gene flow through their populations. A survey of 327 coyotes revealed 32 genotypes and a gene flow so rapid that today's coyotes are moving quickly toward homogenization.[34] The same genotypes, for example, have been recovered from animals as widely dispersed as California and Florida.[35] Nonetheless, genetic evidence shows US coyotes to still cluster in three major groups: western, Midwest/southeast, and northeast.[36]

1.2   Modern wolves

The gray wolf's extensive range gave rise to regional variations in morphology. Dozens of scientific names (many of them synonyms) have been ascribed historically based on coat color, size, skull morphology, geographic distribution, and

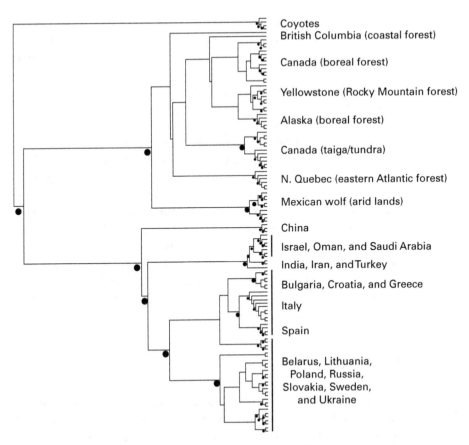

Figure 1.1 Neighbor-joining cladogram for non-admixed wolf populations using a 48 000 SNP data set. Dots show >95% bootstrap support of 1000 replicates. *Source*: vonHoldt *et al.* (2011).

other aspects of natural history and physical appearance.[37] Until recently the high tendencies of wolves to disperse have called into question any notion of long-term restriction to particular localities and subsequent speciation. North American gray wolves have been known to disperse hundreds of kilometers in a few months.[38] Identical genotypes appear in specimens from northeastern Minnesota and Inuvik in Canada's Northwest Territories (3100 km), and from Montana to Nome, Alaska (3600 km).[39] Dispersal distances of Old World wolves are equally impressive (Chapter 5).[40]

Nonetheless, as demonstrated by Bridgett M. vonHoldt and co-authors, gray wolves worldwide, like coyotes in North America, cluster regionally (Fig. 1.1) as assessed using *single-nucleotide polymorphisms (SNPs)*.[41] Partial explanations include habitat-biased dispersal (Chapter 6) and *genetic drift* caused by habitat fragmentation, forcing of wolves into isolated pockets over centuries of persecution.[42] Genetic variability, which is essential for healthy populations, is reduced by discontinuous habitats and low population numbers.[43]

The two populations of wolves in India appear to be genetically unique.[44] A group of about 350 individuals (called here the Indian Himalayan wolf) inhabits the Trans-Himalayan region spanning India's two northernmost states.[45] The other, numbering about 1500 (here called the Indian plains wolf), is found on the arid and semi-arid plains of peninsular India. Both show strong within-group *homogeneity* in having unique *haplotypes* and clustering separately from all other gray wolves including the nearest geographic populations. The Indian Himalayan wolf clustered separately from so-called Tibetan wolves; the Indian plains wolf formed a separate cluster from the so-called Middle Eastern wolf.[46] They appear to be distinct with no overlap in haplotypes with other gray wolves around the world.[47] This population "was found always to be basal to the other major clade comprising all other wolf haplotypes and closest to the jackal, one of the closest ancestral canid species, suggesting them to be the derivatives of a more ancient independent wolf radiation."[48] By this assessment, Indian wolves are the most divergent of the gray wolves, representing a relic ancestral lineage long isolated.[49] If so, their genetic composition could be evidence that wolf-like canids first evolved in Asia. The authors of this study proposed giving them full species status, *Canis himalayensis*[50] and *C. indica*.

1.3   Great Lakes wolf

The heritage of wolves in southeastern Canada and the northcentral and north-eastern United States, already complicated, got moreso in the early 1900s shortly after most wolves had been exterminated and coyotes began expanding east through the Great Lakes states into Ontario.[51] Coyotes were historically restricted to the US south and southwest. Their simultaneous movement into other western regions appears not to have affected the genetics of western gray wolves (see below).[52] Relationships among the canids discussed here and in the next two sections are summarized diagrammatically in Fig. 1.2.

By 1975, before availability of modern molecular techniques, researchers recognized four "races," or "types," of Ontario wolves based on skull morphology: (1) a large, conventional-looking gray wolf (*Canis lupus hudsonicus*) in the northern reaches occupying subarctic *tundra*; (2) a similar animal (*Canis lupus lycaon*) in the boreal forest around Hudson Bay and called the "Ontario type;" (3) a wolf resembling (2) from deciduous forests of the upper Great Lakes (also designated *Canis lupus lycaon*) and called the "Algonquin type"; and (4) a purported *admixture* between the "Algonquin type" and western coyotes called the *Tweed wolf*.[53]

North American wolves had undergone several prior taxonomic revisions based on morphology,[54] but this one stood up well to later genetic testing.[55] An animal from Québec described originally by Johann Christian Daniel von Schreber in 1775 as a separate species (*Canis lycaon*)[56] and later by others as a subspecies of gray wolf (*C. lupus lycaon*)[57] was thought to be synonymous with the "Algonquin type," which supposedly evolved in North America. If true, this

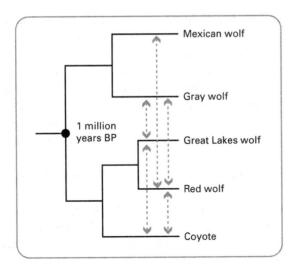

Figure 1.2 Joining tree showing hypothetical admixing (dashed lines) among North American canids.
Source: vonHoldt *et al.* (2011).

would make it North America's only endemic wolf, the ancestors of all others having immigrated from Eurasia. Applicable synonyms are *eastern wolf, eastern timber wolf*, and *eastern Canadian wolf*. Its descendants today, remnants of a unique population in existence before the arrival of Europeans, reside in *Algonquin Provincial Park*, Ontario, and the immediate surrounding area[58] separated by its unique C1 *mitochondrial DNA (mtDNA)* haplotype[59] and an apparent shared ancestry with western coyotes.[60] Return of this population to full species status as *C. lycaon* has been advocated.[61] Whether or not it happens remains to be seen. I doubt whether any admixed canid can properly be labeled a species, the obvious gradation in genomic composition making even the use of "coyote" and "wolf" problematical. Meanwhile, I use *Algonquin wolf* when referring specifically to descendants of the extinct lineage.

The historical range of wolves in central and eastern regions of the US and Canada included Québec, Ontario, parts of Manitoba, the western Great Lakes states (Minnesota, Wisconsin, Michigan), New York, Pennsylvania, New Hampshire, and Vermont.[62] Those occupying the Great Lakes region today (including Algonquin Provincial Park) form a genetically admixed[63] population of western gray wolves, coyotes, and traces of the extinct endemic wolf,[64] and collectively called *Great Lakes wolves*. This heritage separates them from gray wolves occupying the American and Canadian west and Eurasia.

Great Lakes wolves diverge noticeably in appearance from gray wolves, distinguished by: (1) smaller size, (2) darker color (generally gray with dark back and pale undersides grading into fawn-gray), (3) slender rostrum, and (4) long ears relative to body size.[65] In his 1944 review, Edward A. Goldman noted presciently, "Specimens from the Great Lakes region represent a wide range of individual variation in size and cranial details, and grade toward the more robust plains [gray] wolf."[66] Morphology and modern genetics validate his statement: today's admixture, as just noted, carries a heritage of western gray wolves and descendants of historical (i.e. endemic) wolves from the east that retain a coyote heritage.[67] It represents a genotypic/phenotypic cline, coyote-like toward its eastern limit (to about 50%) and increasingly wolf-like (to nearly 100% gray wolf) toward the west.[68] The *genomes* of Great Lakes wolves average about 15% coyote ancestry and >84% wolf, but the Algonquin wolves are 42% coyote, the most of any in the Great Lakes population.[69]

The Great Lakes wolf's smaller size probably explains both its history of breeding with coyotes[70] and confusion about its origin. Through the years it has been considered: (1) a distinct and valid species,[71] (2) a subspecies of gray wolf,[72] (3) a gray wolf × red wolf admixture,[73] (4) a gray wolf × coyote admixture,[74] (5) an admixture of coyote × Algonquin wolf,[75] (6) an admixture of gray wolf × coyote × Algonquin wolf,[76] (7) a smaller gray wolf *ecotype*,[77] (8) *conspecific* with the red wolf (Section 1.4) and both derived from a coyote-like ancestor,[78] (9) a wolf admixture of unknown heritage,[79] and (10) a gray wolf × Algonquin wolf admixture.[80] Hypotheses (6) and (10) are little different because a large part of the Algonquin wolf's genome is coyote. The large wolf component relative to coyote in Great Lakes wolves toward the west suggests extensive crossing back of offspring with wolves but not coyotes.

Admixing between coyotes and gray wolves around the Great Lakes is not entirely a result of coyote encroachment starting early in the twentieth century.[81] Genetic evidence shows the process occurring 546–963 years BP, prior to when Europeans arrived and disturbed the landscape.[82] Pre-Columbian remnants of coyotes have been found in Ontario, Maryland, and Pennsylvania;[83] as mentioned, ancient coyote mtDNA is still detectable in Great Lakes wolf haplotypes.[84] Remains of an extinct coyote-like canid from Québec (400–500 years BP) demonstrates earlier eastern occupation and overlap with wolves now extinct.[85] Coyotes later disappeared from these areas,[86] their descendants not moving north and east again until humans cut down the forests and killed the resident wolves.

Gray wolf × coyote admixtures are notably absent from northern and western North America.[87] Because mtDNA is inherited only from the maternal lineage, the absence in coyotes of gray wolf mtDNA means that female gray wolf × male coyote crosses either do not occur or the progeny fail to integrate into coyote populations.[88] In addition, western gray wolves commonly kill coyotes where the two are *sympatric*, and any close interaction is likely to be tense and unfriendly (Chapter 6). Whereas gray wolves make war on coyotes (Chapter 6), Great Lakes wolves make love to them. Thus gray wolves rarely mate with coyotes, but Great Lakes wolves, by being admixtures, do. As one group of collaborators wrote: "The absence of a Canis [genetic] soup in western North America appears to be attributed to the absence of *C. lycaon* [the Great Lakes wolf], which easily hybridizes with coyotes and can hybridize with gray wolves, thus mediating gene flow among the 3 species."[89] In contrast, coyote genes in Mexican gray wolves, which once ranged into the American southwest and were recently reintroduced there,[90] are barely detectable as genetic background noise.[91] The Mexican wolf is a gray wolf, and its historical reproductive isolation from coyotes is not surprising.

Goldman pointed out the slender muzzles of eastern specimens, their generally small size but grading toward the larger gray wolf, and a resemblance to the red wolf.[92] As mentioned, some authorities see the Great Lakes wolf simply as a gray wolf ecotype or admixture; others disagree and consider it unique. The longitudinal and latitudinal variety expressed by gray wolves inspired several subspecies descriptions. Such variation is common in wolves everywhere,[93] even regions of restricted space. Israel is slightly smaller than New Jersey, extending 418 km at its greatest length. Its northern climate is Mediterranean, and wolves there were historically larger and darker than those inhabiting the arid south.[94] The southern wolves, in adapting to desert conditions, have become smaller, pallid, and able to withstand dry conditions, having been sighted 50 km from the closest source of water.[95]

The Great Lakes wolf genome persists despite rigorous three-way gene flow with *eastern coyotes* (Section 1.5) in the eastern part of its range and gray wolves toward the west.[96] Where admixing with gray wolves it grows bigger.[97] As mentioned, Great Lakes wolves indigenous to Algonquin Provincial Park and vicinity differ genetically from other Great Lakes wolves, and to some authorities this warrants its return to species status as *C. lycaon*.[98] Proponents have argued that the lack of gray wolf mtDNA[99] in pelts of two 1880s wolves, one killed in New York State and the other in Maine, weakens the hypothesis of gray wolf × coyote crosses and strengthens the argument for a North American origin of the Great Lakes wolf (specifically the Algonquin wolf) and its place as a unique historical entity.[100] Whatever the case, the Great Lakes wolf's propensity to interbreed with coyotes is ancient, extensive, and admixing continues.[101]

The percentage of wolves (including gray wolves) carrying coyote genotypes increases from west to east, from zero in Alaska[102] to about 50% in Minnesota and 100% in Québec,[103] but the disparity narrows at latitudes north of central Ontario and Québec. As a result of admixing, the wolves in southern Québec are more similar genetically to Maine eastern coyotes than to other wolves, and gray wolves in northern Québec and Alaska's Kenai Peninsula (4000 km) are more closely related (the *genetic distance* is less) than wolves spanning northern and southern Québec (400 km) are to each other.[104]

Mechanisms perpetuating admixing in these populations are largely unknown. One could be disintegration of the "species recognition barrier" through long-term *introgression* of foreign genes.[105] Viewed from this perspective, the Great Lakes wolf has lost crucial behavioral tools that allowed its gray wolf ancestors to recognize their own kind and reject those unlike them.[106] With continued admixing came a blending and attenuation of species-specific behaviors leading eventually to familiarity.

1.4   Red wolf

Another North American canid, the so-called red wolf, now enters this confusing picture. Admixing with coyotes started 287–430 years BP,[107] well within the time of European occupation and raising the possibility that the red wolf might once have been a distinct genomic entity. Disturbance of the ecosystem that followed culminated in fewer gray wolves and more coyotes. Crossing back of offspring after the initial admixing was predominantly into the coyote population, perhaps because wolves became too scarce,[108] eventually diluting what wolf genes remained. The genome of today's red wolf is 75–80% coyote (Fig. 1.3),[109] calling for a name change to red coyote.

By 1975 admixtures known as red wolves had reached near extinction from interbreeding with coyotes, their range contracted to a few contiguous counties in Louisiana and Texas.[110] The remaining animals were captured in the mid-1970s, and 14 appearing to match the red wolf phenotype – as judged by looking at them – were selected for captive breeding as a "founder" population. Genetic testing was not available at the time, and looks can be deceiving. Twelve of 77 animals captured for the project from 1974 to 1976 and tested years later contained a gray wolf mtDNA haplotype. Of these, one had been identified originally as a red wolf, four as coyotes, and six as admixtures.[111] The initial selection process turned out to be irrelevant. Examination of museum skins of red wolves killed between 1905

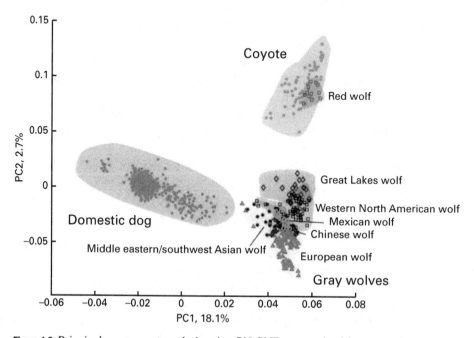

Figure 1.3 Principal component analysis using 710 SNPs ascertained by comparing the dog genome sequence (vonHoldt *et al.* 2010) with that of wolves and the coyote. *Source*: vonHoldt *et al.* (2011).

and 1930 revealed only coyote and gray wolf genotypes.[112] As a result, "captive bred animals are a faithful genetic representation of animals that once lived in the wild and can justifiably be used as a source for reintroduction."[113] That the red wolf was ever a separate species is doubtful. There are now about 100 of them in the wild and many more in captivity across the US. Progeny of the 14 founders were released into eastern North Carolina in 1987,[114] and to the dismay of government biologists they quickly started mating with the local coyotes.[115]

Few would dispute that red wolves carry both wolf and coyote genes or that extant red wolves and coyotes continue to admix.[116] Red wolf vocalizations are apparently distinctive, neither wolf nor coyote but somewhere between,[117] although closer to the coyote's.[118] Red wolves eat like coyotes, focusing on small prey and neither animal declining any known food group. Stomach analyses of specimens killed in the 1930s included rodents, rabbits, birds, carrion, bird eggs, insects, spiders, crayfish, and plant material (e.g. mesquite beans, cactus fruits, persimmons).[119] A list of coyote diets at Lava Beds National Monument (northern California) in the 1930s was similar: rodents, rabbits, birds of more than a dozen species (including domestic turkeys), carrion, bird eggs, insects, badgers, domestic cats (*Felis catus*), reptiles (lizards and snakes), and plant material (grass, apples, wild cherries, gooseberries).[120]

Eight hypotheses have purported to explain the red wolf's origin and status as: (1) a distinct and valid species,[121] (2) a coyote × gray wolf admixture[122] of mostly coyote heritage,[123] (3) a valid species prior to its genome having been diluted by coyotes in recent history,[124] (4) a descendant of a now extinct species of gray wolf,[125] (5) descended along with coyotes from a common ancestor without admixture with gray wolves,[126] (6) a subspecies of gray wolf,[127] (7) the original ancestor of the gray wolf and coyote,[128] and (8) conspecific with the Great Lakes wolf and both derived from a coyote-like ancestor.[129] We now know that (2) is valid, and the red wolf is now – and probably always has been – a coyote × gray wolf admixture without unique genetic components.[130]

A report favoring (8) argued that eastern wolves and red wolves diverged from the coyote line about 150 000–300 000 years BP.[131] The authors proposed synonymy of red and Great Lakes wolves (specifically the Algonquin wolf) and granting the merged entity full species status as *C. lycaon*, this name having taxonomic priority over *C. rufus*.[132] Thus a case was made for the Algonquin wolf and red wolf being the same animal.[133] Additional indirect support of a common origin comes from possible intersecting or overlapping historical ranges.[134] More recent research demonstrates that Great Lakes and red wolves are genetically distinct and unlikely to have shared a common origin: red wolves show close affinity with coyotes, Great Lakes and Mexican wolves more closely resemble North American gray wolves.[135] As mentioned, the genomes of Great Lakes wolves average about 15% coyote ancestry; in red wolves ancestral coyote averages more than three-quarters of the genome.

A major problem for the red wolf as a stand-alone species has been that unlike the gray wolf, Mexican gray wolf, and coyote it has no separate *genetic markers*, no ancient remnant suggesting it was ever unique.[136] If it is now – or ever had been – a separate species there should be genetic material in its lineages distinct from former or current sympatric canids, but none has so far been found.[137] All 14 red wolf "founders," for example, contained a genotype identical to that occurring in Louisiana coyotes.[138]

As mentioned, the red wolf's lineage reveals no history prior to the arrival of Europeans, making it so young that evident mutations have not accumulated since admixing commenced.[139] Nor could the red wolf be a subspecies of the gray wolf. By definition, a subspecies shares special character traits, which red wolves do not.[140] Moreover, the high gene flow that seems standard among canids probably would have engulfed emerging red wolves in a sea of gray wolf and coyote genotypes.[141] Signs of reproductive isolation based on behavioral recognition disappeared long ago, if they ever existed.

The red wolf's convenient size might make breeding easier with both coyotes and gray wolves, thus abetting admixture.[142] Skull comparisons show many putative red wolves to be intermediate between gray wolves and coyotes.[143] Accepting this as indirect evidence of genetic separation requires circular reasoning, because the morphologies of admixtures are typically intermediate.[144] Poor correlation between morphological and mtDNA findings is additional evidence of a muddled inheritance.[145] The red wolf, in other words, is more a mongrel than its nearest relatives, its heritage a blend of genes, a situation that in no way lessens its importance as a top predator in southeastern US ecosystems.[146] However, whether its use of space and other resources differs significantly from the coyote's has not been assessed. If coyotes and red wolves turn out to be ecological synonyms then the red wolf's protected status as a unique biological entity must be questioned.

For its part, the coyote's genes have been barely affected by other canids, indicating sex-biased introgression. Because mtDNA is maternally inherited the coyote genotype has been transferred to Great Lakes wolves but seldom vice versa, evidence of female coyotes mating with male wolves.[147] The offspring might cross back into either species, although genetic evidence favors admixtures later breeding with wolves.[148] If so it means that adult female coyotes could be accepted by wolf packs and allowed to rear young. This would seem to be a rare occurrence among gray wolves, but coyotes are obviously tolerated by Great Lakes wolves.[149] More likely, female coyotes occasionally mated with lone male wolves, either forming pair bonds or rearing their offspring alone.

Wolves and coyotes can easily traverse plains, mountains, and deserts. The lack of historical geographic barriers suggests other reasons why they evidently did not interbreed everywhere. As stated before, some authorities posit that their smaller size makes Great Lakes and red wolves more likely than gray wolves to mate with coyotes.[150] However, the Mexican gray wolf is smaller than other western and northern gray wolves, has coexisted with coyotes throughout its history, and evidence of admixing is barely detectable in its genome.[151]

Environmental barriers that might ordinarily prevent interbreeding are thought to break down during conditions favoring coyotes over wolves. Wolves are affected adversely by a scarcity of large prey, habitat restrictions caused by human encroachment, habitat fragmentation, and declining numbers in a rising tide of coyotes. "Predator control" measures, which typically devastate wolves, can have little effect on coyotes,[152] or actually increase coyote populations except at the very highest levels of mortality.[153]

The *Allee effect* in ecology posits that a species can fail to reproduce successfully when its population falls below a critical number of individuals.[154] In wide-ranging animals like wolves, finding a mate becomes increasingly difficult as the population declines over large areas. As a consequence some think that dispersing Great Lakes wolves mated with coyotes when outnumbered by them and the two species came into frequent contact.[155] The female admixtures later mated with lone wolves too, producing larger coyote admixtures capable of efficiently hunting smaller ungulates such as white-tailed deer (*Odocoileus virginianus*) and perhaps even forming packs. In such situations admixtures filled an ecological space vacated by wolves[156] by retaining part of the wolf genome and becoming wolfish themselves.

What about reverse pairings? Coyote mtDNA lineages isolated so far are remarkably pure,[157] an indication that male coyote × female gray wolf crosses are either rare or the offspring die before reproducing. The fact that mtDNA is inherited maternally is evidence of unidirectional matings; that is, of male wolves mating with female coyotes and female offspring crossing back into wolves to produce subsequent generations carrying coyote mtDNA.[158] Evidence of such admixtures crossing back into the coyote population would be undetectable by mtDNA analysis because of the coyote mtDNA already present.[159]

A reason for the rarity of such pairings could be the size disparity between male coyotes and female gray wolves. "This mating asymmetry may indicate that the smaller male coyotes cannot inspire the larger female gray wolves to mate with them."[160] In fact, genetic evidence accumulated from Ontario wild canids is "generally consistent with the hypothesis that introgression [has been] directional with females of the smaller species historically mating with males of the larger species."[161] Nonetheless, captive canids muster sufficient inspiration to deal with such difficulties. As described by Helenette and Walter T. Silver, "The mixed-breed collie, sire of our first admixed litter, was much larger than the wild female [eastern coyote], and at the time she was bred she stood on a barrel to accommodate him."[162]

When able to function as normal ecological entities, gray wolves in packs commonly kill coyotes (Chapter 6).[163] At *Riding Mountain National Park*, Manitoba, coyotes avoid wolves.[164] Coyotes in Wyoming are less numerous where wolves are abundant.[165] It is unlikely that offspring from a lone coyote × gray wolf pairing would later be integrated into wolf societies (but see below). Even were this to occur, their smaller size makes it doubtful that admixtures could achieve a dominant position in the pack and reproduce with a gray wolf.

Not much sticks to a coyote's genes. Its matings with wolves have left clear heritable markers in Great Lakes wolf populations but little evidence of their own having been similarly affected.[166] Coyotes once coexisted with Mexican gray wolves and red wolves in Texas, and all three species are thought to have been reproductively isolated prior to human encroachment and persecution. Both wolves became functionally extinct, reduced in recent times to captive specimens and small reintroduced populations. Today mostly coyotes remain. If coyote × red wolf and coyote × Mexican gray wolf admixtures had crossed back into coyote populations, genetic evidence should still be apparent in today's Texas coyotes, populations of which rose concomitantly with declines in the others. The effect could have toppled reproductive barriers and increased the incidence of admixing.

Recent experiments tested these possibilities in both maternal and paternal lines of Texas western coyotes using as a control (i.e. genetic "outgroup") western coyotes from a region in Nebraska where only coyotes and gray wolves had lived together in the past.[167] Variability of maternally and paternally inherited markers showed little evidence of increased genetic diversity in Texas coyotes; just one marker contained gray wolf mtDNA, indicating a long-ago mating between a male coyote and a female Mexican gray wolf. Mexican gray wolf mtDNA indicated that at some point in the past a male wolf mated with a female coyote and their female offspring were assimilated into the Mexican gray wolf population, although this lineage has not been found in the remaining few captive specimens.[168]

Both male and female offspring apparently were accepted into coyote and red wolf populations. Red wolves show the most introgression of outside haplotypes and were affected most by admixing. The intermediate-sized red wolf perhaps mediated admixing by mating with both larger Mexican gray wolves and smaller coyotes,[169] a role similar to that of the Great Lakes wolf farther north.[170]

Body size in canids, not necessarily interspecific competition for food, appears to correlate with prey size,[171] accounting to some extent why wolves, which pursue large ungulates preferentially, are bigger than coyotes, which typically feed on rodents, rabbits, lizards, and other smaller animals. This disparity in prey size allows wolves to separate themselves ecologically from coyotes unless large ungulates are scarce or absent.

1.5   Eastern coyote

Eastern coyotes are the animals often incorrectly identified by New Englanders as "coyotes" and "coydogs" (Chapter 2), but they breed reasonably true for external characters.[172] The eastern coyote's range is presently east of longitude 80° and includes New England, New York, New Jersey, Pennsylvania, Ontario, Québec, New Brunswick, and Nova Scotia (Fig. 1.4).[173] Size is 13.6–18.2 kg,[174] although New Hampshire specimens are sometimes bigger (18–20.4 kg).[175] Recent admixing with wolves in the eastern US is unlikely. The last New Hampshire wolf was killed in 1887 in the White Mountains,[176] and coyotes were not recorded in New Hampshire until the 1930s.[177] Wolves in New York State and Maine also had

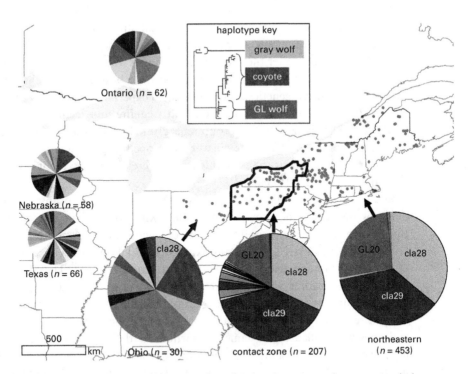

Figure 1.4 mtDNA haplotype frequencies of eastern coyotes and source populations. Sampling localities are represented by gray dots and summarized as large pie charts showing proportions of animals with haplotypes categorized according to positions in the phylogeny.
Source: fig. 2, p. 90 of Kays, R., A. Curtis, and J. J. Kirchman. (2010). Rapid adaptive evolution of northeastern coyotes via hybridization with wolves. *Biology Letters* **6**: 89–93. With permission of The Royal Society.

been exterminated before 1900[178] and were probably gone everywhere in New England by then.[179] However, part of the eastern coyote's estimated Canadian range in 1975 abutted New York State and northern New England,[180] and eastern coyotes appear along an admixed corridor extending south of Algonquin Provincial Park.

White-tailed deer had moved north with clearing of the land,[181] offering a reservoir of protein conveniently packaged. To hunt them effectively requires more body mass, bigger teeth, and stronger jaws than the standard coyote design suited to rabbits and mice. Eastern coyotes differ from western coyotes in both appearance and behavior. Their teeth and skulls are reminiscent of red wolves and small Great Lakes wolves,[182] not scaled-up western coyotes, and the space where jaw muscles attach is 8–15% larger.[183] The heavier jaws and jaw muscula-ture provide added bite strength, adaptations for gripping and subduing adult white-tailed deer and masticating their thick skin and bones.[184] Despite contrary opinions[185] morphologists recognized that such features were unlikely to have resulted from the rapid evolution of western coyote immigrants for feeding on larger prey.[186] Also like wolves eastern coyotes have few primary sweat glands (*eccrine glands*) on their footpads, and thermal stimulation of the pads fails to induce sweating.[187] In contrast, both coyotes and domestic dogs have many more eccrine glands, and under thermal stimulation they sweat readily to cool the skin.

Some of the morphological changes could have been acquired characters, the result of diet and not genetics, as demonstrated experimentally by dividing captive coyotes (related males) into two groups at weaning and feeding them different foods for 18 months.[188] One group was given heavy bones to chew and the other only soft food. The bone chewers developed larger jaw muscles and more prominent *sagittal crests* than the others and were also more adept at consuming rawhide treats and beef shanks.

Body size correlates directly with prey size across all carnivorans: the larger the predator the larger the prey it can capture, kill, disarticulate, and consume.[189] Body size in coyotes increases from west to east across North America:[190] California (10.5 kg), Mexico (11.5 kg), Iowa (13 kg) to 14–18 kg (or more) in eastern coyotes of southeastern and eastern Canada and northeastern US.[191] The eastern coyote preys heavily on adult white-tailed deer, especially in winter.[192] Up to 70% of deer killed in winter by Maine eastern coyotes were healthy.[193] Doe fawns and old deer of both sexes were killed significantly more often; buck fawns and mature bucks and does were killed in the same proportions as their occurrences in the winter herd. The capacity to hunt such large prey efficiently has been acquired either indirectly through natural selection (i.e. *phenotypic plasticity*) or directly from having admixed with wolves.[194] Regardless of the mechanism, eastern coyotes today hunt more like wolves and less like western coyotes.

Eastern coyotes are noticeably bigger than coyotes.[195] Captive coyotes attained adult body mass at about 6 months, at which time they weighed 35–40% less than eastern coyotes the same age.[196] At maturity eastern coyote males were 50% heavier than coyote males, the females 70% heavier.[197] Nearly everything about the coyotes was smaller: bones, paws, nose pads. In addition to their large size, eastern coyotes display several other wolfish attributes: (1) *sexual dimorphism* (males are noticeably bigger than females);[198] (2) the propensity to eat more deer and fewer small mammals;[199] (3) comfortable adjustment to forested habitats;[200] (4) certain behaviors (e.g. refusal to fight with mates) that are more like wolves than coyotes;[201] (5) morphological changes in the jaws and cranium;[202] (6) larger home ranges (Chapter 5) than western coyotes;[203] and (7) attainment of sexual maturity later than coyotes and dogs (Chapters 7 and 8),[204] although females, like western coyotes, can breed before 1 year.[205]

All this confusion calls for a summary. Old and New World wolves differ genetically. Both can be clustered by region and to a lesser extent by habitat.[206] Across Eurasia the separation of newly proposed species in India based on genetic analyses has not been confirmed, and all Eurasian wolves should be considered *C. lupus* until shown otherwise. Wolves in eastern North America are not gray wolves but admixtures in varying proportions of wolf and coyote. The result is a gradation of phenotypes ranging from coyote-like to wolf-like according to which genome predominates. North American carnivorans of the genus *Canis* constitute

six possible groups. (1) The gray wolf (*Canis lupus*) in the west and far north.
(2) The western coyote (*C. latrans*) in three major genetic groups (west, Midwest/
south, northeast), all containing limited introgression of domestic dog genes
(Chapter 2), genes of gray or Great Lakes wolves, or some combination of these.
(3) Wolves of the Great Lakes region called here the Great Lakes wolf (a gray
wolf × extinct endemic wolf × coyote admixture) comprising a graded continuum
of phenotypes becoming smaller in size from west to east and for now including
the Algonquin wolf. (4) The Algonquin wolf, an admixed Great Lakes wolf
population in Algonquin Provincial Park and surrounding area that is nearly half
coyote and contains genetic remnants (C1 mtDNA haplotype) of an extinct
indigenous wolf. Its genome differs in this respect from other Great Lakes wolves,
and some propose reinstating the historical name *C. lycaon*. A few advocate going
further and including the red wolf in *C. lycaon* too.

Gene flow mediated through Algonquin Provincial Park goes in all directions:
north into boreal forest wolves of the "Ontario type," south and east and grading
into eastern coyote, and west into the larger Great Lakes wolf population.[207]
(5) The eastern coyote is a coyote × Great Lakes wolf admixture containing genes
of domestic dogs (Chapter 2) and Great Lakes (specifically Algonquin) wolves.
(6) The red wolf (*C. rufus*) is a coyote × wolf admixture (mostly coyote) that
unjustifiably retains species status. Neither the Great Lakes nor red wolf owes any
distinction in appearance to evolving lineages; instead, variation in external
phenotype has resulted from admixing.[208]

1.6   The color of wolves

The name *Canis lycaon* was given by von Schreber to a live specimen captured as a
pup in Québec, kept chained for a time, and eventually taken alive to Paris by a
French naval officer.[209] There it was seen by the renowned naturalist Georges-Louis
Leclerc, Comte de Buffon, who published a description and illustration of a
"black wolf" in 1761.[210] What became of its remains is unknown. All physical
traces have disappeared, which is unfortunate because a tiny sample of skin might
resolve much of the controversy discussed above.

According to Buffon this animal was smaller than the European gray wolf, with
larger ears. Its tail was also less bushy. When von Schreber began preparing
his massive treatise on mammals of the world in 1774, he gave a brief nod to this
loup noir and reproduced Buffon's color plate, shown here in black and white
(Fig. 1.5). The wolf illustrated is mature and assuredly black, and black Great
Lakes wolves are rare in their eastern range.[211] The descended teats, unless the
result of artistic license, suggest either recent *parturition* or repeated litters,
although I found no record of any offspring.

R. I. Pocock, an expert at the British Museum (Natural History), writing in
1935, doubted that the animal Buffon saw had been a "pure-bred wolf."[212] His
skepticism rising, Pocock mentioned a specimen in the British Museum labeled

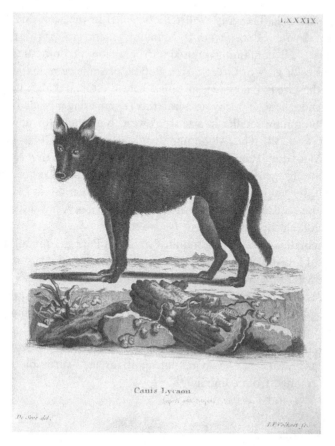

Figure 1.5 Female Great Lakes wolf (*Canis lycaon*) painted in life while on exhibit in Paris. *Source*: von Schreber (1775).

"*Canis lycaon*, N. America," calling it a "so-called 'wolf'" similar to Buffon's and pointing out that its pelt was black too, the attendant skull short, and the teeth small for an ordinary wolf. The pelt had a white patch on the breast, a character that in later gray wolf × domestic dog admixing experiments would be attributed to dog genes. Over several years the Russian geneticist N. A. Iljin produced four generations of captive *wolfdogs* through selective breeding and recorded their characters. Many had white markings that he suspected were derived from dogs, but wrote, "However, the presence of these genes in wolves is also possible, since naturalists have sometimes (though rarely) recorded wolves with white spots on the chest."[213] An early Pennsylvania pioneer noted that wolves "will intermix with dogs,"[214] mentioning "an old she-wolf [that came] into the settlement [to] entice away a number of dogs." Of her six admixed pups, "Two of them had spots on them exactly like one of the dogs." Captive offspring of eastern coyotes captured in New Hampshire were nearly black at birth, not developing the coloration of adult coats until age 3 months.[215]

Maybe Pocock had been right and Buffon's specimen of *C. lycaon* was indeed a gray wolf × dog admixture. White patches on wolves occur, if uncommonly. Some black wolves on the Kenai Peninsula, Alaska, had white chest patches.[216] A lone female gray wolf in Abruzzo, Italy, that had been radio-collared, mated with a free-ranging dog and reared six pups: "These offspring, three of which were radio-collared, behaved like wolves but their appearance was decidedly hybrid; four were black with a white foot."[217] Eastern coyotes crossed with pointer pups produced black pups with white chests and paws.[218]

Black coat color in wild canids has been proposed as evidence of early admixing with domestic dogs.[219] Several putative red wolves (discussed below) killed in the northwestern Ozark Mountains of Arkansas in the early 1930s were black-phase specimens,[220] although even black-phase gray wolves are never truly black, the hairs being banded and simply darker, showing more black and less of the paler undercoat than other wolves.[221] In 1978 it was proposed that genes for *melanism* in coyotes from the southeastern US might be derived from red wolves or domestic dogs.[222] In 2009, researchers published genetic evidence that melanistic gray wolves in western North America, which are more common in forested habitats than anywhere else, derive their black coat color from past admixing with dogs.[223] The same pathway causes melanism in modern coyotes and contemporary Italian gray wolves.[224]

Some black wolves occur in northern Minnesota,[225] the place where gray wolves of western heritage admix with Great Lakes wolves. No black-pelted specimens (or white ones either) have been documented from the population of Mexican gray wolves.[226] Elsewhere black wolves are more common at some locations than others. They were rare at the turn of the twentieth century in the Mackenzie River region of Canada's Northwest Territories.[227] Black wolves occurred in Russia in the early twentieth century, but evidently were not common.[228] A "very large proportion" of the original wolves in *Yellowstone National Park* (hereafter called *Yellowstone*) were black in the 1920s.[229] At Etolin Island in southeastern Alaska, 15 of 18 wolves killed were black.[230] A 1947 publication reported more than half the wolves observed at two of four Canadian Rockies national parks (Banff and Jasper) as black.[231] Black wolves were ordinary at the same time in *Denali National Park and Preserve*, Alaska (hereafter called *Denali*),[232] but only 9% of Denali wolves were black when studied between 1988 and 1994.[233] In contrast, just 13 of 151 wolves radio-collared in southcentral Alaska between 1975 and 1982 were melanistic.[234] A 1968 report based on bountied pelts described the wolves of northern Alaska as predominantly gray (64%) with 29% black; at the crest of the Brooks Range the numbers were 19% black and 72% gray.[235] In the 1980s approximately one-third of wolves on the Kenai Peninsula were black.[236] Litters born to gray parents were entirely gray, but those having a gray mother and black father were 40% black and 60% gray. In parts of Canada and Alaska some populations of wolves follow the caribou herds on their annual migrations from the tundra in summer south to the *taiga* (Chapter 6). These animals are white, or nearly so.[237] Others in the same region are permanent residents of the taiga and their pelts vary from gray through black.

Genotype is difficult to infer from *phenotype* because some gray wolves become paler with age.[238] In the captive wolf colony at Barrow, Alaska, some black wolves turned gray after 4 years.[239] Denali wolves that were gray when young sometimes turned white later.[240] Most of these animals were old with worn teeth when examined. The same pattern was found in Canada's subarctic during the mid-1920s: "Most of the white wolves captured, being aged animals, were found to have bad teeth, with, in some instances, a few altogether missing."[241] Wolves that were old and white have been reported elsewhere from the American west.[242]

2   What makes a dog

We think of other primates as our closest relatives, and in evolutionary terms they are. However, dogs mirror our social patterns in ways no primate can. We recognize in them elements of ourselves, and this permits a certain level of empathy. Selection for *paedomorphism* such as small size, outsized eyes, and soft hair has produced dogs having permanent juvenile features, making them reminiscent of pups in arrested development (Fig. 2.1).[1] Like us, dogs are social with senses attuned to voices, scents, postures, and dependent on familiarity and friendship. A dog growls and we know what it signifies.[2] We shout and the dog understands, if not the words. In behavioral terms, "the primary stimuli are so similar in the two species that appropriate and recognizable social behavior is evoked."[3]

2.1   Domestication

In structure and form the dog is the most variable mammal of all, a situation attributable entirely to humans. Genetic mutations are probably too slow to account for the typically rapid alterations in phenotype.[4] A report on 414 pure-bred dogs of 85 breeds showed that interbreed differences accounted for 27% of the total genetic variation.[5] Western European breed clubs with their attendant standards date from the mid-1800s, and today more than 400 breeds exist.[6] Among the standards adopted was the "breed barrier" rule, which decrees that for a dog to be registered both its parents and grandparents must be registered members of the same breed.[7] The result was to constrict the borders of gene pools through *inbreeding*, making the physical appearance of each breed reproducible. Inbreeding can sometimes have negative effects including reduced incidence of conception, fewer live births, lowered sperm count, and smaller testis volume.[8]

The phenotypic variation so obvious among breeds results from selection, not isolated incidents of wolf domestication.[9] *Domestication* has been defined as "that process by which a population of animals becomes adapted to man and to the captive environment by some combination of genetic changes occurring over generations and [by] environmentally induced developmental events reoccurring during each generation."[10] Domestication implies the subsumation of natural selection by artificial selection; in other words, genetic control over animals

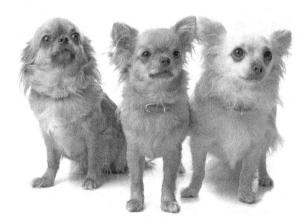

Figure 2.1 Many breeds are selected purposely for such paedomorphic features as large eyes, fine hair, and small size.
Source: Eriklam|Dreamstime.com.

exerted by humans that in the end molds them into new forms that enhance their value to us, functionally or for esthetic reasons. Tameness, a quality often associated with domestic animals, is not exclusive to them because wild animals can also be tamed, and "environmentally induced developmental events" simply hint at evolution, offering nothing specific about domestication.[11]

Domestication of the dog took place multiple times in many places involving any number of wolf lineages,[12] and dogs on all continents have a common genetic origin.[13] Most *modern breeds* are <400 years old and created from common founder stock.[14] The result has been extreme variation in morphology based on a "simplified genetic architecture."[15] Gene flow, of course, "is a force that homogenizes genetic variation."[16] In dogs it has been ancient and extensive, and a dog of any breed, no matter how distinctive it appears, is a mongrel just under the surface. Today's breeds still retain high genetic variability seen as multiple mtDNA sequences,[17] probably because inbreeding is relatively recent, ancestry of the original stock has been blended over thousands of years of *outbreeding*, and several females were used as founders in each case. The use of mtDNA data alone is insufficient to separate dogs from wolves.[18] Add to this the wide geographic distribution of dogs by humans since ancient times.[19]

Evidence of extensive genetic diversity resides in the different haplotypes of modern dogs, and seldom is any specific to a breed.[20] In one investigation more than 95% of haplotypes occurred at the same frequency in dogs tested worldwide: 654 domestic dogs from Europe, Asia, Africa, Arctic America, and 38 Eurasian wolves.[21] Substantial changes in phenotype can be induced without loss of genetic diversity, as shown for eight Japanese breeds.[22] Kintamani dogs of Bali resemble the Chow Chow phenotypically; however, their ancestry shows genetic evidence only of the local street dogs.[23] All this is powerful evidence for domestic dogs having descended from a common pool of genes, one that is ancient and deep.[24]

Breeds are nonetheless identifiable by *nuclear microsatellite markers*. In one study, 99% of dogs screened were assigned correctly to one of 85 breeds, about 30% of the genetic variation being attributed to breed differences.[25] Furthermore, genetic differences between breeds (27.5%) was greater than variation within them (5.4%), and assignment to breed was 99% accurate based solely on DNA profile. Therefore, some dog breeds not only look different, they *are* different. Nonetheless, many European breeds are so closely related that genetic separation is nearly impossible, indicating a recent ancestry shared with dogs of diverse heritages.[26] Another team of scientists traced and reconstructed the collie family tree through a single *allele* inherited from a dog that lived in Great Britain in the mid-1800s before breed standards.[27] Establishing a breed forces a *genetic bottleneck*, reducing haplotype diversity.[28] The Irish wolfhound, for example, has also been squeezed through the narrowest of genetic openings, all of today's breed having descended from a single dog in the early 1800s.[29]

2.2   Early dogs

Eurasian wolves appear to be ancestral to domestic dogs worldwide (Chapter 1),[30] but when and where did the changeover occur, and with which wolves specifically? Domestication took place at least 15 000–40 000 years BP,[31] but how long ago and the locations where wolves were tamed and became actual components of human culture are controversial. A major reason has been the use of mtDNA analysis, which describes only a tiny part of the genome and introduces a strong sex bias (Chapter 1).[32] Add to this problem the extraordinary mobility of wolves and the potential for wolves and dogs to interbreed.[33]

At least five founding dog lineages accompanied late *Pleistocene* humans across the Bering land bridge from Asia and into North America.[34] One estimate of the time needed to acquire the genetic diversity seen in modern dogs placed early domestication events at >100 000 years BP.[35] This has been challenged by newer research[36] and genetic evidence based on analysis of New World fossils suggesting that considerable diversity occurred within just 12 000–14 000 years after the earliest dogs arrived in North America.[37] One team of investigators concluded that dog haplotypes worldwide can be placed into 10 haplogroups, and the only location where all occur is southern China south of the Yangtze River.[38] The mtDNA evidence pointed to a founder population of not fewer than 51 female wolves from this location with domestication occurring at about the same time (no earlier than 16 300 years BP), making it a single event.[39] Another extensive survey replicated this work and found no consistent variation in haplotypes with geography.[40] Using SNPs these other investigators then identified wolves from the Middle East, not southeast Asia, as principal sources of genetic diversity in dogs and no specific location or founder event.[41] Still other investigators pointed to multiple domestication events originating with eastern European wolves.[42] The issue is obviously not settled.

The first domestic dogs to arise in some parts of the world might not have looked like wolves.[43] The Middle Eastern wolf has been proposed as the progenitor of modern small dogs, which are distinguished by the insulin-like gene, growth factor 1, or *IGF1*.[44] Growth factor 1 is associated with body size, and its appearance is rare in large wolf-sized breeds. This mutation is ancient and probably occurred early in the history of dogs.[45] Another approach to isolating when dogs arose assumed an ancient bottleneck during domestication based on a hypothetical population size of 13 000 canids having made the transition from wolf to dog.[46] Using an extensive map of SNPs stretched across breeds, this event was calculated to have occurred about 9000 generations ago (27 000 years BP) with subsequent breed-creation bottlenecks of varying constrictions of 30–90 generations. Breed creations had a far more severe effect on the dog genome than the bottlenecks occurring at domestication.[47]

Still other investigators have studied dog evolution from ancient DNA extracted from fossil bones. According to their findings, salient changes in dog morphology resulting from domestication were abrupt and subsequently became genetically fixed.[48] By about 10 000 years BP dogs were present in Africa, Europe, Asia, and North America. Any future discoveries of fossils far older should therefore surprise no one. Either dogs arose multiple times in diverse locations, or they dispersed with astonishing speed over vast distances.[49] In either case, genetic data collected from ancient bones show that considerable genetic diversity has been lost between the dog's early evolution and dogs of today.[50]

A fossil canid skull found in Goyet Cave, Belgium, in the 1860s has been dated to about 31 700 years BP, or twice the age of the oldest fossil dog skulls aged using methods other than ancient DNA analysis. The Goyet Cave canid was not a form intermediate between wolf and dog, but apparently a *Palaeolithic period* dog, a conclusion bolstered by its skull morphology, and tentatively reinforces genetic evidence of dogs having arisen much sooner than indicated by the fossil record.[51] The unique haplotypes of this specimen and remnants of five others from Goyet Cave are absent in modern breeds, suggesting their origin to be a diverse lineage of wolves long since lost.[52]

Other paleontological evidence exists of the dog's ancient domestication. Deep inside Chauvet Cave, France, are footprints of a large dog along with one of a child, both dated from about 26 000 years BP[53] and tentative evidence that the dog has been a human companion at least since the *Aurignacian period*. The complete skeleton of a dog excavated from a *Mesolithic period* shell midden in Portugal in 1880 dates to about 8000 years BP (Fig. 2.2).[54] Remains from central Europe (Bonn-Oberkassel and Senckenberg) are morphologically more similar to dogs than to wolves and date from about 12 000 years BP.[55] Fragments from Star Carr, Yorkshire, England, are 9400 years old.[56] Dog-like canid fossils from Italy have been aged at 15 000–3000 years BP, although only the most recent are indisputably dogs.[57] The skeleton of an 18-week-old dingo excavated near the Murray River, South Australia, and assembled,[58] represents Australia's oldest known dog (3500 years BP).[59] Ban Chiang in northern Thailand has been

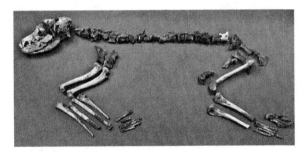

Figure 2.2 Complete skeleton of a canid recovered in the 1880s from the Muge shell-middens, Portugal, and displayed in the Geological Museum, Lisbon. Illustration by J. P. Ruas. Detry, C. and J. L. Cardosa. (2010). On some remains of dog (*Canis familiaris*) from the Mesolithic shell-middens of Muge, Portugal. *Journal of Archaeological Science* **37**: 2762–2774. Reprinted with permission of Elsevier.

occupied continuously for thousands of years. A skull and bone fragments dating from about 5600 years BP to modern times show remarkable similarity to modern Ban Chiang village dogs, which resemble other Asian dingoes.[60] Some of these animals had been eaten;[61] others were buried with humans as grave offerings.

Among the most ancient fossils of domestic dogs yet found are from Russia's central plain in the Dnieper River basin. Two skulls of adults have been dated from the Ice Age at 13 000–17 000 years BP. They were big stocky animals with heads like Siberian huskies except larger and with much shorter muzzles, and they likely descended from subarctic Eurasian wolves.[62] The Natufian culture (13 000–10 500 years BP) in the Middle East is more recent, and fossil dogs from the Levant also appear to have descended from large wolves,[63] calling into question an earlier hypothesis that small wolves must have been the original progenitors of dogs.[64] However, the oldest fossil canid yet found in unequivocal association with humans is not a wolf or dog but a red fox (*Vulpes vulpes*) in the Levant.[65] It had been buried carefully in a pre-Natufian cemetery at Uyun al-Hammam, Jordan, just steps from today's Trans-Jordan Highway, and dates from 17 250–15 350 years BP. Whether there were efforts then to tame foxes is unknown, but this one had been clearly valued for more than its flesh or pelt.

Other fossils of early domestic canids include a jaw from Palegawra Cave, northwestern Iraq dated at 12 000 years BP.[66] An Iranian cave (Ghar-i-Kamarband, or Belt Cave) near the Caspian Sea excavated in the 1940s yielded fossil jaw bones and teeth of domestic dogs from the Lower Mesolithic, Upper Mesolithic, and *Neolithic period.*[67] Carbon dating was inconsistent, but some of these fossils are 8000 years old.[68]

Genetic evidence (mtDNA) from dog lineages through time shows matings of female dogs and male wolves to be rare, the reverse pairings rarer still.[69] Nonetheless, genetic evidence of wolf × dog crosses has been reported from around the world.[70] Although backcrossing with wolves also happens,[71] and dogs and wolves often occur in the same locations, evidence of admixing has been found in only a minority of breeds: basenji (central Africa); Afghan, Canaan, Saluki (Middle East); Samoyed, Alaskan malamute, Siberian husky, American

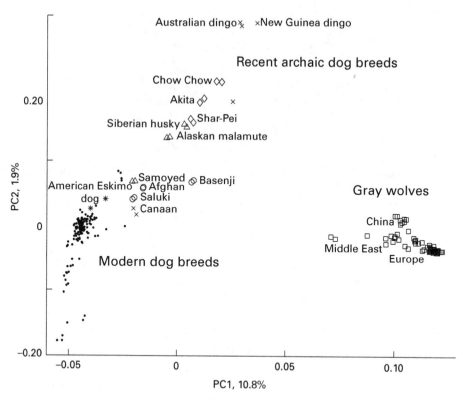

Figure 2.3 Principal component analysis of 48 036 SNPs for two dogs per breed ($n = 171$) and Eurasian gray wolves ($n = 58$). Dogs are readily distinguished, and recent archaic breeds (e.g. Chow Chow, American Eskimo dog) cluster distantly from modern breeds with dingoes demonstrating the greatest separation.
Source: vonHoldt *et al.* (2010). Reprinted by permission from Macmillan Publishers Ltd.: *Genome Research*, advance online publication, 12 May 2011 (doi: 10.1101/gr.116301.110).

Eskimo dog (holarctic and subarctic); dingo (Australia, New Guinea, southeast Asia); Chow Chow, Pekingese, Shar-Pei, and Shi Tzu (China).[72] They arose in far-flung regions of Africa, Asia, and North America long before the advent of breed clubs and display a common heritage brought about by ancient human migrations. These *recent archaic breeds* (i.e. older than 500 years)[73] are probably the closest phenotypic expressions of the ancestral pool of dog genes extant (Fig. 2.3).[74]

Pleistocene hunters crossed the Bering land bridge from Siberia to the Americas between 30 000 and 22 000 years BP,[75] and domestic dogs are known to have been present in North America long before Europeans arrived. Did they accompany early nomadic hunters, or are they derivatives of North American gray wolves? Genetic evidence leans strongly toward the first possibility. Had pre-European dogs in North America descended from local wolves the genetic echo should still be apparent. If, on the other hand, their genetic sequences proved similar to Old World dogs, a likely origin points to Asia. In either case, traces ought to remain in the genomes of their modern descendants, one of which has been around a long time.

In 1571 Francisco Hernández, a physician of King Phillip II of Spain, was dispatched to the New World in search of medicinal plants. Among the native dogs he encountered in Mexico was a breed completely devoid of hair.[76] The Xoloitzcuintle, as the Toltecs called it, was sacred and evidently has been distinct for at least 2000 years.[77] The Spaniards had taken along their own dogs, which mated with the native breeds, and any unique New World characters faded quickly into the background.[78] The Xoloitzcuintle was nonetheless preserved in remote parts of the country because of its religious value and today retains the original morphological features.

Even the Xoloitzcuintle displays Old World haplotypes.[79] Tissue samples from modern specimens were compared with those of 27 populations of wolves from Europe, Asia, and North America and 67 recognized dog breeds.[80] Seven haplotypes could be sequenced, none unique to the Xoloitzcuintle or New World gray wolves, including the Mexican wolf. One of the most common haplotypes also occurs in wolves native to Romania and European Russia. In other words, genetic sequences discovered in this unique New World dog are identical to those of Old World breeds, further evidence that North America was originally colonized by numerous dogs of genetically diverse ancestry. Mitochondrial DNA from the remains of pre-European dogs as widely dispersed as Alaska and Peru demonstrate this Old World heritage too.[81] Thus New World and Old World dogs have a common ancestry, and modern genetics has confirmed what was long suspected.[82]

Domestication of wolves by mobile hunting societies seems a logical step. Wolves, like the humans who tamed them, hunt large game in groups, and combining skills might have benefited both.[83] Whether this ever happened is purely conjectural, but the possibility is intriguing. Philip Tome and his friends hunted deer using trained dogs in the northern Pennsylvania wilderness during the early nineteenth century. At times wild wolves participated in the chases, and Tome and his companions left them shares of the kill to keep them around.[84]

Northern Ice Age dogs appear to have been selected for large size and perhaps served as beasts of burden. We know they were eaten: one of the two Dnieper River skulls mentioned previously has a hole cut into the side so the brain could be removed.[85] Besides being sources of labor and food, some early dogs were evidently kept as pets. A Natufian tomb unearthed in northern Israel from about 12 000 years BP revealed the skeleton of an adult hunter-gatherer whose left hand rested on the skeleton of a dog or Middle Eastern wolf of 4–5 months, "proof that an affectionate rather than gastronomic relationship existed between [the animal] and the buried person."[86]

According to one hypothesis, modern dogs derived from at least five genetic lines of female wolves.[87] The unknown factor is whether gray wolves were tamed at various locations at different times, or if the event happened about the same time at different places with later occurrences of wolf × dog admixing.[88] Domestication likely occurred numerous times in many locations,[89] but in either case data attempting to stamp the time and place are inconclusive.[90] It can be stated only that the origin of dogs is diverse, included more than one wolf population,[91] and there was substantial crossing back of dogs with their wild ancestors.[92]

So far only groups of wolf populations have been identified. They comprise North America, the Indian subcontinent, the Himalayas, and the remaining parts of Eurasia.[93] Haplotypes of Indian plains and Himalayan wolves do not occur in dogs,[94] which leaves only Eurasia exclusive of these other two regions.[95] More specifically, genetic evidence identifies eastern Asia as the region where dogs, including the dingo,[96] were first domesticated.[97] These were not just the earliest tame dogs, but supposedly the first animals of any kind to come under domestication.[98]

2.3   Coydogs and wolfdogs

The prevalence in our fields and backyards of first-generation coyote × domestic dog admixtures, or *coydogs*, is itself an admixture of fact and urban legend.[99] Captive coyotes mate with domestic dogs,[100] but such events are rare in nature as inferred by studies of comparative reproductive biology[101] and demonstrated both by mtDNA[102] and nuclear microsatellite analysis.[103] Traces of ancient American Indian dogs have been recovered from coyote skulls dated to 481 years BP.[104] Modern coyotes throughout the US contain fractions of dog genes, but <10% in all cases as revealed using the canine SNP microarray.[105]

When admixing does occur, matings between male domestic dogs and female coyotes are more likely than the reverse situation because male dogs are fertile all year (Chapter 7). Male coyotes, in contrast, produce sperm only during the breeding season. As a consequence, any male coyotes encountered by an estrous dog might be out of reproductive phase and therefore infertile.[106] As a further detriment, first- and second-generation male coydogs born and raised in captivity provided no paternal care (Chapter 8),[107] meaning that female coydogs, like free-ranging dogs, would be left to rear their offspring alone.

Most animals identified by sight as coydogs are simply dogs. As one observer wrote in 1942, "hybrids between dogs and coyotes are occasionally reported in North America, but for most of these the paternity is assumed from the appearance of the young rather than definitely known."[108] This assumption of parentage based on appearance seems to be common,[109] and at least some specimens in the northeastern US declared to be western coyotes or coydogs might have been misidentified eastern coyotes (Chapter 1).[110]

Modern genetic analysis has shown coydogs to be rare. Data from the mtDNA of 686 eastern coyotes, for example, turned up only a single partial sequence of a "dog-like" haplotype from a Vermont specimen.[111] Another report found a dog haplotype in southeastern coyotes, evidence of a single long-ago mating.[112] Finally, true coydogs (i.e. first-generation admixtures) are unlikely to be recognized as such.[113] Breeding experiments show them to resemble dogs more than coyotes, making them indistinguishable from other mongrels.[114]

According to a New York State biologist writing in 1974, "Over the past half century, wild canids bearing a resemblance to coyotes have been encountered with increasing frequency in New York, particularly in the Adirondack region."[115] He went on to say that many of the specimens were admixtures. All had been shot or trapped by bounty hunters or state game wardens and their skulls examined by anatomists who detected elements of both coyotes and dogs. Comparing skulls can suggest admixing, but never demonstrate it.

By the mid-1940s some of these intermediate specimens had begun more and more to resemble coyotes, with most specimens subsequently classified either as domestic dogs or coyotes, but seldom admixtures. Into the 1950s literally hundreds of "coydogs" killed by hunters were turned in at deer-checking stations in the Adirondacks. Experts examined a few, but no skulls or skins were kept. Maybe these were free-ranging dogs, as one specimen proved to be. Perhaps some were actually later-generation admixtures crossed back into the coyote population, or simply coyotes without dog genes at all. Then again, maybe they were eastern coyotes.[116]

Admixing occurs most frequently along advancing fronts of the invading species. As eastern coyotes crossed the St. Lawrence River from Canada into New York State, first-generation "coydogs" were reported as most common along the periphery, eventually disappearing as true coyotes increased in number and took charge of the ecological space.[117] In most reports the mothers were "coyote-like" and elusive. Admixed offspring were easily trapped and shot, perhaps a liability of their domestic heritage, but the coyotes themselves were wild and wary. Mere visual inspection of a dead specimen is unreliable, and many of the purported admixtures were undoubtedly dogs.

Regardless of the breed of dog involved in such matings, the first-generation admixtures seldom resemble coyotes. After examining progeny from known crosses of captive eastern coyotes with several breeds of domestic dogs, Silver and Silver wrote, "none of the hybrids, at any age, were distinguishable from domestic dogs by casual observation."[118] They looked intermediate between the parents. Coydogs produced by Lee R. Dice had wider muzzles and shorter faces than coyotes, their skulls broader and ears typically lopped instead of erect like a coyote's.[119] The coat might mimic the parent dog's in being spotted or mottled with shorter hair. All are phenotypic characters of domestication.[120] Offspring of eastern coyote × purebred dog crosses looked like lop-eared mongrel dogs.[121] This is not surprising because coat color, coat pattern, and morphology of wolfdogs render them easily mistaken for mongrel dogs too.[122]

Domestication, whether through admixing or captive breeding of wild canids selected for tameness, eventually results in distinctive, predictable changes in morphology.[123] Foremost are shortening and broadening of the snout and palate[124] causing crowding of the teeth and a reduction in tooth size,[125] a steeply rising forehead and wider posterior cranial vault,[126] and differences in the position and angle of the orbits.[127] These features are used in attempts to distinguish fossil dogs from fossil wolves.[128] A kinked tail or tail that is curled forward,[129] lopped ears,[130] and color or pattern of the coat[131] are other indicators of domestication. Dental overlap, especially of the lower fourth premolar and lower first molar, is a less reliable indicator.[132] Reduction in body size, another feature of canid domestication,[133] is unreliable in the case of fossils; for example, wolves and northern Ice Age dogs were similar in size.[134]

Changes in the brain also occur during domestication. *Tameness*, the absence of conflicted behavior (Chapter 3),[135] probably preceded the selection of traits for appearance. It seems reasonable that dogs in primitive human societies were first kept for food or other utilitarian purposes, and to be useful they had to be tame to some extent. If tameness is a behavioral trait derived from wildness then patterns of *gene expression* in the brains of dogs ought to differ from the conserved ancestral expressions in their wild relatives. Tests of comparative *messenger ribonucleic acid* (*mRNA*) expression levels in dog, wolf, and coyote genes show that selection for behavior has modified the mRNA expression patterns in the dog *hypothalamus*, and that the hypothalamus of coyotes and wolves displays a conserved expression profile in comparison.[136]

As mentioned, natural admixing between wolves and domestic dogs is rare. According to one survey, none of 350 wolves from 26 locations throughout their worldwide range had an mtDNA genotype common in domestic dogs.[137] Genetic sampling of ancient dog remains has yielded little evidence of female gray wolf lineages,[138] and today's North American gray wolves seldom admix with dogs despite their occasional proximity.[139] Nonetheless, dogs of North American Plains Indians commonly associated with wolves early in the nineteenth century. One chronicler wrote, "in shape they differ very little from the wolf, and are equally large and strong ... Their voice is not a proper barking, but a howl, like that of the wolf, and they partly descend from wolves, which approach the Indian huts, even in the daytime, to mix with the dogs."[140]

Pliny reported how the Gauls tied estrous dogs to trees so they might mate with wolves.[141] Evidently this technique strikes a universal chord. Early explorers wrote that Eskimos occasionally staked out sled dogs in heat hoping wolves would mate with them, thereby enhancing the hardiness of their breed.[142] To quote Glover M. Allen: "There is much evidence, though of a somewhat uncertain character, that wild male Wolves will breed with female Eskimo Dogs at proper seasons, and the northern Indians are said to encourage such occasional crosses."[143] However, as Raymond and Lorna Coppinger pointed out, "but what possible wolf trait would anyone want to add to a sled dog team? Wolves are not faster or stronger, nor do they have more stamina than sled dogs."[144] They also take commands poorly. Even the wolf expert Erik Zimen was unable to train a group of five young wolves to pull a sled. They consistently refused direction, often fighting or lying down in their traces.[145] Still, wolves have been trained to perform this function,[146] as have wolfdogs.[147]

Allen also quoted an 1829 report in which Sir John Franklin mentioned the Cree Indian dogs. According to Franklin, in March the female wolves "frequently entice the domestic dogs from the forts, although at other seasons a strong antipathy seemed to subsist between them."[148] In fact, at other times wolves in the vicinity of Hudson Bay commonly killed and ate Eskimo dogs.[149] Plains Indians were said to stake out estrous dogs to mate with male coyotes, and many early writers considered Indian dogs in general to be tamed coyotes. Allen found no physical evidence of coyote influence from skulls he examined.[150]

North American Plains Indians once used dogs as pack animals, and each was said to carry from 16–22 kg in backpacks, or pull tent poles used as *travois* loaded with goods.[151] Later "the horse replaced the dog as a beast of burden and the man's legs for chasing buffalo."[152] Some of these dogs were used for hunting, reportedly driving deer into water[153] and keeping them trapped there until the hunters arrived.

Admixing events might be more common in Europe, where wolf populations are small and fragmented[154] and mates scarce or absent,[155] making the Allee effect more likely. However, fears that Old World wolves are losing genetic integrity by admixing with dogs[156] are largely unfounded.[157] Such events happen rarely in Spain and Italy, for example.[158] There appears to be no instance of Spanish male wolves admixing with female dogs and the offspring crossing back with wild wolves.[159] Furthermore, when female gray wolves disperse they attempt to find a permanent mate and form a new pack, a task for which male domestic dogs are poorly suited. Dogs are not monogamous, and males do not help rear the pups (Chapter 8). Consequently, pup mortality could be higher than when young are raised by wolf pairs. Even for survivors inadequate socialization makes later integration into a wolf pack unlikely.[160]

Admixing among canids, as determined by mtDNA analysis, occurs in one direction (i.e. is asymmetric).[161] Because mtDNA is inherited maternally, an mtDNA test of wolves for admixing can identify offspring only from matings of female dogs and male wolves and their back crossings. Eastern and Great Lakes wolves, for example, express coyote mtDNA haplotypes, but the coyotes that coexist with them display only their own.[162] Microsatellite data show the same thing.[163] Therefore, either such matings are exclusively female coyote × male wolf or the offspring do not cross back into coyote populations. Italian female wolves that mate with male dogs are probably not accepted into their natal packs.[164] Any surviving offspring might not be acceptable to the pack either, making back crosses unlikely.[165]

Wolves and coyotes breed once annually at a specific time of year, but domestic dogs have no season (Chapter 7). Thus a female dog in heat can mate with a wolf or coyote only during the male's limited breeding period, but a male dog encountering a female wolf or coyote in estrus is prepared to mate at anytime. Admixing between wolves and dogs, and between coyotes and dogs, is thought to be further hampered by this *reproductive phase shifting*, especially for first-generation admixtures, and the resulting offset breeding cycles might prevent admixed offspring from crossing back into wild populations of coyotes or wolves.[166] Such animals experience a shift of 3 months to an earlier breeding cycle. Captive coydogs were noted to mate once annually in late autumn instead of the typical February breeding time of coyotes.[167] Comparable observations were reported for coyote × wolf[168] and wolf × dog[169] crosses and their offset breeding cycles.

Another detriment to such crosses is behavioral. As mentioned, male dogs, unlike male wolves and coyotes, rarely provide paternal care (Chapter 8). Any admixtures they might father with female wolves, coyotes, or eastern coyotes would likely receive care only from the mother, thus lowering their chances of survival.[170] The effect could be worse if parturition occurred in midwinter instead spring.[171]

2.4   Dingoes

Dingoes evolved in southeast Asia as semi-domesticated dogs and arrived in Australia about 5000 years BP during human expansion through the islands of southeast Asia.[172] The founding population was small, perhaps just one pregnant female, and dingoes remained isolated from other dogs until the arrival of Europeans.[173] Testing of modern Australian dingoes suggests the ancestral loss of genetic variation through one or more bottlenecks even before their arrival. Australian and New Guinea dingoes (Fig. 2.4) share alleles not found in Bali street dogs, which are among the world's most genetically diverse, suggesting that the Australian dingo might have come from New Guinea and not Indonesia.[174]

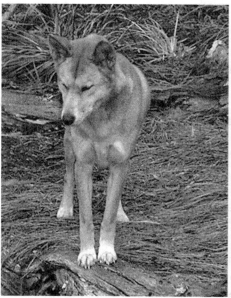 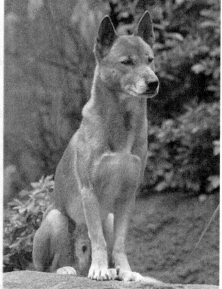

Figure 2.4 *Left*: Australian dingo. *Right*: New Guinea dingo, also called New Guinea singing dog.
Source: (Left) David Croft, Industry and Investment of New South Wales. (Right) Michael Elliott|Dreamstime.com.

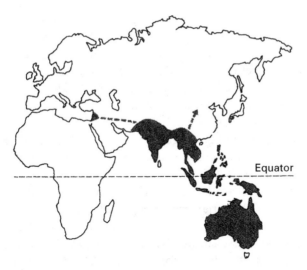

Figure 2.5 World range of dingoes with broken lines indicating probable distribution. From *Proceedings of the Ecological Society of Australia*. This material is reproduced with permission of John Wiley & Sons, Inc.
Source: Corbett (1985).

Morphologically, the dingo is considered "a distinctive feral domestic dog,"[175] and the domestic dog itself is too close to the wolf genetically to warrant separation. Dingoes and domestic dogs readily interbreed, no doubt because dingoes are dogs too.[176] This makes the term *dingo-dog* an obvious redundancy. Still, it offers a convenient way of separating them for conversational purposes. Dingoes and similar dogs occur from Israel across southeast Asia (Fig. 2.5).

Dingo-dogs are impossible to identify without genetic testing because dingo skeletal morphology, coat color, and other characters overlap those of dogs. When the two interbreed their progeny typically display blended characters.[177] Attempts to classify Australian free-ranging dogs into dingo, dingo-dog, and free-ranging domestic dog based on morphology or external appearance[178] have been notoriously unreliable,[179] and genetic studies have been few. Dingoes have been thought to have longer muzzles, larger *auditory bullae* and *carnassial teeth*, more slender canine teeth, and flatter skulls with larger *nuchal crests*, but otherwise little distinguishes them morphologically from ordinary dogs.[180] Dingoes also have erect, pointed ears and bushy tails.[181] Despite having been ascribed several color morphs (e.g. ginger, black-and-tan, brindle, white, patchy, sable), "pure" dingoes everywhere were probably ginger at one time,[182] which can range from sandy to nearly red, sometimes lighter on the underside and insides of the legs (Fig. 2.4).[183] Ginger is therefore regarded as "the basic dingo coloration."[184] White on the feet and tip of the tail are typical of Australian animals,[185] but not Thai dingoes.[186] Variation can be expected between individuals and among populations.[187] However, coat color and pattern, like skull conformation and other physical features, are unreliable diagnostic characters.[188] Black dingoes were reported by early European explorers and settlers, including some in Queensland with white chest patches.[189] Today black dingoes are rare. One thing is certain: after collecting, processing, and evaluating all these data, no one knows which combination – if any – represents the unadulterated dingo. Admixing was recognized early. Gerard Krefft, writing in 1866, stated that "neither the strychnine of the settlers, nor the guns or spears of the Aboriginals could exterminate the breed: which no doubt is also maintained by stray shepherds' dogs – not all the so-called Dingos being of the pure 'Warrigal' blood."[190]

Matings in Australia between free-ranging male dogs and female dingoes were projected as more likely than the reverse pairings because female dogs might have difficulty rearing pups alone.[191] This viewpoint is questionable for two reasons: (1) free-ranging female dogs around the world routinely rear litters, often in harsher conditions than the Victorian eastern highlands; and (2) dingo males are very likely inattentive fathers, no different than males of free-ranging domestic dogs (Chapter 8). Even if my assessment is wrong the pivotal point still holds true: admixed offspring make up the driving force behind further admixing, and the process accelerates as additional fertile admixtures enter a breeding population.[192] This would be the case anywhere in the world, whether the original pairings involved wolves, coyotes, dogs, or dingoes.

3   Visual and tactile communication

Behavior, which is a phenotypic *trait*,[1] can be defined as everything an animal does, but such a bland statement has no functional value. To make the term relevant I shall paraphrase a definition used by John Paul Scott and Emil Fredericson: *behavior* is the attempt by an organism to adjust to changing conditions.[2] Note that behavior is not a response to an *existing* condition, but to a *change* in conditions. *Communication*, a form of behavior, is an association between the sender's signal and the receiver's behavior as a consequence of the signal.[3] It can therefore be defined as the process of influencing others.[4] I define *signal* as a specific stimulus used in communication; alternatively, a semiotic sign (see below).[5] The *receiver* is the individual receiving a signal, the *sender* (or *signaler*) the one transmitting it.

3.1   Metaphors and semiotics

A term parasitized by many definitions turns stale and ultimately worthless with metaphorical use,[6] becoming a "dead metaphor." In trying to compare current usage with the original definition, we generally find language and culture to have changed and the relationship no longer relevant. Manufacturing metaphors for scientific purposes is not dishonest, merely hopeless. The conviction that they capture some essential element of nature is "no more important in the interpretation of metaphorical claims than ... in the interpretation of literal claims."[7] Their application in scientific description devolves ineluctably into discussions about whose metaphor is the most literal and thus closer to real explanations of nature. Unfortunately, metaphors that are only partly metaphorical are as rare as dogs that are only part mutt.

Attempting to define and describe animal communication is fraught with problems, many caused by our inability to banish the metaphors common to linguistics. Among the most prominent of these is the *conduit metaphor*,[8] which identifies the flaw in thinking of communication as a form of "representational ideation" linking sender and receiver; that is, the sender's signal as *encoded* in a message transmitted through a "conduit" directly to an expectant receiver's nose, ear, or eye pressed against the other end. The receiver supposedly *decodes* the message and "retrieves the relevant representational content."[9] Explicit is the notion of language in which both communicants experience a shared system of mutual mental representations and the presumed *intentionality* of signalers to inform receivers; that is, a *theory of mind*, something no nonhuman animal possesses.[10] Only humans have language, accounting for the inability to set aside our own theory of mind in trying to understand how other species communicate without it. At 7 months old, human infants already attribute goals and intentionality.[11] They assess the beliefs of others and retain them as alternative representations of the mental environment.[12] These achievements far exceed the capacities of any adult animal.

Without theory of mind, communication is unbalanced, or asymmetric, rather than modulated by mutual mental representation. The result is absence of intentionality by signalers and none of the referential aspects of language necessary to actually inform receivers.[13] The implication is extraordinary: *information is neither transmitted nor received.*[14] The same holds true for human communication. The notion that information is transmitted among individuals or stored in books and bytes is an illusion. Metaphors like "I can *read* your mind" and "learn to *speak your mind*" have encouraged the mistaken belief that "information" is actually contained inside "messages" and transmitted directly as a stream of packages. *Only signals are mobile; nothing else can be transmitted and received.*

Communication is far more versatile among humans because we have a theory of mind. Animal A, being unable to predict animal B's mental state, sends a signal, not for the purpose of establishing two-way communication but simply to influence B's behavior. At the receiving end, B interprets A's signal and responds independently or not at all. These events can be subtle and complex, offering the illusion of "conversation" accompanied by understanding, yet neither party in this example has understood the other's state of mind.[15] Conversely, when you say to a friend, "I smell coffee," he understands.

Like gold prospectors in a landscape where only pyrite has been found, animal behaviorists still seek the elusive proof of intentionality and representational symmetry in animal signals. Recently, however, the effort has been camouflaged beneath a startling rubric called "functional reference," which attempts to preserve the notion that such signals are indeed referential and therefore analogous to language even if the putative "information" transmitted is unintentional,[16] as it could only be in the animal world. Ambiguity fills spaces where clarity has departed, resulting in models of compromise. These are seldom effective as testable hypotheses, and the suggestion accompanying "functional reference" that "meaning" in animal signals exists along a continuum motivationally bounded at one end and functionally referential at the other is no exception.[17] Nikolaas Tinbergen warned that "teleology ... in which function was given as a proximate cause ... may well be a major stumbling block to causal analysis in its less obvious forms."[18]

It was long assumed that communication by humans and other animals involved the exchange of information, but what exactly does this mean? In fact, what does *mean* mean? Using only simple dictionary definitions, a message received and understood contains *information*. This seems transparent enough at the surface, but the epistemological barriers are deep and turbid. A *message* by definition makes sense to a receiver provided the information is understandable, and also presuming messages received but not understood, or not received at all, are either nonsense or irrelevant. If we eliminate these last possibilities the remainder is a tautology: information and message are inseparable.

The conduit metaphor necessitates encoding signals for receivers to decode. To *encode* is to convert information into *code* for transmission. The fallacy is in thinking something actually changes. A code is simply a relationship between two systems. As Reddy stated, "it does not 'change' anything into anything else."[19] Nothing except the signal actually travels anywhere. Anyway, why would the "coding" of metaphors be useful, much less necessary, when they already defy description? A wolf baring its teeth sends a signal to another wolf. The receiver interprets this gesture easily because wolves evolved as social animals, their signs interpreted and reinforced through every generation by *learning* and experience. To insert decoding into the sequence requires the existence of a message with its implication of *meaning*, sometimes defined as a message intended, expressed, or signified. We have no evidence that messages are even passed during communication, much less with intentionality. In any case, a signal is assuredly not a message.[20]

It should be obvious that our present epistemology of animal communication is a loose, infinitely regressive system of circular definitions placed in overlapping layers of reductionism. At the surface of this edifice lies the most primitive and presumably least confusing of ethology's methods: observational data transcribed by hand, intuitively pleasing but mostly numbed by dead or vacant metaphors. Data at the bottom layer where new growth occurs have been reduced to molecular chemistry accompanied by disarming promises of old metaphors newly distilled, decanted, and now rendered literal.

Because discussions about animal communication center on definitions and their philosophical and empirical foundations, valiant attempts have been made to rectify (and often justify) loose-fitting terminology. I start using semiotics to set conceptual boundaries before eliminating tautologies and stripping out descriptive terms based on metaphors long deceased. Think of it as a simplistic exercise and nothing more. Some will accuse me of sweeping troublesome linguistic problems under the carpet then jumping up and down on the lump to lower its profile, and they might be correct. Nonetheless, I believe parsimony has a useful place in structured thinking, and semiotics provides a flat surface on which to stretch out and examine, if only superficially, terms too amorphous and flaccid to be useful.

Semiotics is the study of signs and their meanings (Fig. 3.1). At one corner of the semiotic triangle is the *sign* itself (also called the *signifier*) conceived as an object or sensory stimulus; that is, a signal transmitted by a sender. In human terms it could be the odor of coffee brewing or a flashing traffic light. A semiotic sign is something palpable: a landmark, sound, odor, gesture, or posture. The visible signs of wolves and dogs include specific body postures, facial expressions, and vocalizations used alone or in combination. All apparently relate to increasing, decreasing, or maintaining distance from one or more conspecifics.[21] A *snarl* (Fig. 3.2) is defined

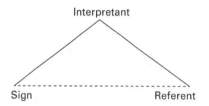

Figure 3.1 The semiotic triangle.
Source: Spotte (2006).

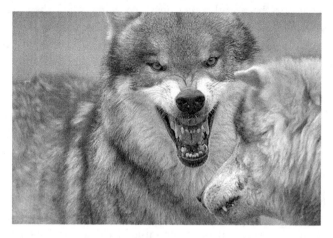

Figure 3.2 Snarl.
Source: Christian Schmalhofer|Dreamstime.com.

by two signs, one auditory (a growl), the other visual (a characteristic facial expression of lips retracted with *teeth-bared* and nose wrinkled). Consciousness – as in self-awareness – need not be involved. However, the capacity to display most signs, visible or otherwise, sometimes follows an ontogenetic progression. Thus signs might become functional only at specific developmental stages. Wolves, for example, lack any change in facial expression until about age 3 weeks and "prior to this time the face [has] a 'mask-like' appearance."[22] Nor are ear movements apparent until after age 3 weeks.

The sign is linked to the *interpretant*, which is the object or property being signified. The interpretant is what a sign represents to the receiver, or what it signifies: anger, uncertainty, fear, lust, dominance, submission. To qualify as a semiotic sign, a signal must possess qualities needed to be interpreted by the receiver.

At the remaining corner of the triangle is the *referent* "to which the interpretant both refers and serves as mediating agent with the sign."[23] The referent can be indirect (a memory of drinking coffee) or direct (seeing a coffee shop). Other examples are watching snow fall and feeling cold, hearing rain and glancing at an umbrella in the corner; in other words, experiencing a connection at least vaguely familiar. In primitive organisms sensory perception alone can select for referents.

The dashed line in the figure connecting sign and referent emphasizes increased conceptual distance and often lack of a clear connection. This is because signs – words, for example – are neither parts of things nor do they consistently imply things with which we make them correspond; *we can only impute an association between a sign and its referent*. White-tailed deer show little fear of humans where they have not been hunted in many years. This trust dissipates quickly if hunting resumes, at which point: sign (humans) → interpretant (danger) → referent (ancestral memory of predation). Humans have now become associated with predators, although exactly how this links with the sign – how a deer actually recognizes a predator *as such* – is unknown.

An individual can obviously work through a semiotic sequence alone, but where communication is involved at least two are required, a sender and a receiver. The referent has a long history of confusion in animal communication, some claiming its origin must be exclusively external, others willing to include the signaler's behavior too.[24] Much of it seems misplaced when reduced to semiotics. As mentioned, a signal of any kind is a sign to which the associated referent is tenuous. Defining the referent in terms of signaling behavior confuses the issue further. W. John Smith wrote, "if a signal provides information about (refers to) a signaler's behavior, yet behavior cannot be called a referent, how do we express the relationship?"[25] Here three obvious sources of confusion arise. First, the interpretant, not the referent, *refers to* the sign (the signaler's behavior noted by Smith) and serves as its mediating agent. A male bullfrog's vocalizations – its behavior in this situation – are signs, not referents. A female hearing his call receives the signal, interprets it, and makes an appropriate response or no response at all. Second, from a receiver's standpoint a signaler's behavior at the instant of signaling *is* the sign and therefore can never be the referent. Third, processing a message (the interpretant) is internal, devoid of overt behavior. This is true even if signal and response seems nearly instantaneous to a third-party observer. Between them must be an interpretant. A housefly standing on a kitchen table perceives sudden movement from above (sign) and nimbly avoids the fly-swatter (response). Wedged between these events was the interpretant (impending doom). The sign and referent (innate predator avoidance) were obviously connected, but the fly's decision was effected by the interpretant's mediating action.

The terms information, message, meaning, encode, and decode all crowd together in semiotic confusion, and none is actually necessary for purposes here. The next step is to examine these words and how they relate to one another. The most salient and misleading is information, a classic dead metaphor. Some investigators advocate abandoning the concept of information in animal communication and replacing it with "influence."[26] This is a radical idea, but not radical enough. Removing information narrows the focus of how animals actually communicate while forming a needed alliance with neurobiology (see below). However, the notion of a transmitted message with its attendant meaning should also be eliminated. Two inseparable ideas (information and message), one scarcely different from the other, present a potential tautology, especially considering that information is sometimes defined as meaning.[27]

If any of the terms mentioned so far in discussing signal → response fail to fit the semiotic triangle, are they necessary? A purely mechanistic signal can be described qualitatively without resorting to the "code" word even if reduced to a molecular level (Chapter 4). Thinking of a wolf as "encoding" the neurological steps involved in baring its teeth before bundling them into a visual signal and sending it off toward a receiver is distracting and unnecessary. We know because this behavior can be described adequately without the encoding metaphor. *The receiver is not waiting at the other end to "decode" the signal but to interpret it.* Putting aside the linguistic metaphor omits nothing we could salvage by keeping it.

A message without meaning is gibberish, and meaning requires a message to exist at all. So where does meaning reside? Inside the information, according to the conduit metaphor, which itself is contained inside and inseparable from the message. Message, information, and meaning become a purée once stuffed inside the metaphorical conduit. Choose any of them. My choice is none. Message brings along a disconcerting and incestuous tie with information, and meaning, even if dissected out carefully, will always require the caveat that its application not be confused with meaning in semantics, although even there it seems inseparable from a semiotic sign. Linguistic meaning in semiotics is imputed by the broken line connecting sign and referent (Fig. 3.1), personal but simultaneously communal because it can be recognized by others. *In communication what the sender transmits is a signal, not meaning wrapped inside information wrapped inside a message.* The receiver simply interprets the signal. Assessing the interpretant is the receiver's task alone. A female bullfrog hears a male's croak (the sign) and perceives it to be what we would term a mating call (the interpretant). The sign, mediated by the interpretant, is now linked vaguely to an ancestral "memory" of reproduction (the referent), a bullfrog's equivalent of smelling the coffee.

3.2   Signal and response

Whatever a howl signifies to the wolf emitting it, to a listening wolf things are obviously more complicated. *The capacity to influence is always greater for the sender than the receiver.* This is because interpretation is not required of the sender, only the receiver. Also, interpretation of a specific signal is hindered by simultaneous information arriving from other sources, and by corruption of the signal during transmission. All this incoming data constitutes noise, whether its source is acoustical, chemical, visual, or haptic, and each signal received needs to be interpreted before being placed in order of importance.

Functionally, *noise* is any interference in the background that disrupts a receiver's ability to discriminate a signal of any kind. Clearly, noise is not just an acoustical property when the context is communication, but rather the property of a specific communication channel that opens according to sensory modality. One of these is visual, in which case a sequence of flashing lights might constitute noise by disrupting the visual communication channel. Thus a *communication channel* represents the sum of all paths by which a signal is transmitted to specific sensory receptors of the receiver. Similarly, substituting deodorant for showering offers hope of introducing less disagreeable and confusing noise into the olfactory channels of anyone sitting beside you on the subway.

A signal can be made distinct from channel-specific background noise in three ways: (1) increase its intensity, (2) reduce its variability by making it stereotyped, or (3) render it more complex to form a distinctive pattern.[28] All are used by canids in one form or another. The use of chemical cues to signal estrus, for example, employ them all (Chapter 4), as do the body postures signaling dominance and submission to be described shortly.

Descriptions of behavioral interactions often exclude temporal elements, as if events happened in a dimensionless universe. Simply connecting signal with response omits the step necessary for assessing how different behaviors factor into the time budgets of social animals. The transmission of a discrete signal is easily observed and measured, but its effect on the receiver could be subtle, prolonged, and much more difficult to assess. If stereotyped, a signal's effect on the receiver can be cumulative; alternatively, the receiver can become habituated, the initial stimulatory effect tapering off to indifference.

Much of behavior results from learning, which involves associating familiar signals with remembered responses. One way of retaining something learned (i.e. of remembering) is by reinforcement (see below). We might begin a behavioral experiment by identifying and isolating a *primary signal* (the *releaser* of classical animal behavior), S_1, which elicits a specific – and automatic – response under given conditions. This short unidirectional sequence of signal $\rightarrow$ response provides a narrow but reliable measure of behavior enabling us to state that if we apply a primary signal, S_1, in defined and restricted circumstances the probable (and statistically predictable) result will be the *primary response*, R_1. This is true provided the receiver has experienced it before, learned what it signifies, and remembers.

Suppose we keep experimental conditions the same and change only the signal. Instead of applying the primary signal, S_1, we use a different one, a *secondary signal*, S_2. The expected response will be no response at all (R_0) because the receiver is unable to make the association (i.e. has not yet learned to associate S_2 with S_1). By subsequent application of the primary and secondary stimuli together ($S_1 + S_2$) we consistently elicit the primary response, a procedure known as *reinforcement*. After the animal has learned the new association by repetition we can omit S_1, apply just S_2, and still elicit R_1. Our experimental animal has adjusted to a *change in conditions* from no response, R_0, to the primary response, R_1, in the presence S_2.

To invent an example of how this works, picture a young dog with limited social etiquette badgering an elder trying to sleep. The old dog turns without warning and gives the surprised youngster a gentle nudge (S_1), inducing a primary response (R_1) of abruptly stopping the torment and stepping away. The minimal pain is soon forgotten, and the young dog again pounces on the older one. This time the old dog growls (S_2), a meaningless gesture to a receiver without experience of such signals. Finally, having suffered enough, it growls while simultaneously administering a gentle nip ($S_1 + S_2$). The young dog demonstrates the primary response, R_1, once again stopping its activity and moving away. Having now reinforced that a growl is likely to be followed quickly by a nip, on the next occasion the old dog needs only to growl – that is, apply the secondary signal, S_2 – and the young receiver recognizes this behavior as preceding a nip and backs off. It has learned and adjusted to the change in conditions.

A secondary signal, if used alone repeatedly without reinforcement, will eventually cause the primary response to attenuate and degrade toward R_0. If reinforcement is eliminated the eventual consequence is complete loss of the response (reversion to R_0) and *extinction*. The saying in conservation biology that extinction lasts forever does not hold true in behavior. A sequence of $S_2 \rightarrow R_1$ can be exhumed after sufficient time has passed and resuscitated by reinforcement. This Phoenix-like quality is evidence of permanent association.[29]

3.3   Agonistic behavior

Communication necessitates that both signal and response be recognized. Among the most extensively described behaviors of canids are *dominance* and *submission*,[30] thought to maintain stability by stiffening the social order.[31] In displaying certain facial expressions and postures recognized by subordinates a dominant animal confirms its rank in a hierarchy, and the rest acknowledge their lesser positions by showing appropriate expressions and postures both they and the dominant understand. A *dominant wolf* (also called the *alpha wolf*) is a socially superior animal in its pack that usually breeds.[32] Domestic dogs and wolves have evolved a greater range of facial and body expressions than more solitary canids.[33]

Dominance is supposed to maintain social order from the top down while submission reinforces it from the bottom up,[34] although neither is necessarily permanent. It bears emphasizing that dominance "is not an individual trait but a reflection of an asymmetrical and dynamic relationship between two individuals that could vary over time and ... context."[35] The same, of course, can be said of submission, and in neither case is it necessary that dominance and submission even involve the same two individuals.

The qualities of dominance can erode in special circumstances. A dominant wolf captured and radio-collared on the Kenai Peninsula lost his status and upon being released became a subordinate.[36] This wolf dispersed soon after and formed a new pack. Under similar circumstances a captive dominant male was deposed after having been separated briefly from the group.[37] *Dominance behavior, therefore, is attributable to ascension in rank and not to any individual trait.*[38] A previously subordinate wolf, having suddenly assumed the mantle of emperor, instantly acts the part.

Agonism, or *agonistic behavior*, conceptually tethers submission with dominance so that each can be interpreted and reinforced by the other.[39] In doing so, a directed signal and the elicited response are simultaneously linked and reciprocal. One does not exist apart from the other. Consequently, all behaviors requiring adjustments to change by the participants can be "packaged" in context. Patterns of agonistic behavior have been considered essential for living in large groups,[40] and agonism encompasses conflicting aspects of social competition. It is not a synonym of *aggression*, which is unidirectional and makes up just one element of dominance behavior.[41] The evolution of agonistic behavior is considered tied to social living because most of its elements are abbreviated or nonexistent in foxes, coyotes, and jackals, which are more solitary.[42] The consequence is social stability passed along through generations, resulting in "relatively constant selection pressure over long periods of time."[43]

The important functional aspect is that agonism is bidirectional, occurring when one animal shows dominance toward another, which might respond by submissive behavior (e.g. running away, flopping onto its back). Sometimes a subordinate displays submission to a dominant without having been cued first, which the higher-ranking animal can then ignore or acknowledge with a reciprocal display of dominance. *Subordinance-acknowledging, in other words, is not always prompted by dominance-confirming, and either of them can serve as signal or response.*

Aggression, when teased out of this entanglement, is seen to be a component and not the endgame.[44] Dominance hierarchies are thought to establish ordered access to resources among individuals.[45] Arguments that they promote social stability typically take this form: dominance hierarchies reduce incidences of aggression because subordinate animals do not fight dominants. The part about fighting has been called a "solecism,"[46] but a bigger problem is circular reasoning built into the notion itself. As a hypothesis the concept is self-fulfilling and not falsifiable: remove the dominant animal and subsequent aggression subsides only after another becomes dominant.[47]

Aggression takes two basic forms.[48] *Competitive aggression* is aimed solely at the other participant over a tangible object (i.e. is object-directed).[49] Competitive aggression, in other words, seems to occur "only when possession of the object can be assured."[50] For example, a squabble over food usually ends when the dominant animal takes possession.

In general, aggression is most violent and extended in the absence of competition; that is, when fights between combatants are *noncompetitive* (i.e. not object-directed). This is true of many species including captive mice[51] and captive wolves.[52] Its agonistic component includes behaviors of both the dominant animal and a subordinate that might be trying to escape. Such an encounter is often prolonged,[53] and if escape is impossible the outcome can be serious injury, even death.[54] Noncompetitive aggression in captive animals might actually represent attempted displacement of the receiver to gain undisturbed living space, a result of the inability to disperse.[55]

Dominance and submission, seemingly easy to categorize, actually exist on a continuum. We could, in a slightly different context, interpret this unbroken line as extending from seriousness to playfulness.[56] Furthermore, the facial and postural displays we identify and label probably convey different signals when used in different combinations and sequences.

From here on I present the dominance ↔ submission association with a two-way arrow to emphasize its reciprocal nature, similar to a reversible equation in chemistry. Feedback is continuous in both directions. A dominant animal (the sender) might direct a signal at a subordinate (the receiver), but when the receiver gives its response the arrow reverses and sender and receiver exchange roles. Now the subordinate animal's response becomes a signal directed toward the dominant, which assumes the role of receiver.

Learning within the context of dominance ↔ submission takes three forms.[57] The first is trained winning or losing in which individuals learn to behave as dominants or subordinates during new encounters based on personal history of having previously won or lost. Identities of past and present opponents are irrelevant, and an animal with a history of submissiveness (or dominance) is likely to display these traits in future encounters with conspecifics.

The second form, like the first, involves training and depends on a previous history of winning or losing, with this difference: interactions take place between two individuals known to each other. Such a situation obviously requires mutual recognition. Third is site-specific learning, which is purely situational. An animal is dominant when defending its territory (Chapter 5), but might switch to submissive mode at other locations. As with the first form of learning the identities of opponents are irrelevant.

Learning as an effect variable is usually ignored in tests of dominance. We can assume that canids recognize others of their species as individuals and that outcomes of dominant ↔ subordinate interactions are not only remembered by the participants but predictable to all. In other words, each animal gravitates to its place in society regardless of whether the predicted response is learned or innate.[58] During an experiment hungry mice fought over food. When tested at satiation they still fought, but control mice did not.[59] Just one trial induced this effect. A similar situation of learned behavior is seen in groups of domestic dogs, which typically fight over food even if not hungry.

3.4   The physiological stress response

The main physiological stress response in mammals is nonspecific. In other words, regardless of the origin and nature of the stress factor the response it triggers is essentially the same each time. Adrenaline released into the blood raises heart and breathing rates in seconds. Blood pressure rises, and energy stored in the tissues is released for immediate use. *Corticosteroid hormones* (*corticosteroids*) secreted by the *adrenal glands* also enter the blood during stressful times. The result is to temporarily divert energy, making it instantly available for self-defense or escape. The long-term effects of either repeated spikes or sustained elevated concentrations of corticosteroids are harmful, having been implicated in growth reduction, impairment of digestion, reproductive failure, immune suppression, disruption of brain function, and reduced life span.[60]

The physiological stress response is well-documented, its validity not in doubt. Of interest here is how individual members of wolf societies are affected. From early experiments on aggression using laboratory rodents (essentially gladiator contests in a restricted space) came the idea that only subordinate animals suffer the physiological consequences of stress.[61] Dominant social canids, however, feel the pressure of high status more than subordinates. With authority comes stress.

Wild dominant gray wolves and African wild dogs have elevated corticosteroids more often than subordinates, indicating a metabolic cost associated with high social rank.[62] Frequency of agonistic and aggressive behaviors among wolves does not correlate with corticosteroid concentration, nor do dominants engage in either behavior more often than subordinates do with each other.[63] Moreover, corticosteroids of dominant Yellowstone wolves were consistently higher than those of subordinates.[64] Concentrations of corticosteroids are more elevated in dominant than in subordinate African wild dogs not just during the breeding season, but all year round.[65]

The effect of elevated stress can also be detected behaviorally. A dominant and a low-ranking subordinate wolf were separated from a captive group, placed in separate cages, and their activities compared.[66] The dominant spent less time sleeping, more time in the part of his cage nearest the main group, and his stereotyped pacing was more intense than the subordinate's. The dominant wolf had also been more active prior to separation.

Confirmation that subordination is not always stressful can be seen when lower-ranking wolves actively solicit domination, approaching a dominant and annoying it until receiving the expected response.[67] On many occasions a subordinate's actions are simply ignored. Altercations are likely to be more intense and impose a heavier social burden on the dominant animal, which might be required to defend its position while lower-ranking animals might be content where they are.[68]

3.5   Visual and tactile signaling

Most behavior termed communication in ethology is better described simply as interaction. Even visible routines amenable to consistent labeling often have undemonstrated functions. Linking simple cause–effect relationships into predictable behavioral sequences leaves a feeling that something truly important has been missed. Here I repeat what the literature offers. Interpret it with circumspection, because much of what we see is not necessarily as it seems.

Wolf societies evidently are held together by affection among individuals and a hierarchy based partly on mutually recognized signs of dominance ↔ submission.

Living in a society requires interaction among its members, and canids do this in various ways. Vision, scent, taste, hearing, and touch are important, but the most obvious class of canid behaviors – at least to us – involves elements of vision and touch. The correlation of facial expressions, body postures, and touch during social interaction has been studied extensively in captive wolves.

Among the first to document and attempt to interpret these signs was Rudolf Schenkel. His most extensive work, published in German in 1947, was followed by a shorter English version 20 years later. Many of his original observations and interpretations, and later ones by Michael W. Fox, apparently remain valid in descriptive contexts, and I reprise some of them here.

Schenkel and subsequently others saw in captive wolves dominance hierarchies comprising rank orders that were often bilinear, one male, the other female. An individual's rank could be challenged, a dominant usurped. Subordinates formed shifting alliances, and battles apparently over status were sometimes violent, even fatal. In reading these reports it seems as if nature might indeed be ruled by fang and claw, until you consider that zoo enclosures are unlike nature; that is, unnatural.[69]

In the ensuing discussion descriptive terms for visual and haptic agonistic behaviors have been hyphenated to emphasize their specific qualities. I have defined them in Table 3.1 but not in the Glossary.[70] A subordinate wolf might only appear to challenge a dominant, and to an uninitiated observer it would seem that the roles are even reversed. The subordinate animal sometimes grips the muzzle of the dominant gently in its jaws (*muzzle-grab*) (Fig. 3.3) or paws its face (*face-paw*) (Fig. 3.4) then perhaps throws a foreleg over the dominant's neck (*foreleg-over*)[71] and pushes down (*push-down*).[72] Lois Crisler mentioned the foreleg-over several times when describing how captive wolves interact with each other and with dogs. She interpreted it as a sign of friendliness,[73] but the gesture can be agonistic if the subordinate's attempts at push-down persist. The dominant usually resists. It growls, maintains a rigid upright posture or *walks stiff-legged* holding the head high (*head-high*), keeping the ears erect (*ears-erect*), and the tail elevated or at least horizontal (*tail-high*) and sometimes wagging slightly (*tail-wag*).[74] All are signs of authority, and the composite pose incorporating these features is *stand-taut* (Fig. 3.5).[75] During *stand-over* a dominant animal stands-taut while straddling a subordinate lying on its side or back.[76] In *stand-across* the dominant stands-taut with its body perpendicular to the subordinate's (Fig. 3.5). A consistent variation of *pin-down* was displayed by captive eastern coyotes when the dominant animal placed its forepaws on the shoulders, chest, or abdomen of a prone subordinate.[77] Adult pairs often interacted this way, not necessarily during the breeding season, and the animal being pinned was not necessarily one sex or the other.[78]

Alternatively, the subordinate wolf faces the side of the dominant's neck with teeth-bared and growls. The dominant once again stands-taut or lowers its head slightly (*head-low*) and growls back. In another configuration the subordinate crouches slightly (*crouch*) and stands parallel to the dominant with *tail-low* (drooping or between the legs) while growling with teeth-bared. In all situations the dominant

Table 3.1. Wolf visual and haptic agonistic behaviors. DOM, dominant; SUB, subordinate. Various sources.

Behavior	Description
clasping (hugging)	SUB sits or crouches facing DOM, wraps both forelegs around DOM's neck; thought to be a friendly gesture
crouch	SUB lowers head and body nearly horizontal to the ground, tail-low
ears-erect	DOM's ears stand erect
ears-flat	Ears stand out flat to sides of head; seen in both DOM and SUB
ears-folded	SUB folds ears to side of head and backward when facing DOM
face-paw	SUB crouches and paws DOM's face
foreleg-over	SUB attempts to force DOM to the ground by placing a foreleg over its neck
French-kiss	SUB licks inside of DOM's mouth while DOM stands-taut and holds mouth open
genital-sniff	SUB lies prostrate in passive submission while DOM sniffs its genitals
group-ceremony	SUBs surround DOM licking-up, face-pawing, tail-wagging
head-high	DOM holds head high while in posture like walking stiff-legged, stand-across, stand-taut
head-low	SUB approaches DOM with head lowered
lick-up	SUB crouches before DOM and licks DOM's mouth
mount	SUB attempts to mount DOM, often from the side, as if attempting sexual penetration
muzzle-grab	Usually performed by SUB, which takes DOM's muzzle gently in its jaws
nose-push	SUB sits or crouches before DOM and pushes up DOM's muzzle so it points skyward; considered a friendly gesture
pin-down	DOM pins SUB to ground by neck or chest using one or both forelegs
push-down	SUB attempts to push DOM to the ground using foreleg-over
snarl	DOM wrinkles nose with teeth-bared and growls
stand-across	DOM stands-taut in a position perpendicular to the SUB
stand-over	DOM stands-taut with genitals above recumbent SUB in passive submission, which sometimes sniffs them
stand-taut	DOM stands erect, unmoving, ears-erect, tail-erect or slightly elevated, and receives SUB's behaviors
stare	DOM stares at SUB, forcing it to look askance.
submissive-grin	Facial expression by SUB when threatened by DOM; lips retract horizontally in what appears to be a grin
tail-high	DOM holds tail high or horizontal
tail-low	SUB holds tail low or between legs
tail-wag	Performed by DOM or SUB and considered a friendly gesture; can also signal excitement
teeth-bared	DOM or SUB bares its teeth without growling; visual signal of aggression or fear during which the nose wrinkles and the lips retract
tongue-flick	SUB flicks the tip of its tongue quickly in and out; thought to be an anxious or nervous gesture
walking stiff-legged	DOM walks slowly with an exaggerated stiff-legged gait

poses with ears-erect and tail-high, the subordinate with tail-low and ears folded back against the head (*ears-folded*). Sometimes a subordinate wolf faces a dominant, crouches, and puts both forelegs around the dominant's neck (*clasping*).[79] This is ordinarily considered a friendly gesture.[80] *Tongue-flick*, when the tip of the tongue

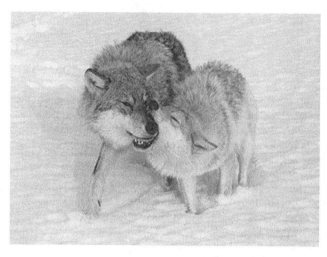

Figure 3.3 Muzzle-grab.
Source: Vladkiselev|Dreamstime.com.

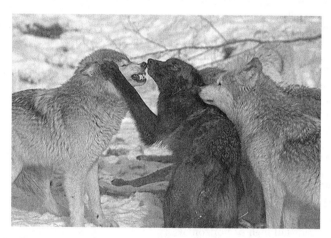

Figure 3.4 Face-paw.
Source: Outdoorsman|Dreamstime.com.

moves rapidly in and out of the mouth like a snake's (Fig. 3.6), has been inter-preted as a sign of submission[81] but also as evidence of stress, fear, apprehension, or pain.[82]

Schenkel proposed two categories of submission, active and passive.[83] Others later labeled the accompanying displays of both as "ritualized conflict,"[84] which seems appropriate mainly for captive wolves. Conflict implies a state of dishar-mony, not unusual among wolves in zoos. Within stable societies such "rituals" are thought to place limits on disharmony instead of reinforcing it, which occurs when each flash of agonism by a sender likely elicits a counter display from the receiver. Dominance ↔ submission has been reported when strange wolves meet in the wild,[85] but agonistic behavior among pack mates is much rarer in wild

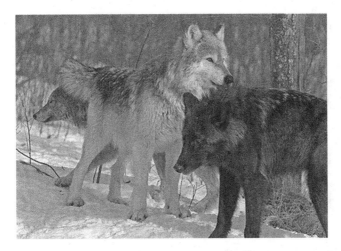

Figure 3.5 Stand-taut.
Source: Outdoorsman|Dreamstime.com.

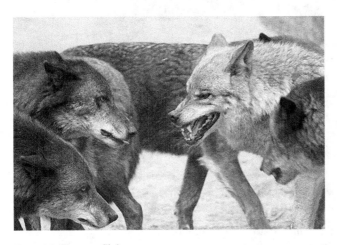

Figure 3.6 Tongue-flick.
Source: Mayerberg|Dreamstime.com.

wolves,[86] evidence that such "rituals" seldom devolve into aggression under normal living conditions.[87]

During *active submission* the subordinate is slightly crouched, tail-low, ears-folded. Friendliness, not hostility, is now evident, as the subordinate attempts to lick the dominant's mouth, called *lick-up*[88] (Fig. 3.7). The dominant animal usually stands-taut with *ears-flat* (ears flattened and extended perpendicular from the sides of the head)[89] and lips pulled back slightly,[90] although a submissive animal displays similar behavior if it feels an immediate threat (Fig. 3.8).

Alternatively, the subordinate might push up the dominant's muzzle with its own (*nose-push*), sometimes until the dominant's nose points skyward,[91] then licks-up. The nose-push and face-paw are thought to be both submissive and

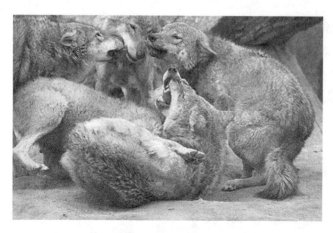

Figure 3.7 Lick-up.
Source: Gea Strucks|Dreamstime.com.

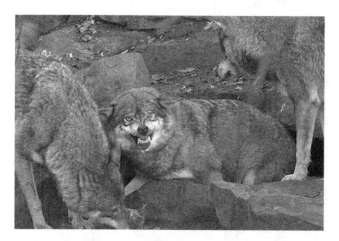

Figure 3.8 Ears-flat demonstrated by a subordinate wolf.
Source: Renier Vervaart|Dreamstime.com.

friendly gestures.[92] As part of either sequence the subordinate might gently muzzle-grab, following up by face-pawing or performing little dance steps with the forepaws. These activities are usually accompanied by deferential tail-wagging. Some of these behaviors are also seen during courtship (Chapter 7). Subordinates often approach a dominant sideways, head-low, crouched, tail-low, tail-wagging, face-pawing, and licking-up. On occasion subordinates even *mount* the dominant either from the back or side.[93] When directing a submissive greeting the eyes of the subordinate narrow, the eyebrows drop, the lips retract horizontally in the *submissive-grin*,[94] and the ears rotate to ears-flat or ears-folded (usually the latter).

During any of these displays the dominant animal, if feeling intolerant, turns toward the subordinate with a snarl or simply teeth-bared, eliciting avoidance and a submissive-grin. At this point the dominant might pin-down the subordinate

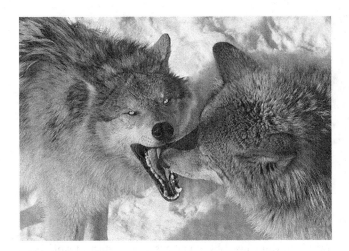

Figure 3.9 French-kiss.
Source: Denis Pepin|Dreamstime.com.

and muzzle-grab it.[95] A dominant can end all interaction by stand-taut and staring at the wolf causing annoyance (*stare*) until the subordinate looks askance.[96] Even from a distance the subordinate usually avoids eye contact. With ears-folded it sometimes cringes, whines, displays tail-low, or slinks away in a crouch.[97] Subordinate members of a wolf pack look at the dominant animals more often than their looks are returned.[98] As experienced dog handlers know, staring at a strange dog usually elicits the submissive responses just described or an attack. *Piloerection* (hair standing up) is evident on the tail, back, shoulders, and rump during agonistic encounters[99] and can be expressed by both dominant and submissive animals.

Lick-up is evidently an important feature of dominant ↔ subordinate interactions. Another behavior, termed *French-kiss*,[100] occurs when a dominant animal growls while permitting a whining subordinate to lick the inside of its mouth (Fig. 3.9).[101] Fox reported this behavior in the context of *ambivalent aggression* (I find *conflicted aggression* more descriptive) during which a subordinate approaches an unthreatening dominant and attempts a muzzle-grab. When the dominant subsequently snarls the subordinate face-paws then licks-up or French-kisses.[102] Conflicted aggression has also been described as consisting of mixed signals conveying both dominance and submissive components and believed to derive from motivational conflict.[103] An example of *conflicted behavior* is expressed when a wolf is approached unexpectedly by another wolf or human (Fig. 3.10). The typical response is a blend of dominant ↔ subordinate visual signals: piloerection, head-low, tail-low, ears-erect.

Schenkel also used active submission to describe what he called the *group-ceremony* (Fig. 3.11).[104] Here, the pack gathers around the dominant animal, subjecting it to friendly and excited nose-pushes, lick-ups, and muzzle-grabs. These few moments involve much crowding together and tail-wagging. Group-ceremonies often occur in captive packs if the dominant has been absent (e.g. removed for experimental purposes or veterinary care).[105] In the wild they

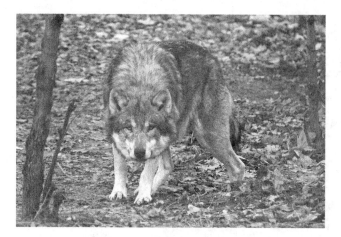

Figure 3.10 Conflicted behavior caused by apprehension in a startled wolf. Notice the semi-crouch, ears-erect but tail-low, and piloerection on nape of the neck. *Source*: Dawid Baøuch|Dreamstime.com.

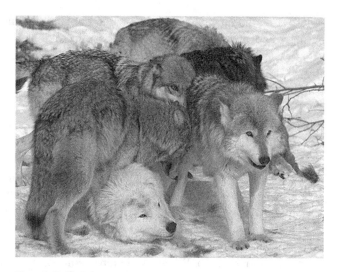

Figure 3.11 Group-ceremony.
Source: Outdoorsman|Dreamstime.com.

are seen when the pack wakes up or before leaving on a hunt (Chapter 6)[106] and in the latter case might involve assembling nose-to-nose and tail-wagging before setting out.[107] Fox observed a *contagious effect* among young captive wolves during the group-ceremony. They became excited, performing tail-wags and lick-ups directed toward each other that demonstrate reciprocal active submission, and then breaking into bouts of play.

During *passive submission* the subordinate lies on its side but twisted so that its chest and sometimes part of the abdomen are exposed, a sort of upside-down prostration.[108] Forelegs are retracted, ears-folded, the tail bent inward or even placed between the thighs. In this configuration the subordinate remains motion-less while the dominant sniffs its genitals (*genital-sniff*).[109] In another version the subordinate crouches, tail-low and ears-folded, while the dominant stands-taut, muzzle-grabs, and growls.[110]

Attempts to interpret the facial expressions and postures just described without rigorous hypothesis testing are numerous.[111] These have at least two serious defi-ciencies: (1) all are intuitive and lack quantification, and (2) all assume that our interpretations of the expressions and postures observed correlate directly with the subject's *affective* (i.e. emotional) *state*. Construction of behavioral models based on observation of expressions and postures can only be arbitrary and heuristic.[112] In addition to these difficulties are emotional interpretations of our own that inevitably creep in. As John C. Fentress wrote, "in many respects . . . the wolf has a Mona Lisa quality in which expression varies as a function of the observer."[113]

Affective state can be short, lasting as long as the behavior seeming to express it, or longer, as in *mood*.[114] A trait is a more permanent individual characteristic.[115] Similar to dominance ↔ submission, expression of an affective state must be defined within the context of a directed signal and the receiver's response, although it extends deeper.[116] Dominance ↔ submission describes a visible reci-procity, but affective state ↔ response allows us to see only the response, the observation of which is far less complex. Thus a response can remain constant while the affective state that stimulates it ebbs and flows in unknown ways.[117]

The dominance ↔ submission link is best assessed from the receiver's response and not the sender's signal. As a measure of affective state the signal is the less reliable, partly because interpretants are more nuanced, allowing greater flexibility about the extent and direction of the "negotiation" momentarily in flux. Attempts to quantify facial expressions and postures of wolves without regard to affective state have cast doubt on early interpretations. Ordination of data collected from observing captive wolves has tentatively shown, for example, that ears-flat and head-high, both presumed signs of aggression, failed to cluster with any other component of dominance, as did tail-wag and the composite feature stand-taut.[118]

Other forms of aggressive behavior displayed by captive wolves are apparently decoupled too, tacit evidence that the agonistic component of dominance is driven by more than aggression.[119] Threat and assault, for example, apparently are not indica-tors of general dominance but of dominance that varies temporarily with the situation, meaning that either behavior can be directed by a dominant or subor-dinate at any member of the pack without upsetting the hierarchy, and, if directed by a subordinate toward a dominant, usually without being punished.[120] When the setting is competitive and food is involved an "ownership zone [is retained] around the mouth of each wolf."[121] Wolves can attempt to steal food from each other, but every individual, regardless of rank, has the apparent right to retain it. A subordinate wolf is often intolerant of a higher-ranking individual attempting to take its food, and that this is respected by the dominant and not punished.

Also falling into this category is the apparent dominance of breeding females over all other pack members until pups leave the den (Chapter 8).[122] Mech discussed what he called "exceptions to dominance privileges"[123] and gave as an example an incident he witnessed at a zoo. The female of a wolf pair had recently given birth. When her mate of three years or more approached her, "the female instantly charged him in a dominant posture, and the male ran off submissively in an attitude very rare for him."[124] In a more developed form, Jan A. R. A. M. van Hooff and co-authors, in studies of captive wolves, termed such reversals of the normal order *situational dominance.*[125]

Muzzle-grab, face-paw, mount, and bark appear to be weakly associated with dominance.[126] Repeatedly licking the lips has also been labeled a conflicted signal in wolves[127] and domestic dogs,[128] but *tongue-flick* probably indicates nervousness. Conflicted behavior is reportedly common among captive wolves of all social ranks, and when expressed by dominant wolves has been interpreted as evidence that dominance ↔ submission should be considered apart from aggression.[129] Much of this had been anticipated in the 1960s based on primate studies.[130]

The question posed is whether agonistic behavior might be a poor predictor of dominance in wolves. In the opinion of Randall Lockwood, agonism "represents the type of behavior that the existence of a dominance hierarchy should prevent."[131] Whether such a stasis could evolve – much less persist – without reinforcement then becomes the issue. It actually did evolve and indeed persists, with minimal reinforcement among wild wolves.

Should we accept the obvious agonistic components of dominance ↔ submission as the principal forces maintaining social order? Probably not. The use of social signaling to curb aggression and the subsequent injury and disorder it brings (Chapter 9) is hardly evidence of such a function being served. The idea of *dominance style*[132] among primates has been adapted to canids in interesting ways by Roberto Bonanni and colleagues, mainly by broadening our perspective of dominance behavior's more subtle and tolerant aspects.[133] Dominance encompasses far more than agonism. Reports of extreme incidents of dominance ↔ submission described later (Chapter 9) come from observations of captive wolves and present a distorted picture of canid societies.[134] The dominance style among wild wolves and free-ranging dogs is practiced within a framework that makes peaceful group living possible. It takes into account non-dispersive methods of settling conflicts while still reinforcing social status. Frans B. M. de Waal's primate work led the way, and he warned about emphasizing the outcome and rewards of dominance instead of the costs of social conflict.[135]

These insights are equally true of wolves and dogs in which outright fighting is ordinarily mitigated by unidirectional expressions of social status leading to reduced prospects of aggression. The process consists of an abbreviated display of active submission, here called *paying homage.* A wolf or dog paying homage ordinarily initiates this act of obeisance, the analog of kneeling before the emperor and kissing his ring. A subordinate executes a relaxed, unidirectional, abbreviated sequence of behaviors requiring only that approaching the dominant animal be conducted appropriately with head-low, ears-folded, tail-wagging, and initiating physical contact by licking-up or nose-pushing (Fig. 3.12). A dominant accepts

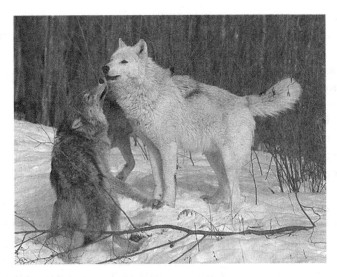

Figure 3.12 Active submission.
Source: Outdoorsman|Dreamstime.com.

this tribute solemnly, *receiving homage*.[136] It stands-taught, ears-erect, tail-erect and wagging. In being universal the submissive's signals are unambiguous. The dominant is never confused and thus unlikely to attack. By each party acknowledging the other's social position the dominant's status is not contested. In more aggressive displays of dominance ↔ submission the subordinate avoids eye contact, lowers its head and tail, folds its ears, and perhaps rolls onto its back in passive submission. If feeling directly threatened it yelps, withdraws slowly, or runs away with tail-low.[137]

Dominance ↔ submission and seriousness ↔ playfulness, as the arrows indicate, are reciprocal. In pups especially, play-fighting, chasing, biting, and so forth can slide easily into agonism; conversely, the direction is reversible and what had been dominance behavior one moment turns abruptly into play.[138] This is evident when the pups of wolves and domestic dogs play-fight. One pup flops to the ground and rolls onto its back while the other stands-over. They jaw-wrestle and nip each other, and what is generally considered a dominance ↔ submission episode now has different meaning. It becomes especially clear when the pups exchange positions and play-fighting continues uninterrupted.

With age comes a tightening of certain associations and a loosening of others, and most become fixed in wolves during the first several weeks.[139] Smoother integration enlarges the repertoire of visual signals as maturing wolves become adept at blending these components into expanded sequences. The result is facile communication through a subtle visual system of mutually recognized signals and responses.

During communication each component – that is, each facial expression, posture, or haptic contact – sets the stage for a specific interpretation; combinations of signals, or suites of them in combination, increase the array of possible interpretants.[140] Different signs might share the same interpretants, in which case they would not be used together. One signal could override another, and some (e.g. tail-wag) that in McLeod's experiments did not cluster with others might serve as "metastimuli" topping off the hierarchy of signals used in visual communication.

The notion of dominance and submission has undergone intermittent reassessment, so far without emergence of a clear paradigm.[141] Experiments based on faulty assumptions are partly to blame. Paired food competition,[142] for example, is a doubtful test of dominance because it assures that one animal will reach the food first and be "nominally dominant" over the other,[143] and because the experimenter is not actually in control. Place a cookie in the middle of a small room and release two dogs, Bowser and Fido, into the space simultaneously. Assume each has been starved for the same length of time and that other known variables are accounted for. Both rush toward the cookie, but Bowser gets there first and eats it. This brief sequence has been completed without aggression, yet only one dog got the treat. Repetitive trials are likely to give similar results, enough to reveal statistical distinctions, and Bowser is declared dominant over Fido. Is he? The dogs actually produced the result themselves by having "learned to learn this type of problem efficiently."[144] The hierarchy is false in being caused – not revealed – by the participants. Bowser and Fido have trained each other. Fido trained Bowser to be dominant in these trials, Bowser trained Fido to be subordinate, and reinforcement of the status quo was hardened by repetition. If placed with strange dogs they would probably retain their current status.[145]

Social hierarchies are established and sustained within an intricate web of context and circumstance. Animals, like experimenters who watch them, base predictions of future behavior on observations made in the present and assessed using the data to establish historical patterns. After studying captive baboons, Thelma E. Rowell concluded that submission correlates better with rank than dominance, and "subordinance hierarchy" might be more accurate than "dominance hierarchy" considering that responses come mostly from submissive animals. She remarked, "you cannot chase someone who doesn't flee."[146] This idea is especially appealing when space is not limiting, simply because animals can avoid each other, a reasonable alternative to conflict. In such instances the subordinate simply avoids the dominant, rendering the latter's *motivational state* irrelevant.[147] An equally appealing explanation is the inevitable disconnect between sender and receiver in the animal world, the sender having transmitted a signal to influence a receiver with which it has no representational parity.

I suppose if behavior is defined as anything an animal does, doing nothing qualifies too. However, if demonstration of rank is measured as direction and frequency of a response, the animal that actually does something (e.g. runs away) is the more reliable marker. Subordinate animals thereby maintain the hierarchy. Moreover, it is often a subordinate's initiation of submissive behavior – cringing, running away, fear-grinning – that elicits the dominant's response.[148]

Hierarchies are nonetheless most clearly delineated in captive animals where space is restricted and dispersal impossible (Chapter 9). Here expressions of submission are heightened in both frequency and duration, usually more so than reciprocal expressions by the dominant individual. Hierarchies among rhesus macaques (*Macaca mulatta*) become more fixed and intense as competition heats up. This rarely occurs in wild troupes, but is common in macaques confined to cages, free-ranging but fed by humans, and living in urban areas.[149] Common squirrel monkeys (*Saimiri sciureus*) and white-fronted capuchin monkeys (*Cebus albifrons*), which have no hierarchies in nature, can be induced to form them in captivity by restricting their space and making them compete for food.[150]

Selective breeding has drastically altered the morphology of domestic dogs, probably introducing behavioral disadvantages. One consequence has been selection for such paedomorphic features as both eyes directed straight ahead, making it impossible to look askance safely while avoiding eye contact. In fact, most dog breeds have paedomorphic body shapes compared with the ancestral wolf, posing the question of whether such forced deviation affects visual signaling.

Basic visual communication in wolves and dogs is the same.[151] Tail position and movement (tail-high, tail-low, tail-wagging) are among the most consistently reliable stimuli used to express agonistic behavior in captive wolves,[152] and even from a distance the dominant wolf in a wild pack can be discerned by its elevated tail.[153] Not surprisingly, long tails are more effective than docked tails at transmitting visual signals between dogs, and tail docking appears to hinder intraspecific communication.[154] Tail-high signals dominance, tail-low submission, and tail-wag is a sign of friendly interaction.[155] A dog minus its tail has lost an important appendage for communicating.[156] Other features thought to be attractive to dog fanciers have resulted in breeds with teeth exposed in a fixed snarl and others unable to bare their teeth.[157] Some have permanently wrinkled foreheads and noses, both signs of aggression.[158] Still others have ears too deformed for useful signaling.[159]

Is deviation from a wolf-like morphology detrimental to visual signaling? Apparently so. Adult behaviors and postures in dogs develop early and many are in place, at least in rudimentary form, by the age of 8 weeks (Chapter 9). Because paedomorphic changes amount to arrested physical development we have no reason to assume that visual signals used among wolves during agonistic encounters have passed intact to domestic dogs. Most of those identified in 10 highly selected breeds having limited repertoires paralleled those of wolves only up to age 3 weeks.[160] Selective breeding, it appears, has led to comparable behavioral stunting, and the most paedomorphic breeds express only the infantile behavioral patterns of wolves.

Breeds least resembling the wolf morphologically also had the fewest wolf-like patterns of agonistic behavior. As seen in Fig. 3.13, of the six breeds expressing seven or fewer signals, one (or none) were among those associated with submissive behavior in wolves. Three of four gun dogs tested (cocker spaniel, Labrador

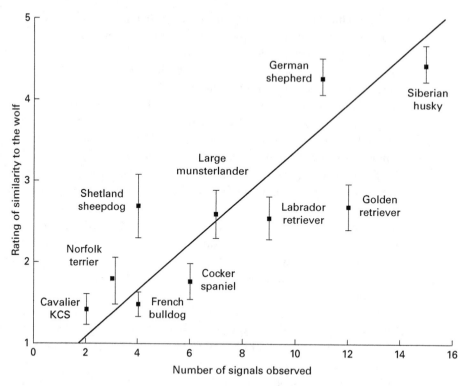

Figure 3.13 Relationship between number of signals performed by each breed with its degree of similarity in appearance to the wolf (average of eight characters). Values depicted are means (±SD). From Goodwin, D., J. W. S. Bradshaw, and S. M. Wickens. (1997). Paedomorphosis affects agonistic visual signals of domestic dogs. *Animal Behaviour* **53**: 297–304. Reprinted with permission from Elsevier.

retriever, golden retriever) kept more wolf-like behaviors than indicated by appearance. Despite its wolfish morphology, the German shepherd expressed fewer wolf-like behaviors than the Siberian husky and golden retriever. Results of tests from the two herding breeds (German shepherd, Shetland sheepdog) infer that "once a behaviour has been lost from the repertoire it cannot be reconstructed merely by altering the physical appearance of the breed."[161]

The protean range of dog behaviors (e.g. pointing, retrieving) has been produced by selection and training, variation resulting from "exaggeration or suppression of patterns of behavior already present."[162] However, the underlying behaviors before modification are tangible evidence of wolf ancestry. Dogs, like wolves, also communicate using tail-high, tail-low, and tail-wag.[163] The amplitude of tail-wag (how widely the tail sweeps predominantly left or right) expresses *affective behavior*, indicating the tendency to approach or withdraw from a presented signal, although its symmetry is context-dependent.[164] When isolated dogs were shown approach signals they wagged their tails significantly more to the right (left brain activation). These stimuli, in declining strength of amplitude, were their owners, a human stranger, and a cat. When shown a withdrawal signal

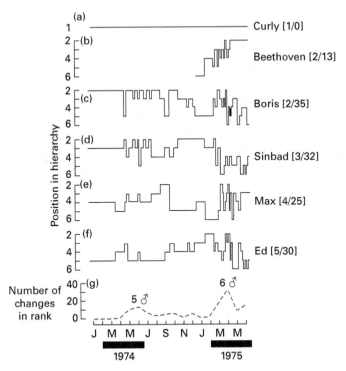

Figure 3.14 Fluctuations in the social rank of six adult male dingoes, (a)–(f), in captivity. Shown in brackets is a dingo's usual rank followed by the number of times his rank changed (e.g. Beethoven usually ranked second but he changed rank 13 times). Monthly changes in rank of all males are shown in (g). Solid bars = breeding seasons.
Source: Corbett, L. K. (1988). Social dynamics of a captive dingo pack: population regulation by dominant female infanticide. *Ethology* **78**: 177–198. This material is reproduced with permission of John Wiley & Sons, Inc.

(a dominant dog) they wagged their tails significantly more to the left (right brain activation).

Nearly all the 90 or so visual and tactile behaviors documented for wolves also occur in domestic dogs,[165] an exception being the pinning of a subordinate to the ground, which evidently only wolves do.[166] However, many of these behaviors seem to be absent in highly paedomorphic breeds, the number lost correlating directly with deviation from wolf-like morphology.[167] Of 10 breeds tested for successful use of 15 agonistic signals, 1 acoustical (growl) and the others visual (e.g. stand-taut, teeth-bared), the Siberian husky executed them all, the cavalier King Charles spaniel just 2.

The only comprehensive investigation of captive dingoes shows their dominant ↔ subordinate relationships to be similar to wolves[168] with a notable exception: pups started participating in disputes with adults at 6 months, perhaps a manifestation of their earlier maturation. Agonistic postures appeared in captive dingo pups at 4 weeks and slightly later in wild ones.[169] Postures and facial expressions were the same as in wolves: teeth-bared, stare, and all dominant behaviors reported for wolves were enacted by dingoes, as were features defining active and passive submission. During tail-erect the tail was sometimes curled over the back. There was evidence of rank order with the dominant male ranking above all others, the dominant female just below him and dominant over the rest, subordinate males generally dominating their female counterparts, and pups ranking lowest. Same-sex ranks were fluid, and individuals often switched places in the hierarchy, especially males and particularly during the breeding season (Fig. 3.14). A male named Boris changed ranks 35 times over 18 months, but usually ranked second. Curly, the dominant male, never lost his rank. Most aggression occurred within the sexes. As in wolves, "active submission may have been an indicator of rank stability within the pack."[170]

4   Olfactory and vocal communication

Our fascination with minutiae is associated with the search for distinctions. Nowhere is this better exemplified than by the recently discovered genetics of scent reception. Scent-related genes make up the largest family in the mammalian genome.[1] Visual and auditory stimuli might seem complex, but future research is likely to reveal them as abbreviated and clumsy compared with the subtle emission and reception of odors.

The canid nose is finely tuned to scent reception.[2] However logical it seems that air-borne compounds in the glandular secretions, urine, and feces of wolves and dogs contain important (and presumably) intraspecific signals,[3] the current evidence is overwhelmingly observational. Simply watching how a dog behaves after sniffing urine or feces, for example, does not establish a causal link. Conclusions based solely on behavior are inferential until validated physiologically. Between signal and response must be evidence of specific chemical compounds produced by senders that subsequently bind to identified receptors in neurons of receivers.

4.1   Odor and pheromone reception

Reception at a molecular level involves *olfaction* (the detection of odorant molecules),[4] possible detection of pheromones, and taste (gustatory reception). *Odorants* taken in from the external environment consist mainly of volatile compounds. *Pheromones*, which are excreted into the environment in fluids like urine or retained on the emitter's body (e.g. in sweat or saliva), are discrete compounds or blends of compounds serving as chemical signals among conspecifics to elicit sexual and social changes in behavior and physiology.[5] Pheromones are mainly nonvolatile and require direct contact with sensory cells to stimulate detection.[6] In other words, *pheromones are both excreted and taken up as fluids, not aerosols*. Their uptake by rodents after arousal is mediated by pumping action of the vomeronasal organ (see below). Because each sensory neuron expresses just one allele on a single receptor gene, the connection between emission and reception becomes fused only when the appropriate molecules bind to their specific receptors. The result is a signal sent to the central nervous system culminating in a sensation of smell (odorants) or some behavioral or physiological change (pheromones). Olfaction and taste are not easily separable, odorants and pheromones even less so.

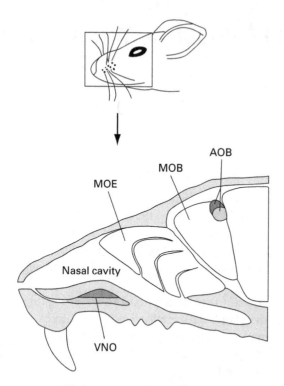

Figure 4.1 Chemosensory organs of the mouse. MOE, main olfactory epithelium; MOB, main olfactory bulb; AOB, accessory olfactory bulb; NC, nasal cavity; VNO, vomeronasal organ. *Source*: Ferrero, D. M. and S. D. Liberles. (2010). The secret codes of mammalian scents. *Wiley Interdisciplinary Reviews: Systems Biology and Medicine* **2**: 23–33. This material is reproduced with permission of John Wiley & Sons, Inc.

Most four-legged animals have two separate olfactory systems (Fig. 4.1). The larger is the *main olfactory system (MOS)* comprising the nasal passages and *main olfactory bulb (MOB)* where signals from odorant molecules detected by the *main olfactory epithelium (MOE)* are conveyed to the brain.[7] The MOS-expressed *odorant receptors (ORs)* are sensory neurons located in the nasal passages that sense odorants in the influent air.[8] An odorant molecule has a unique signal allowing it to be accepted by a matching neuron for further transmission, similar metaphorically to a bar-scan. Signals from these neurons are relayed sequentially to the MOB, from there to the brain's olfactory cortex, and finally to other cortical areas involved in perception and discrimination of odors.[9]

There are two families, or repertoires, of genes, one expressing ORs,[10] the other *trace amine-associated receptors (TAARs)* used to detect volatile odorants and some pheromones (Table 4.1).[11] Mice TAARs recognize volatile amines in urine, one of them associated with stress; two others identify putative pheromonal compounds in urine of both sexes. For simplicity I combine these gene families into ORs. Each OR probably recognizes a specific molecule shared by many complex odorants, and in this capacity a single OR can accept more than one.[12]

Table 4.1. Olfactory and pheromone gene repertoires compiled from animals for which adequate genomic data are available. Blank spaces indicate no data. Sources: information in Grus and Zhang (2008 and references), Grus *et al.* (2005), Olender *et al.* (2004), Quignon *et al.* (2005), Rouquier and Giorgi (2007), Young *et al.* (2005). Gene counts vary slightly by source. Data for V2Rs adjusted (Young and Trask 2007: 213, table 1); TAARs data from Liberles and Buck (2006).

	V1R functional genes	V1R pseudo-genes	V2R functional genes	V2R pseudo-genes	OR functional genes	OR pseudo-genes	TAARs
Pipid frog (*Xenopus tropicalis*)	21		249		405		3
Chicken (*Gallus gallus*)	0		0		77		3
Platypus (*Ornithorhynchus anatinus*)	270		15		261		4
Opossum (*Monodelphis domestica*)	98		89	81	871		21
Dog (*Canis lupus*)	8	54	0	10	1094	~223	2
Mouse (*Mus musculus*)	187	165	123	160	~1500	~300–500	15
Rat (*Rattus norvegicus*)	106	110	87	157	1493	291	17
Cow (*Bos taurus*)	32	41	0	20			
Human (*Homo sapiens*)	4	194	0	20	960	~610–660	
Chimpanzee (*Pan troglodytes*)	0	102	0	18			
Rhesus macaque (*Macaca mulatta*)			0	12			

The other system comprises the *vomeronasal organ (VNO)*,[13] a tubular structure positioned at the bottom of the nasal cavity above the roof of the mouth, and the *accessory olfactory bulb (AOB)* (Fig. 4.1). The VNO is separated both anatomically and physiologically from the MOS but opens by means of a small duct into the nasal cavity, mouth, or both,[14] depending on species.[15] In carnivorans the anterior VNO opens into a duct connecting the oral and nasal cavities and ends blindly at the posterior end.[16] The VNO actually serves a peripheral sensory function to the AOB[17] through which its signals are relayed to the *amygdala* and hypothalamus, regions of the brain associated with olfactory and pheromone-induced endocrine and behavioral responses.[18] The VNO and AOB in combination form the *accessory olfactory system (AOS)*.

At one time the functions of the MOS and AOS were thought to be mutually exclusive, the MOS detecting environmental odorants drawn into the nasal passages and the AOS devoted to pheromone detection. Many functions are now known to overlap. Because the MOB and VNO can both detect volatile and nonvolatile compounds, the original model is no longer correct.[19] Overlap leans heavily toward the MOS, which is much more general than the narrowly channeled AOS and can process some of the same compounds.[20] The reverse situation does not hold up as well, and odorant receptors are expressed less often by vomeronasal receptor genes (see below).[21] The mouse VNO is exceptional: its neurons respond to very low concentrations of both odorants and pheromones.[22] Neither system alone perceives a single class of cues, although signal transduction remains separate.[23]

Animals must be able to identify conspecifics and recognize age and sex differences[24] in addition to processing signals identifying reproductive status of prospective mates and eliciting the appropriate behavioral responses.[25] Pheromones have been thought to control these processes in mammals, as they do in insects, by transferring specific chemosensory signals from sender to receiver,[26] although here a problem arises: the existence of mammalian pheromones is problematical except in rodents and some marsupials.[27]

The original definition of pheromone proposed in 1959 by P. Karlson and M. Lüscher applied to hormone-like compounds but with an important difference: "Unlike hormones ... the substance is not secreted into the blood but outside the body; it does not serve humoral correlation within the organism but communication between individuals."[28] They noted that according to the definition then in use, hormones are produced by endocrine glands, and "this should not be lightly expanded and diluted." They defined pheromones as "substances which are secreted to the outside by an individual and received by a second individual of the same species, in which they release a specific reaction, for example, a definite behaviour or a developmental process." Karlson and Lüscher clearly separated pheromones from odorants and suggested that pheromones might also include "the territory-marking substances of the Carnivora, though here much remains to be solved." This is still true more than 50 years later.

Karlson and Lüscher used insects as examples, but no invertebrate has a VNO. Insects and vertebrates thus express odorant receptors differently.[29] Insect pheromones are discrete compounds or blends of compounds, and their functions are usually direct and specific.[30] So-called mammalian pheromones are largely undefined, and those of cockroaches and mice might require different definitions. I therefore call the receptors of mammals *vomeronasal receptors* (*VRs*) instead of pheromone receptors.[31] Chemical signaling is undoubtedly common among mammals, but the notion that vertebrates excrete exclusively intraspecific molecules into the environment to serve just these specific functions is controversial,[32] especially when none has yet been identified unequivocally.

If pheromones by the original definition are species-specific,[33] what are we to make of identical compounds in the urine of wolves, dogs, coyotes, probably other canids, certainly other mammals, and supposedly serving pheromonal functions (Chapter 7)? Either pheromones are not what we thought they were, or species boundaries need to be expanded and redefined. Broadening what we call a pheromone to include a suite of compounds instead of just one is not the answer. Mammals excrete hundreds – perhaps thousands – of different chemicals in urine, glandular products, and feces, and the more of them we throw into a basket labeled "pheromone" the more our collection resembles the original uncharacterized substance.[34]

A recipient's behavioral response to an olfactory or pheromonal signal, like any sensory response, can be overridden or masked by external phenomena, and behavior therefore constitutes the last and loosest link in a sequence that until then is completely mechanistic. Think about a male dog sniffing urine left by an estrous female and intent on following her until distracted by a car horn and frightened away. Here an auditory signal supplanted a predictable response by altering the recipient's anticipated behavior and reducing the olfactory signal to secondary status. The observed behavior was fright, not at all related to courtship and reproduction.

The evolution of primates has been accompanied by deterioration of the olfactory system. *Pseudogenization* (deactivation of functional genes to *pseudogene* status) of OR genes and loss of olfactory function progresses from prosimians and New World monkeys (~15–20% pseudogenes, or comparable to the mouse) through Old World monkeys (~30%), apes (~45%), and humans (~65%),[35] perhaps tracking the acquisition of trichromatic vision.[36] This, along with development of stereoscopic vision in primates and also carnivorans, is believed to have compensated for the loss of odorant reception.

Two repertoires of VRs found in the VNO, labeled *vomeronasal receptors 1* and *2* (*V1Rs, V2Rs*), detect intraspecific signals including putative pheromones.[37] Because each repertoire is activated by distinctly different compounds[38] they are related only distantly.[39] Expression in both cases, like that of OR genes, apparently involves a negative feedback mechanism: expression of a VR triggers a signal preventing transcription of other receptors in the repertoire.[40] Individual V1R genes expressed in sensory neurons of the VNO epithelium are located apically. The V2Rs express differently and are concentrated in the basal part of the epithelium. Dogs lack functional V2Rs (Table 4.1), but high divergence and *polymorphisms* (i.e. diversity of form) across alleles are displayed in rodents like wild mice that retain working copies.[41]

Rodents and marsupials are likely the only mammals with functional V2Rs.[42] A VNO exists in most amphibians and reptiles, is absent in birds, and has mostly disappeared in primates except for rare fetal vestiges.[43] These are probably nonfunctional.[44] In other mammals the VNO's complexity varies, as do the repertoires of V1R and V2R receptor genes (Table 4.1) Both are indicators of a species' probable use of pheromones, and the history of evolutionary VNO reception through time is indicated by the prevalence of pseudogenes. In any case, odorant detection by the MOE[45] might be required to initiate sampling by the VNO, even in rodents.

As mentioned, the MOS and AOS are separate systems isolated from each other except for limited access through the roof of the mouth. The VRs are not exposed to air passing continuously through the nasal cavities, and a signal is necessary to activate them. A distinctive facial expression (the flehmen response) is thought to be a mechanism for driving pheromones into the VNO, but if so they would be aerosols. Although common in ungulates, cats, and some other mammals a flehmen response has not been described in dogs. This fact, along with the small repertoire of V1R and V2R genes and thin VNO epithelium, indicates a deterioration of VNO function.[46]

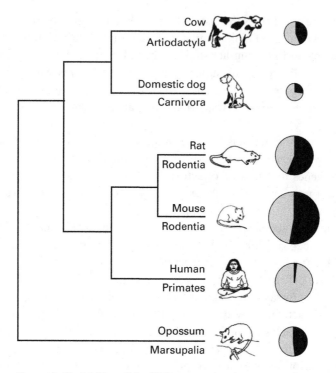

Figure 4.2 Variability of the V1R repertoire size among six mammalian species. Pie graphs represent complete V1R repertoires corresponding to each species and their sizes to number of V1R genes. Black and gray indicate potentially functional V1R genes and pseudogenes, respectively.
Source: Rodriguez, I. (2005). Remarkable diversity of mammalian pheromone receptor repertoires. *Proceedings of the National Academy of Sciences* **102**: 6639–6640. Copyright (2005) National Academy of Sciences, U.S.A.

Male canids often lick urine deposited by females in heat, making "chomping" motions with their jaws to supposedly waft pheromones into the VNO.[47] However, the VNO could be involved only if liquid urine actually touches it, leaving olfaction and taste as the remaining possibilities. Zimen's male wolves picked up and chewed urine-covered snow left by an estrous female, and "for a few seconds their eyes were directed into the void in characteristic fashion."[48] If wolves can literally taste pornography then humans might not be the more exalted species after all.

Evidence of pheromone use among mammals is strongest in rodents, which possess the most highly developed VNOs and most numerous VRs.[49] Putative pheromones in mouse urine mediate individual recognition, block pregnancy, jump-start early puberty, and control certain behaviors (e.g. maternal aggression).[50] Variation in size of the V1R repertoire across representatives of five orders of placental and marsupial mammals is large, the implications provocative. Just eight complete V1Rs and 22 V1R pseudogenes have been found in dogs (Fig. 4.2), and whether more will be discovered is doubtful. The cow has 32 functional V1R genes to go with 41 pseudogenes, numbers that might change as more data are posted. Neither the dog nor the cow comes close to the mouse (187) or rat (102) for numbers of functional V1R genes. Shaded areas of the graphic show dogs to have lost many formerly functional ancestral genes. Sizes of both dog and cow V1R repertoires are substantially smaller than those of rodents and primates. Modern humans have only four functional V1R genes, but inclusion of pseudogenes raises the total to about 200. The opossum VNO contains 49 apparently functional V1R genes.

Vomeronasal function in dogs is minimal, and any pheromonal activity in the VNO is likely to be minimal too. The dog's evolution is too recent for domestication to be the cause.[51] Moreover, evidence of pseudogenization would still remain in the genome. Nor could the dog's small V1R repertoire be bolstered by V2R function, remnants of which are pseudogenes, the same as in all mammals not rodents or marsupials. In terms of possible pheromone function rodents are the exceptions among mammals, not better equipped examples of the rule.

Carnivorans in general might be especially deficient in V1R function. The sensory epithelium of their VNOs is much thinner compared with rodents.[52] That of the male European polecat (*Mustela putorius*)[53] could be typical of a carnivoran pattern. Its VNO is rudimentary and polecats, like wild canids, undergo seasonal reproductive changes including gonadal recrudescence (Chapter 7).[54] Furthermore, the MOS, which is well developed, and not the AOS, is required for mate identification among polecats.[55] A classification of VNOs from most complex (A) to simplest (E) placed dogs in (C) along with polecats, ungulates, prosimian primates, and New World monkeys.[56] Complexity of the VNO thus correlates with the number of intact and working V1R genes and "may be used as a proxy for the sophistication of pheromone communications within species."[57] *If mammalian pheromones exist, their role in the lives of canids appears very limited.* Assuming they do exist – and pheromones really are species-specific – then barriers to prevent between-species reproduction must be firmly in place before they can operate effectively. In other words, for reproductive pheromones to work each species must recognize only conspecifics as suitable mates and reject all others, presumably because detection and response to a pheromone is limited to its own kind. Reproduction is flexible within the genus *Canis* (Chapters 1 and 2), "species" of which interbreed without apparent difficulty.

Dogs, like rodents, are considered *macrosmatic* (scent-oriented) animals. The dog's capacity for scent discrimination is superb,[58] its olfactory receptor repertoire impressive, but neither matches that of a mouse or rat. The ORs of dogs demonstrate high polymorphism at up to seven sites and allelic variants indicating breed specificity, genetic evidence that some breeds are better "smellers" than others.[59] These characteristics could account for refined odor discrimination, a capacity affected not just by selective binding affinity at reception sites but concentration of the odorant.[60]

Three possibilities suggest reasons for the large size discrepancies in functional AOS repertoires between rodents and dogs.[61] First, V1Rs actually do signify an expanded range of specialized functions in rodents, perhaps even permitting the

AOS to accept volatile odorants and overlapping the MOS. Second, many VRs in rodents are redundant and overlap each other, the extra genes providing only a minimal boost in range of functions. Third, other gene repertoires in the dog MOS might function as pheromone receptors. This possibility presumes limited usefulness of the dog VNO, thus obviating any need of a functioning AOS, and it depends on the MOS to operate fully at dual capacity.[62]

What we typically call *taste* is actually *flavor*, the combination of true taste, olfaction from the influence of volatile molecules in food, and somatosensory perception (e.g. texture, pain).[63] It starts at the *taste papillae* distributed in and around the inside of the mouth, principally the tongue and palate. A papilla holds one or more *taste buds*, structures shaped like onions embedded in epithelium. Each contains about 100 cells including *taste receptors* (*TRs*), which were not discovered until 1999.[64] The TRs detect *tastants* (the gustatory equivalent of odorants) in food and relay signals to the brainstem and *thalamus*, but unlike OR and VR neurons these have no direct connections in the brain.[65] Taste stimulates the digestive response in dogs less effectively than the sight of food or its odor.[66]

4.2   Scent-marking

Most mammals have scent glands that produce substances used to scent-mark objects in the landscape. These can be deposited by rubbing or, in the case of glands near the anus, by defecation. Volatile urinary compounds are believed to constitute most olfactory signals in scent-marking by canids. *Scent-marking* is the initial or repeated urination, defecation, or rubbing of scent glands on objects, which leaves volatile olfactory signals recognizable by conspecifics.[67]

At least one aspect of scent-marking seems counterproductive by potentially making ungulate prey more difficult to hunt. The odor of fresh cougar (*Puma concolor*) and wolf feces puts elk (*Cervus canadensis*) on high alert, triggering increases in heart and respiration rates,[68] and semi-wild kangaroos (*Macropus* spp.) avoided feeding troughs where dingo urine had been placed.[69] Tasmanian red-bellied pademelons (*Thylogale billardierii*) and brush-tailed opossums (*Trichosorus vulpecula*) in Tasmania fled when encountering dingo urine even though dingoes are not indigenous.[70] The odors of wolf and dog feces, caused mainly by fatty acids, are effective sheep repellents.[71] The compound Δ^3-isopentenyl methyl sulfide[72] isolated from red fox urine effectively kept away introduced brush-tailed opossums in New Zealand and diminished the damage they cause to vegetation.[73] This substance and others appear to be sex attractants among canids (Chapter 7). The elevated concentrations of urinary sulfurous compounds from a meat-eating diet are also repellent to herbivores.[74]

Several intraspecific functions have been attributed to scent-marking by canids, including to: (1) reinforce dominance,[75] (2) establish and strengthen pair bonding,[76] (3) indicate sexual status or establish "reproductive synchrony" in breeding pairs,[77]

(4) mark territorial boundaries as a putative warning to intruders,[78] (5) announce identity,[79] (6) provide olfactory landmarks for orienting and navigating within territorial boundaries,[80] (7) make acquaintances,[81] (8) recognize sex differences,[82] and (9) identify empty food caches.[83]

Some, such as marking territorial boundaries (Chapter 5), seem to have more support than others. Nonetheless, wolves trespass deep into the territories of their neighbors.[84] In doing so they might make their visits discreet: a nonbreeding pair at *Isle Royale National Park*, Michigan (hereafter *Isle Royale*) that lived almost completely within the territory of a larger pack did not scent-mark.[85] Scent-marking is perhaps not used in agonism because "its efficiency simply lies in the avoidance responses which are shown by the intruding individuals."[86] This notion dominates the canid behavioral literature and still has little empirical support.

Wolves sometimes urinate on emptied food caches, the conjecture being that it constitutes a form of "bookkeeping" by letting other pack members know the site's status.[87] It presupposes that only the urinating wolf knows the stores have been depleted, not considering that any wolf so inclined could easily find out for itself by taking a few sniffs. A more reasonable signal might be the odor of decomposition.[88] Captive wolves in Spain urinated on leftover food and dead rats.[89] Dogs will urinate on certain objects too: old diapers, fresh fried chicken, old fried hamburger, and especially old broiled fish.[90] The behavior could also indicate propriety: a captive wolf has been seen urinating on its food then standing guard over it.[91]

I found no evidence that domestic dogs recognize scent-marks as territorial boundary markers (Chapter 5), and it seems that every dog over-marks the urine of previous visitors with its own.[92] The strength of a deterrent scent-mark among wolves has not been put to a rigorous test. What we have instead is a literature filled with reports of scent-marking by wolves and other canids and anecdotal agreement on what it means, hardly a substitute for empiricism. Neither avoidance nor attraction is simply a reflexive response to olfactory signals, but rather the culmination of a complex process of identification and interpretation offering a choice of several possible actions.[93]

Wild canids, with their long narrow faces, have large MOBs compared with cats and other carnivorans that have shorter faces.[94] The MOBs of canids are also sophisticated, giving them an excellent sense of smell. Sniffing in mammals (including humans) induces the MOB to oscillate. The *frequency* at which it oscillates (number of oscillations per unit of time) then activates the *piriform lobe* (a section of the brain associated with smell).[95] Sniffing an object, in other words, alerts the brain's sense of smell to an impending signal from the olfactory bulb, and the intake of odorants requires sniffing. The efficacy of olfaction is diminished by overheating.[96] Wolves and dogs pant when hot, and panting causes a decline in sniffing rate. These actions are impossible to perform simultaneously.

According to one hypothesis, evolution of the MOB of carnivorans coincides with foraging and monitoring large home ranges (Chapter 5), and an analysis of 146 species showed direct correlation between olfactory bulb size and size of the home range.[97] This association presumably enables a canid to orient itself and navigate through familiar terrain (Chapter 5), and to monitor and evaluate the movements of known and strange conspecifics by using olfaction (scent-marks). Scent-marks thus make up an intricate system of olfactory signs allowing those able to read them a clear method of navigating and processing social signals.

Wolves have a scent gland on each side of the anus. Most compounds produced are by the wolf itself, although some apparently are generated by microbes normally found in the *anal glands*.[98] Wolves can voluntarily control the deposition of anal gland excretions, allowing or not allowing them to be deposited with feces.[99] Captive adults of both sexes and all hierarchical ranks including adolescents can deposit anal-gland excretions, with dominant males doing so most often.[100] Although a captive dominant female urinated in a flexed-leg posture (see below), the rate at which she deposited anal gland excretions was no different from that of her subordinates. In an earlier study compounds produced by the anal glands of beagles and coyotes varied in concentration from one sample to the next, and no consistent differences were found between the composition and concentrations of these substances and sex, species, and state of estrus except that beagles produced greater concentrations of volatiles than coyotes.[101]

Four functions for anal glands of canids have been proposed: (1) sexual attraction, (2) marking of territorial boundaries, (3) individual recognition, and (4) in response to alarm.[102] None has been convincingly affirmed or refuted. The first is doubtful: male dogs are reportedly attracted to urine and vaginal excretions from estrous females (Chapter 7), but not to compounds taken from their anal glands.[103] The second has not been tested. The strongest possibilities seem to be the last two. As to (3), from the frequency and regularity with which social animals sniff specific sites on conspecifics where scent glands are located it is reasonable to think they could function in individual recognition.[104] As to (4), captive wolves sometimes deposited anal gland excretions independently of defecation, seemingly when frightened.[105] At other times they defecated when excited or aroused, and these scats were not marked with scent-gland excretions. Fear and excitement evidently induce separate responses to different stimuli, anal-gland excretions in feces signaling fear or alarm.

Defecation without accompanying excretions might be used for delineating territorial boundaries in the manner of *urine-marking* (one form of scent-marking) and perhaps even signaling identity, sex, or social status.[106] For example, the scats left by the dominant pair of a wolf pack can contain higher levels of corticosteroid and sex hormones, possible indications of status and perhaps serving a scent-marking function.[107] Wolves leave aggregations of scats surrounding their dens and rendezvous sites (Chapter 8) and on conspicuous objects.[108] Elevated locations are sometimes chosen preferentially,[109] and junctions and crossroads were especially popular places to defecate.[110] This behavior, in combination with the strong odor of wolf feces, lends credence to the hypothesis that volatile fecal compounds are visual and olfactory social stimuli and probably functional scent-marks even without accompanying anal-gland excretions.[111] Whatever these substances contain, their odors are irresistible: fresh scats and urine make effective lures used to trap wolves.[112] Dingoes defecate throughout their home ranges, putatively as a means of scent-marking,[113] but this hypothesis remains just as vague and untested.

Male canids lift a hind leg to urinate starting at sexual maturity (e.g. 4–9 months in domestic dogs and wolfdogs),[114] but the behavior can be induced at 2 months in dogs by administration of testosterone.[115] Urine leaves a strong odor, and usually a squirt or two is sufficient to mark an object.[116] During *raised-leg urination* (*RLU*) a scent-marking adult male canid typically directs his urine at *scent-posts*, conspicuous vertical objects (e.g. tree trunks, tufts of grass, snow banks, fence posts, rocks).[117] In urban and suburban landscapes these can include trees, lamp posts, fire hydrants, the tires of parked motor vehicles, and one time the leg of a chair in which I was sitting. When urine-marking, a dominant female wolf squats and elevates one hind leg slightly (RLU), but more commonly bends a hind leg under her body and performs a *flexed-leg urination* (*FLU*).[118] For simplicity I shall use only FLU when describing dominant females. Some investigators consider urine-marking to be different from straightforward urination,[119] which would be true if composition of the urine differs. We have no evidence that it does.

Immature and subordinate males often spread their legs apart and urinate in a posture of *standing-urination* (*STU*), and confining a mature dog in a tight space or frightening it sometimes causes reversion to this posture.[120] Females, some immature males, and pups use *squat-urination* (*SQU*), spreading the hind legs and lowering the hindquarters to just above the ground.[121] Of these postures RLU (dominant males)[122] and FLU (dominant females) are used in scent-marking, STU and SQU during regular urination.[123] Social stature and not just age influences which of these positions is used. A previously subordinate male wolf seen using STU switched abruptly to RLU 5 days later when he took over a nearby pack without a dominant male.[124]

Injection of male and female hormones seems to have little predictive effect on the urination posture of male dogs.[125] Some dogs castrated as neonates displayed the RLU posture as adults[126] but others retained the SQU posture of pups,[127] and RLU is not necessarily extinguished by castration in adulthood.[128] Females retain the same SQU posture whether intact or spayed,[129] and intact females administered testosterone from the first day of birth exhibited RLU as adults.

The RLU posture of domestic dogs is unrelated to social status, not justifying the conclusion that by raising its hind leg every male dog "considers itself alpha."[130] In a wolf pack only the dominant pair urine-marks,[131] the frequency of which increases during the winter breeding season,[132] especially in males.[133] Alternatively, it can be the dominant male's exclusive purview. Incidences of urine-marking by captive dominant males increased with rising testosterone concentration, both variables peaking in winter. Subordinate males had testosterone concentrations that were just as high, but did not urine-mark.

During the breeding season reproductive status and frequency of FLUs correlate directly.[134] However, the rate at which captive dominant females urine-marked also rose and fell synchronously with testosterone but not estradiol concentration, indicating that social factors and not just hormones exert a strong influence.[135] As further evidence, outside the breeding season dominant males had low testosterone concentrations and showed no interest in females induced into estrus. Scent-marking in wolves is nonetheless hormone-driven, because it is not seen until after puberty. That social bonds are strong among wolves was demonstrated in this captive group after the death of the dominant female. Her mate retained his social status but ceased urine-marking and abandoned other behaviors associated with high rank (e.g. tail-high).

Urination (especially RLU) and sometimes defecation is occasionally followed by *ground-scratching*.[136] Some authorities consider this behavior a form of scent-marking, claiming volatile compounds are transferred to the ground by putative "interdigital glands" in the paws.[137] To my knowledge canids do not have such structures[138] unless reference is to *apocrine sweat glands* in the footpads that possibly generate scents. These are present in western coyotes, but investigators have been unable to find them in North American wolves, domestic dogs, and eastern coyotes.[139] The function of the eccrine glands is to cool the skin, making them unlikely sources of scent. I therefore consider ground-scratching an auxiliary behavior associated with scent-marking but having no (as yet) demonstrated function.

Wolves often leave evidence of ground-scratching along trails.[140] During vigorous scratching "a wolf paws the ground with alternate motions of the stiffened right and left forelegs, each combined with a similar movement of the rear leg on the opposite side."[141] Generally, only dominant wolves ground-scratch after scent-marking, and the grass and dirt thrown up are rarely deposited on top of the new mark.[142] Untested functions of ground-scratching other than scent-marking have been suggested. Ground-scratching could carry a visual assertion of dominance, reinforcing an RLU,[143] or a visual signal of some other kind.[144] Stanley P. Young declared, "the scratching by the wolf after defecating or urinating is possibly the vestige of a former habit of burying the dung or urine."[145] To Crisler it was seen as a display of defiance.[146] One investigator noted that his captive wolf ground-scratched after defecating only if the location was strange to him.[147]

Why wolves and dogs roll on objects or rub against them (usually stinky ones) is unknown. A captive wolf that had just caught a vole rolled on it but did not eat it;[148] other wolves (whether captive or wild is unstated) have been seen rubbing and rolling against ungulate carcasses before starting to eat.[149] A captive wolf rolled and rubbed his neck on smelly objects such as old bones,[150] and male wolves are reported to roll on rat and impala feces.[151] A tame wolf that was free-ranging while the Crislers lived on the Brooks Range returned now and then to visit them. On entering their tiny cabin, "he tried to roll in the Ivory soap, the coffee, the bacon wrapper."[152] When Chris Crisler "sprinkled Quelques Fleurs on his palm ... the wolf rolled on that." Captive eastern coyotes rolled or rubbed their faces and shoulders on meat, toys, and carrion.[153] Unlike dogs, wolves and eastern coyotes are attracted to perfume.[154] Several hypotheses have been proposed to explain this behavior,[155] four of them untested: (1) to familiarize the unfamiliar, (2) to reinforce self-assertion or highlight identity by soliciting attention and investigation from other group or pack members, (3) to impart personal odor to the object as a means of scent-marking, and (4) to derive pleasure (response to a pleasant signal).

Hypothesis (1) seems the best candidate to me with (4) the runner-up. In my opinion familiarity is the one factor a social canid values most. It wants familiar companions and familiar spaces. Marking the world is one way of keeping it unremarkable. As to (4), apparently all canids display what Fox termed the *consummatory-face* when eating, urinating, defecating, and rolling or rubbing in a strange odor, during which "the ears were partially flattened and the eyes either narrowed or completely closed, or open and fixed in a 'middle distance' stare or 'glazed daydream'."[156] These expressions of contentment seem little different from those of a harried father who has locked himself in the bathroom with the sports pages.

Three tested hypotheses are (1) response to a novel odor, (2) response to a familiar scent that has been altered, and (3) response indicating strong aversion or attraction.[157] Captive wolves rubbed against locations marked with perfume most often. Also popular were motor oil and feces of other carnivorans: cougar and black bear (*Ursus americanus*). Food odors (tuna oil, salt pork) and herbivore feces (Aoudad sheep, *Ammotraqus lervia*, and Sable Island horse, *Equus caballus*) were ignored except for the salt pork, which was rubbed once. Novelty was less important than the odor itself. Odors tasted and rubbed correlated inversely.

These experiments, although interesting, were descriptive, and the motivation behind rubbing and rolling on scented objects remains unknown. As a marine biologist I participated in the necropsies and dissections of many sea mammals that had died and washed ashore, including whales. Nothing in my experience smells worse than a decaying animal the size of a modest ocean-going vessel. At times when the wind died it took intense concentration not to gag. Sometimes colleagues brought their dogs to the beaches where these events took place. They appeared stunned at first, overwhelmed by ancestral olfaction myths about Dog Heaven suddenly come true. I can state with certainty that nothing seems more joyful to a dog than taking a good roll against the collapsed carcass of a putrid whale.

That wolves and dogs typically sniff an object before marking it suggests detection of a previous mark. However, sexually experienced adult male dogs made *anosmic* (unable to smell)[158] showed only slight reductions in scent-marking and no changes in the incidence of ground-scratching afterward.[159] Anosmic wolves scent-marked with urine, anal-gland secretions, and feces,[160] evidence of a decoupling of signal from response. Female wolves seemed less affected than males by anosmia.[161] In fact, other than impairment in three factors associated with reproduction (male sexual behavior, urine-marking by females, and pair bonding; Chapter 7), all other social behaviors of male and female wolves seemed unaffected, raising the question of how important olfaction and taste actually are in everyday interactions among social canids.

A group of free-ranging dogs in Alaska's interior routinely urinated on scent-posts of coyotes while ignoring those of foxes.[162] In contrast, scent-posts of wolves – and even wolf trails – drew excited interest, inducing the dogs to ground-scratch where wolves had urinated and to over-mark these locations with their own urine. Occasionally they rolled in the wolf urine. Wolves in turn have shown interest in dog scent-posts.[163] In evident contrast with other canids, wolves (females especially) commonly defecate in response to odors of strange conspecifics,[164] and male wolves over-mark the urine of strange wolves with their own.[165] When wolves approach a scent-post marked by another wolf pack there is much excited urination and defecation.[166] Other observations point to spontaneous urination as a sign of agitation, fear, or excitement. David Freeland Parmelee and a colleague encountered a pair of wolves on northern Ellesmere Island where humans rarely ventured in the 1950s. One kept its distance, but of the other Parmelee wrote: "Frightened no longer the wolf became curious, approaching me within four feet. It sniffed the ground where I walked, ran off, urinated frequently, returned and sniffed again."[167] As discussed previously, dogs can detect the odor of human footprints, and wolves probably can too.

Scent-marks made with urine are often marked repeatedly whether left by the same or different animals, and fresher marks are more likely to stimulate over-marking than old ones.[168] Over-marking tends to be especially prevalent along territorial boundaries: "In effect, each territory is an olfactory 'bowl' with the edges composed of high rates of the resident pack's marking interspersed with high rates of the neighbor's marks."[169] Scent-marks at the peripheries of territories are about twice as common as marks near the center (Fig. 4.3).[170] Wolves traveling at their usual speed of 8 km per hour[171] "would encounter and produce an olfactory sign about every 2 minutes, including an RLU every 3 minutes."[172]

By using the largely invisible olfactory map of its territory a wolf is presumably oriented at all times, never lost, and knows its boundaries exactly. But how do animals actually make use of their own scent-marks to orient themselves inside a home range or territory? According to one suggestion they can judge the age of a scent-mark, which allows them to know when others have passed through.[173] A model has been proposed based on a "radial olfactory gradient field."[174] Among its assumptions is a gradient diminishing from the core outward, or the opposite of how things work in canid territories, which are marked more strongly from the boundary inward. The reasoning remains unchanged because of another assumption: animals scent-mark as they move, and they tend to move where they have scent-marked previously, over-marking older scents and thereby establishing a pattern of space use. The model permits a hypothetical animal to navigate through its home range using gradients of *its own* olfactory intensity, establishing an archive of checkpoints analogous to an array of GPS coordinates.

If scent is so important, how does anosmia affect behavior? Is a wolf made anosmic a lesser wolf than before? As mentioned, this surgery has been performed on captive wolves with interesting results.[175] In short, wolves compensate, females more competently than the males. Anosmic wolves eat normally and maintain

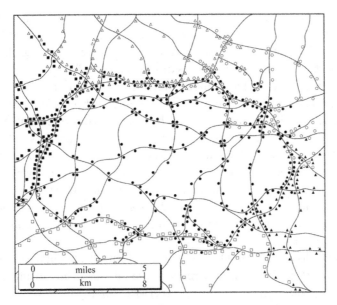

Figure 4.3 Hypothetical model of urine-marks made by a resident wolf pack throughout its territory (solid circles), which adjoins the territories of packs represented by the rest of the symbols. Notice that most marks occur at territorial boundaries and that only those made by the resident pack's own members occur inside the boundaries.
Source: From *The Way of the Wolf* by L. David Mech. Copyright 1991. Reproduced with permission of Voyageur Press, Inc.

body weight despite being unable to detect meat by smell, nor can they detect urine, feces, or anal gland excretions. Dominant wolves continued to urine-mark, but not as often. Despite the futility all surgically altered animals "investigated" the environment by sniffing. Reproductive physiology seemed unaffected. Hormones cycled on schedule and at normal concentrations, ovulation and sperm production were unremarkable, the dominant wolves reproduced, and a subordinate even became dominant. Sexually inexperienced males, however, showed no interest in estrous females, but an experienced male mated successfully. The authors wrote: "Chemosensory priming from female urine during the protracted proestrous phase, as well as urinary and vaginal odors during estrus, appear to be critical for induction of full sexual potency in sexually naive males."[176] There was also evidence that compromised mutual scent-marking as a result of anosmia might have inhibited formation of new pairs.

4.3   Vocalization

In contrast with visual, tactile, and olfactory communication, vocalization provides instant data that are functional up close or from a distance. Animal vocalizations influence the behavior of listeners, which interpret them to represent their environment.[177] Nothing about this process is analogous to spoken words, and references to the "language" of dogs or "speaking dog" are vacuous metaphors. Still, animals make sounds that tease us with hints of hidden meaning, challenging our objectivity by "wreathing themselves in the living fire."[178]

Casuistry erodes what we know about animal communication, too often attributing intentionality and understanding when neither has been adequately demonstrated (Chapter 3). Motive and referential behavior are discerned where the data show only pattern. In fact, a receiver replying to a conspecific's call does so without perceiving the sender's mental state (Chapter 3). Eavesdropping, we might think of the sound as plaintive, lonely, sad, but these interpretations would be ours alone. Unlike us, animals are unable to recognize the mental states of others.[179] Consequently, senders in the animal world *do not intentionally signal to inform others*, and receivers interpret a sender's signal *without recognizing it as reflecting what the sender knows.*[180]

These crucial distinctions hold true for every form of communication among animals. As to uttered sounds, they render false all statements of intentionality about animal vocalizations until proven otherwise, forcing us to reexamine their functional value too. For example, "a wolf barks *to warn its pups*" is a false statement; "wolves howl *to let other pack members know their location*" is another; "a dog barks *to attract its owner's attention*" still another. During the breeding season a male wolf might "solo-howl" for hours without receiving a response,[181] but claiming he does this *to attract a female* has no empirical basis and is teleological by stating explicit intentionality and purpose. To further claim that any female within hearing distance *understands* what the male knows is equally explicit and just as false. Even assuming vocalizations serve these communicative functions, evidence of function is still not evidence of intentionality.

And function is seldom obvious. Traits accumulate over time, meaning that conditions favoring a trait during its original evolution are not necessarily the same as those now maintaining it.[182] Take, for example, wolf barks that serve the putative function of warning pups of nearby danger. Either of two hypotheses – or both together – has been used to explain the adaptive nature of such *alarm calls*: (1) signaling discouragement to predators; and (2) signaling a warning of danger to conspecifics, kin in particular.[183] The wolf's bark seems to be used most often near dens and rendezvous sites,[184] and in canids generally the young hide on hearing it.[185] More likely the utterance is an affective startle response, not a "warning" signal or anything else so narrowly directed or referential. The pups' response is to be startled too.

Suppose a wolf's bark indeed warns pups of danger. If so, indirect benefits of kinship resulting from their survival might be expected to enhance inclusive fitness of the group (Chapter 8). However, studies of other mammalian species suggest that alarm signals (including calls) reduce the caller's own risk instead.[186] We would also expect social species living with kin to be the most common users of alarm calls, but this was only marginally true when 209 species of rodents were assessed. Because neither hypothesis has yet been falsified in canids, neither can be considered viable.

The majority of animal vocalizations are affective; that is, expressions of the sender's emotions (e.g. fear, arousal), and those of canids are not exceptional.[187] Affective state sets the intensity of a subsequent behavior and consequently differs from *motivation* (*motivational state*), which results in such behavioral patterns as foraging that are truly function-specific.[188] Few animal vocalizations are actually referential by denoting some immediate property of the environment (Chapter 3). Observations of captive wolves, for example, indicated that the acoustical composition of a howl is unrelated to simultaneous behavior such as pacing. *To qualify as referential a signal must be context-specific. Affective signals are nonreferential.*

Vocalization can theoretically be affective, potentially referential, or both.[189] Different acoustical signals (or variation in segments of graded signals along a continuum) can derive from the same affective state, which then motivate the sender to choose an interpretant.[190] Most work in this field has been done with nonhuman primates. Chimpanzees produce "rough grunts" associated with feeding, emitting different acoustical patterns when encountering different foods.[191] A group of captive chimps at a Scotland zoo preferred bread to apples. Recordings of "rough grunts" made while the group fed and later replayed to one of its members seemed to show that foraging chimps recognize acoustical differences in these sounds and use them in locating favored foods.[192] If true, nuances in the grunts function referentially by being context-specific; that is, denoting specific foods in the context of foraging.

Research on canid vocalizing has consisted mostly of identifying and categorizing sounds and patterns of sounds (e.g. barks, howls) and attempting to correlate subsequent expressions of behavior with affective or referential state. Little of this work has shown unequivocal links. One problem has been failure by investigators to recognize that although the sender's signal influences a receiver, the receiver's perspective might be very different.[193] Another has been inconsistent standards and definitions used to name and describe types of calls,[194] some being simply onomatopoeic labels.[195] This last is evident in some of the sound types made by canids: whines (including yips, yelps, and whimpers), screams, barks, *growls*, coos, howls, mews, and grunts.[196]

Ronald M. Schassburger identified 11 discrete sounds made by wolves, some with two or three categories: *whine* (whistle-whine, full-whine), *whimper* (whistle-whimper or squeak, full-whimper), *yelp, growl, snarl, woof, bark, moan* (harmonic, intermediate, noisy), *whine-moan, growl-moan, howl.*[197] They are defined acoustically in Table 4.2. The presumed function or affective state of some sounds is summarized in Table 4.3. Schassburger classified them into three types on the basis of fundamental frequency range: *whine-like, growl-like,* and *moan-like*. In addition, wolves combine one or more of the 11 principal sounds to produce *mixed sounds*. These take on nuances of their own. A *graded sound* is the gradual morphing of one discrete sound into another culminating in a mixed sound; *transition* is a sudden and recognizable changeover from one discrete sound to another.

Placed in a behavioral context, wolf sounds were considered to be of two kinds. Nonaggressive (those in response to pain and fear, greeting, frustration, and

Table 4.2. Fundamental frequency ranges of major vocalizations made by wolves.

Vocalization	Fundamental frequency range, Hz	Sound type, Hz
Whine	440–680	
Whimper	575–645	Whine-like (380–780)
Yelp	380–555	
Howl[a]	150–780	
Growl	70–145	
Snarl	145–170	Growl-like (70–170)
Woof	90–120	
Bark	145–170	
Moan (harmonic)	185–215	
Moan (intermediate)	75	
Moan (noisy)	80–105	Moan-like (75–665)
Whine-moan	305–665	
Growl-moan	90–165	

[a] From Theberge and Falls (1967).
Source: Schassburger (1993).

Table 4.3. Presumed links between specific vocalizations of wolves and affective state. Information in Schassburger (1993).

Vocalization	Presumed function or affective state
Whine	frustration/anxiety, submission/appeasement, sexual arousal
Whimper	frustration/anxiety, greeting/greeting-ceremony, desire to socialize, friendly approach
Yelp	fear/pain, expression of submission
Growl	warning/threat, prelude to attack, defense, expression of dominance, expression of increased aggressive arousal
Snarl	warning/threat often with growling and barking
Woof	warning, protest, often a prelude to barking, low-intensity protest
Bark	warning, threat/attack, protest, often associated with growl and woof
Moan, whine-moan, growl-moan	agonistic expression of conflict, expression of play mood
Howl	expression of affective state

anxiety), and submission and appeasement sounds. They might be accompanied by visual displays. For example, greeting involves tail-wag, nose-push, face-paw, and muzzle-grab (Chapter 3). The associated sounds are mostly *harmonic*. As to the other kind, aggressive sounds, uttered during social displays of dominance (e.g. stand-taut, tail-erect) and threat and attack (e.g. piloerection, teeth-bared), are mostly noisy. Behaviors that seem conflicted are typically associated with intermediate vocalizations. Thus motivation correlates crudely with acoustical structure.

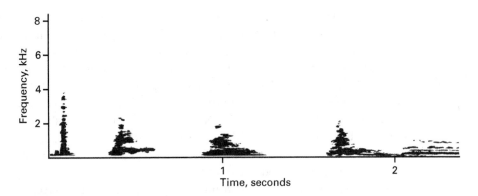

Figure 4.4 Spectrogram of a wolf's bark, which is harsh, low-pitched, noisy, and produced by the abrupt expulsion of air through the open mouth. Amplitude is represented in black. Duration is 0.25–0.4 s, the fundamental frequency 145–170 Hz.
Source: Schassburger, R. M. (1993). *Vocal Communication in the Timber Wolf*, Canis lupus, [*sic*] *Linnaeus: Structure, Motivation, and Ontogeny*, Advances in Ethology No. 30. Berlin and Hamburg: Paul Parey. This material is reproduced with permission of John Wiley & Sons, Inc.

Vocalizations can amplify visual signals or substitute for them;[198] their effectiveness in combination with haptic and olfactory signaling is unknown. As described previously, limited tests with anosmic canids indicate a reduced role for olfaction during normal social interaction and courtship. The apparently good association between certain vocalizations and visual signals[199] is intriguing but still not evidence of substituted, additive, or synergistic function because no combination of signals has yet been assessed in isolation. Nor can it be said at this time that one or the other induces – that is *causes* – an identical response from the receiver under the same conditions. Schassburger introduced the term *functional summation* to describe "the overlap of meanings and functions between sounds within a major sound type ... since the motivational balance being expressed is not that between conflicting dispositions, but rather between complementary and additive ones."[200] This might make sense for function, but without agreement on what is meant by "meaning" even in our own species any useful transposition to another seems unlikely.

The assessment of animal sounds is made difficult by subtle variations in frequency, *tonality*, *amplitude*, and *duration*. Add to these variables the measurable differences among individuals. For example, frequency characteristics, which are controlled by anatomical nuances of the vocal apparatus, are diagnostic of individuality[201] including the whistle-calls of dholes.[202] Individual wolf howls are best distinguished by their frequency discontinuities and frequency *modulations*.[203] Those with frequency discontinuities are of longest duration. *Barks* are considered *noise* (auditory definition) by being deficient in *harmonic overtones* (Fig. 4.4). Any *tonal frequencies* are usually swamped by dominant atonal ones. Barks, in other words, typically lack a *fundamental frequency* and are *broadband*, having frequencies that extend across the acoustical spectrum.[204] These acoustical features, which are shared widely among vertebrates, "are ideally suited for capturing and manipulating listener attention and arousal."[205] They work so well for capturing the attention of humans that "dog-appeasing pheromone" and other compounds of doubtful utility are marketed to discourage the relentless barking of owned dogs.[206]

The *pitch* of a bark varies by species, size, age, breed (domestic dogs), and other factors. In relative terms the amplitude of barks is generally loud, abrupt, and of short duration. Consequently, barks work most effectively at short range where random fluctuations in amplitude are less likely to interfere with signal reception. Social birds that communicate over short distances also rely on broadband sounds with sharp-amplitude modulations.[207]

Stereotypical vocalizations, by being repetitive, increase the perception of loudness in noisy environments.[208] Relentless group barking in kennels has long been considered "an attention-getting device," which is probably true but not for the reason most think. A signal must be detectable against background noise, which is made more difficult if they happen to be similar.[209] Stereotypical barking is also thought to increase during times of unstable social relationships,[210] which typifies kennels.

Nearly all vocal signals, even short ones like grunts and barks, are graded, or emitted along an acoustical continuum without measurable breaks, and most (if not all) are affective.[211] Categories of vocalizations (e.g. barks, growls) expressed by domestic dogs can be partitioned acoustically into subtypes and tested for context-dependent motivation.[212] To qualify as referential an acoustical signal must satisfy four criteria: (1) pattern varies by context, (2) prerecorded signals elicit different responses when played back, (3) altering the referent alters the signal, and (4) affective state remains constant while vocalization varies.[213] Wolves and dogs growl when making threats, guarding food, and during play.[214] Growls of domestic dogs supposedly meet all requirements when tested under these conditions.[215] Playback experiments of food-guarding growls, for example, kept dogs away from a bone more effectively than threatening or play-growls.

Before these results are accepted at face value a comment is warranted about criterion (4). In an essay titled "What Is It Like to Be a Bat?", the American philosopher Thomas Nagel argued that we can never know how it might feel to be another species.[216] Even after identifying every possible requirement of bats we could still never know what *being* a bat is really like. Questions such as Nagel's fall within the realm of ontology, not animal behavior. Nonetheless, before the affective state of a dog could be measured and deciphered the investigator must first know *what being a dog is like*, obviously impossible unless you are one. Consequently, criterion (4) is essentially opaque to empirical investigation by humans, and by dogs too. Before a dog could devise and test hypotheses it would have to become human, at which point the affective states of dogs would once again be a mystery.

Some vocalizations are elicited by several stimuli, others by only one. The narrower the range over which a signal is effective the more predictive it is and the greater its potential influence. A signal's specificity depends on how tightly

Table 4.4. Motivation-structural rules for close-contact sounds made by animals.

Low-frequency sounds warn that the sender will attack if the recipient comes closer

High-frequency tonal sounds indicate that the sender is submissive to the recipient or is afraid of the recipient

Frequency and tonality blend on a continuum: the higher the frequency the more fearful (or friendly) the sender, the lower the frequency the more hostile; and the greater the sound's noise component the greater the aggressive motivation, the more tonal the more fearful (or friendly) regardless of frequency

Sounds rising in frequency indicate falling hostility and rising appeasement (or fear); sounds decreasing in frequency indicate hostile motivation

Sounds that rise and fall more or less equally in frequency or have a nearly constant mid-range frequency indicate conflicted motivation (i.e. the animal is undecided whether to approach the stimulus or withdraw from it)

Social species display a prevalence of high-frequency sounds compared with species that generally avoid contact with their own kind

The more complex the society the greater the range of signals

The higher the frequency of an alarm sound the more an animal is likely to withdraw

Source: Information in Morton (1977).

signal and response are linked (influential value) and how much variation can be tolerated to still elicit the response (referential specificity).[217]

Eugene W. Morton proposed the *motivation-structural hypothesis* for animals in close vocal contact: "birds and mammals use harsh, relatively low-frequency sounds when hostile and higher-frequency, more pure tonelike sounds when frightened, appeasing, or approaching in a friendly manner."[218] He noted, "in animals that are 'face to face,' the possibility and consequences of attack, escape, or association are immediate, and [natural] selection will favor sound signals that express current and rapidly changing motivational states."[219] Proximity, he pointed out, lessens the difficulties of communicating, although not the immediate consequences. His main points are outlined in Table 4.4.

Morton's hypothesis is supported more strongly for low-frequency sounds; variation in acoustical structure within the high-frequency context conforms less well.[220] The idea is intuitively satisfying because it also applies to us. We humans, when speaking "baby talk" to infants and pets, raise our voices to a higher frequency where it sounds appeasing or friendly. A female wolf often squeaks when entering her den containing young pups,[221] and captive eastern coyotes commonly whined and squeaked when their young pups strayed.[222] The howls of wolves perceiving a threat are low-pitched and harsh.[223] A domestic dog might bark relentlessly in its owner's absence, but it seldom whines (appeasement, friendliness) unless someone is there.

Mouse-like social squeaking is part of the vocal repertoire of adult wolves[224] and eastern coyotes,[225] but not dogs. A wolf raised among people and farm animals emitted high-pitched squeaks when greeting persons he knew, pup dogs, and when visiting captive wolves at the zoo.[226] Squeaking might be associated with establishing contact or simply with pleasure; when greeting familiar persons this wolf also behaved submissively, tail-wagging enthusiastically and sometimes rolling onto his back. However, he also squeaked and growled if his owner tried to take away his

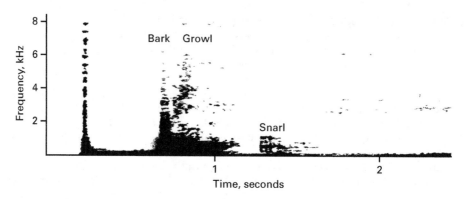

Figure 4.5 Spectrogram of a linked sequence of bark–growl–snarl in a wolf. Amplitude is shown in black.
Source: Schassburger, R. M. (1993). *Vocal Communication in the Timber Wolf,* Canis lupus, [*sic*] *Linnaeus: Structure, Motivation, and Ontogeny*, Advances in Ethology No. 30. Berlin and Hamburg: Paul Parey. This material is reproduced with permission of John Wiley & Sons, Inc.

food bowl, indicative of conflicted aggression. Placating, high-frequency whines are often made by submissive wolves[227] and by wolves in frustrating or conflicted situations, as in one instance when wanting to attack a large boar but uncertain whether to do so.[228] Wolves make any number of soft and varied utterances while interacting in a friendly way with pack mates and humans they know.[229] At the opposite pole are low-frequency aggressive sounds: barks, growls, and snarls are more broadband with less tonality (i.e. are harsher) than high-frequency appeasing or friendly sounds, and they often grade into one another (Fig. 4.5).[230]

If we accept that certain dominant postures like stand-taut, stand-over, and piloerection serve to exaggerate size, and that postures of submission such as crouching and cowering with tail-low serve to lessen it,[231] then size perception has social relevance. Canid barks are similar acoustically. Each species barks within its own acoustical range because intraspecific variation in body size and shape is limited, and these factors place restrictions on sound-making anatomy (see below).[232] A receiver hearing the vocalization of a conspecific might be able to judge whether its sender is large or small. This could be true if the source is nearby, low-frequency, and broadband (e.g. growling, barking), and provided vocal tract length correlates directly with body mass.[233] Dogs can apparently evaluate low-frequency signals (growls) of other dogs and adjust their own behavior based on feedback of perceived size of the sender relative to their own.[234]

Harmonic vocalizations of dogs and wolves are thought by some to be less ambiguous than noisy sounds. As a corollary the noisy part "is more elaborate and therefore more expressive of subtle motivational fluctuations."[235] This makes sense in terms of Morton's motivation-structural hypothesis because many such sounds are complex and carry less well, making them useful only in close contact. However, just because howls can be mixed with other discrete sounds and vary in characteristics such as frequency, intensity, and duration does not necessarily make them long-distance "potential codes," nor can this be said of other harmonic vocalizations (e.g. whine, whimper, yelp). In fact, the parsimonious position should be that no discrete or mixed sound – or sound of any kind – can be considered anything but affective at the pragmatic (functional) level, and that the semantic (meaning) level is unattainable except by humans.[236]

For those who believe animals to be much more, this is not so bleak as it seems. The emotional range of dogs and wolves is unquestionably broad, intricate, and replete with fleeting and fragile subtly. For example, sound frequency could influence interpretation by a receiver if the harmonics correlate with the sender's affective state. This notion is reinforced by the motivation-structural hypothesis. Certainly, the ontogeny of vocalization shows direct correlation between complexity of sounds and developmental stage (Chapter 9). Having mastered how to emit and interpret all the discrete sounds, and with maturation of the vocal tract, adult wolves and dogs can use gradation and transition to mix them in combinations offering remarkable complexity. A quick calculation shows that just the 11 discrete sounds reported by Schassburger have 110 combinations; in multiples of 3, 990 different ones are possible. Can adult canids make use of them all? That remains to be shown.

Sound generation works as follows. Sounds produced at the glottis pass up the vocal tract through a resonating column of air. Certain frequencies are filtered out while selected others pass into the environment via the mouth and nose. These specific resonances are called *formants*. Stated differently, formants represent the varying energy levels of harmonic overtones. Dispersions inside a tube are smaller because spacing between resonant frequencies decreases with increasing tube length. During growling, for example, a dog's mouth is closed (or nearly so), and the entire vocal tract is used. Dogs seem able to change the shape of the vocal tract by adjusting the mouth opening to produce variable sounds; further modifications can be made by use of the tongue, repositioning the lips, altering placement of the larynx, and so forth.[237] A wolf's howl can achieve different timbres described as a "mournful plangency."[238] X-ray images of anesthetized dogs show that vocal tract length varies considerably but correlates directly with body mass, from 6.9 cm in a Yorkshire terrier to 22.4 cm in a Rottweiler.[239] Vocal tract length increased and formant dispersion decreased with body mass when these dogs were induced to growl. Therefore, as in other canids the signals sent by dogs are reliable indicators of body size.

The fact that barking is widespread in birds and mammals[240] has resulted in much speculation about its function, but no animal has generated more interest than the domestic dog, which seems to bark for any reason or none at all.[241] A dog's barks have been ascribed variously to: (1) paedomorphism,[242] (2) alarm,[243] (3) excitement,[244] (4) announcements of territoriality,[245] (5) play solicitation,[246] (6) reflections of affective state,[247] (7) conflicted behavior,[248] (8) attention-seeking,[249] (9) signals co-adapted with humans,[250] (10) the result of *social facilitation* (e.g. the barking of other dogs),[251] and (11) artifacts (i.e. *hypertrophied traits* in this case and having no specific functions).[252]

Throughout their history dogs have been bred for many qualities, but tameness in particular. Accordingly, some consider the heightened tendency of domestic dogs to bark as resulting from relaxed selection pressure to remain silent.[253] If dogs are fed and protected through many generations they might lose the need of silence to avoid predators or frighten away prey. However, if barking evolved as a contact response to humans[254] then other domesticated canids should bark more too, assuming barking to be a byproduct of tameness.

The only canid other than the dog that qualifies as domesticated comprises several lines of "silver" foxes at a Siberian fur farm.[255] Starting in 1960 the Russian geneticist Dmitry K. Belyaev bred them selectively for tameness and no other quality.[256] In 1970 he initiated another line that has since been bred only for aggressiveness. Investigators recently chose 25 foxes each from groups bred for tameness (40–45 generations), aggressiveness (30–35 generations), and no particular quality (control group) and described their vocal responses toward humans.[257] Only 2 of the 75 ever barked during nearly 13 000 recorded vocalizations, both from the aggressive group. Foxes not included in the experiment could be heard barking in contexts other than human contact. The group bred for tameness indeed vocalized differently, but its human-associated sounds were cackles and pants, not barks. Domestication therefore does not always induce hypertrophied barking in canids, and the development of human-associated vocalizations is probably species-dependent.

Acoustical equipment can distinguish dogs individually by their barks and also categorize barks accurately as being stimulated by disturbance, isolation, and during play with a human or another dog.[258] *Disturbance-barks*, such as elicited when a doorbell rings, are harsh, low-frequency, and without modulation. In comparison, *contact-barks*[259] and *play-barks* are more modulated with greater tonality and higher frequency. As responses these different barks appear to be referential by denoting consistent links to context-specific stimuli, thus functioning in different situations.[260] Maybe so, but the associations could be entirely affective, the distinctive acoustical patterns caused by differing levels of excitement. Certainly the progression indicates a gradation of emotion consistent with the motivation-structural hypothesis.

Referential content in contact-calls of canids and primates has yet to be demonstrated convincingly. As mentioned, wolves are thought to use howling as a means of establishing contact with pack members[261] or as signals to assemble,[262] but are they? Baboons dispersed over a large area bark frequently, giving human observers a false impression of informing others about their locations; in other words, that the barks are referential. However, no call – not even in response to vocalizations from their own infants – induces contact-barks from dispersed females. Instead, females emit these calls when they sense *themselves* becoming isolated from the group.[263] Their vocalizations are not referential at all, but entirely affective. The persistent barks of a dog chained alone in a yard could also be affective expressions of isolation and nothing else.

Another possibility, the *co-adapted signaling hypothesis*, proposes that dogs and their human respondents mutually reinforce barking, the incidence of which attenuates without direct human contact.[264] That free-ranging dogs rarely bark[265] is thought to have survival value by not drawing attention.[266] Groups of free-ranging dogs in Italy mostly limited their barking to two situations. The first was while assembling for a trip to the local dump to scavenge; the second occurred during agonistic encounters with other groups and involved a "bark-off" until one group retreated. The same behavior has been reported in dogs foraging at a dump on a Navajo reservation.[267] In both cases they mirrored the howling of wolves in similar situations.[268] Like wolves, most free-ranging dogs hunt silently,[269] although a group having hound ancestry vocalized loudly while pursuing or trailing prey.[270]

Confinement and isolation are what make the owned dog's situation different. Anecdotal reports suggest a relationship between human contact and the maintenance of barking. Darwin claimed that progeny of dogs left in isolated places parts of the world ceased to bark.[271] Descendants of those abandoned on Juan Fernandez Island became dumb within 33 years, but specimens taken from the island acquired the capacity to bark when once again in contact with humans. The propensity to bark spontaneously and in varied circumstances might indeed be a trait of extended domestication.

Many earlier breeds (if they were breeds) could only howl. The Hare Indians of Canada's Northwest Territories kept a type of dog that "at some unusual sight . . . would make a singular attempt at barking, commencing with a peculiar growl and ending in a prolonged howl."[272] Domestic dogs bark far more often than they howl. Wolves are the reverse. They emit acoustically similar barks over a range of conditions,[273] but evidently not during play.[274]

Variation in the barks of domestic dogs appears to be minimally context-dependent with detectable acoustical distinctions associated with disturbance, isolation, and play.[275] Dogs can evidently tell the recorded barks of other dogs approached by a strange human from those of a dog left alone tied to a tree[276] and also distinguish the barks of other individuals,[277] giving varied responses not just to different barks but to the barks of different dogs.[278] Dogs can therefore distinguish barks both from the same individual in different contexts and different individuals in the same context.[279] If true, then barks reveal something about the sender's identity and affective state in very restricted context-dependent situations. None of this is evidence of between-dog communication or even that barking is a primary mode of communication.[280]

4.4 Wolf howls

Howling is part of what wolves do, and it starts early in life. Pups howl at 28–62 days,[281] although a pup eastern coyote howled on day 15 and chorus-howled at 2 months.[282] Wolves in the wild howl both night and day,[283] and their sounds show little variation with region: howls of wolves from North America and the Iberian peninsula are nearly indistinguishable.[284] Speculation attributes howls to any of at least seven functions: (1) affective responses,[285] (2) *vocal signatures*,[286]

(3) announcements of location,[287] (4) calls to link scattered pack members,[288] (5) calls to assemble,[289] (6) calls to increase distance between adjacent packs,[290] and (7) maintenance of territorial boundaries.[291] All hand-waving to "functional reference" aside, none has been validated, and all except the first two are doubtful in these stated configurations by implication of intentionality and assuming the receivers understand the senders' mental states.

Howls might simply be emotional release or *vocal signatures*; that is, putative calls of identity of individuals or packs. The howls of individual animals are unique, making them potentially recognizable by conspecifics. Howls could transmit individuality better than barks and growls because vocalizations having *narrowband frequencies* are easier to distinguish.[292] For howls to serve this function requires recipients to recognize them as such. Human technology can assign nearly 85% of howls to the correct wolf.[293] Whether wolves can exceed this accuracy or even use howls in recognition is unknown. Wolf pack A howls. At the receiving end, pack B processes the signal, interprets it (or not), and howls back an affective message of its own. If the signal received triggers a purely affective response then interpretation might be minimal or unnecessary. Although packs A and B are linked momentarily by a communicative event, "it is not necessarily so much *what* is communicated that is of significance, but rather *how* it is communicated."[294] *Whatever triggers the sender to vocalize stands apart from any effect it has on a receiver.*[295]

Frequency modulation, if used in signaling, would appear to work best at long range. Amplitude modulation, in contrast, requires repetition "to counteract the accumulation of random fluctuations and reverberations."[296] Among the sounds canids make only howls carry long distances,[297] at least 9 km in wooded areas[298] and perhaps 16 km on open tundra.[299] *Howls* are distinguished acoustically from other vocalizations by their tonality, modulated frequencies, and extended duration (Fig. 4.6).[300] Recorded howls have lasted up to 11 seconds.[301] Pitch can change several times, but amplitude is generally constant.[302] Acoustical equipment can separate and identify howls of individual animals despite their considerable variability,[303] and perhaps wild canids can too.

Most problems involving vocal signaling occur at the receiving end when the receiver: (1) fails to detect a signal, or (2) is unable to separate signal from noise.[304] Errors of the first type are confined to the communication channel through which a signal arrives, and they occur because other perturbations in that channel are similar. This is a problem when signals are weak; that is, one of declining signal-to-noise ratio.[305] Repetition is a way of overcoming it by focusing attention, dampening noise in the channel, and building up a cumulative effect until a threshold level is attained in the receiver.[306] Errors of the second type, which like the first are affected by attenuation and degradation during transmission, occur because the receiver is unable to detect important variations in the signal, a worsening situation with increasing distance.

The most effective signals are directional, but this might be irrelevant where wolf howling is concerned. A wolf's low-frequency howl travels farther than one

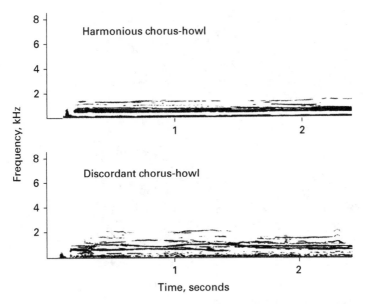

Figure 4.6 Spectrogram of the chorus-howls of a group of captive wolves. Howls can be harmonious or discordant. Discordant howling is more likely if the wolves are young or when howling by the pack is not part of the group-ceremony. Amplitude is shown in black. *Source*: Schassburger, R. M. (1993). *Vocal Communication in the Timber Wolf*, Canis lupus, [*sic*] *Linnaeus: Structure, Motivation, and Ontogeny*, Advances in Ethology No. 30. Berlin and Hamburg: Paul Parey. This material is reproduced with permission of John Wiley & Sons, Inc.

of higher frequency, but its transmission is less directional. If aimed at the receiver a more narrow-beamed source increases the intensity of the sound and thus the range of detection, provided the environment is not scattering. However, wolves seldom know the locations of other wolves, assuming the howls are for their benefit.

The environment strongly affects acoustical emissions, howling in particular. Attenuation and degradation of signals transmitted through the atmosphere limits acoustical communication. Sound is attenuated by: (1) absorption (atmosphere, objects in the environment), (2) the ground, (3) deflection of sound waves by stratified objects (vertical layers of leaves), and (4) scattering of directed sound.[307] My discussion is limited to *sonic frequencies*.

Ground attenuation at the receiving end of an acoustical signal is caused by interference between direct and reflected sound waves.[308] Among other factors, its severity depends on height of the source. Attenuation is greater for frequencies below about 1 kHz than at medium frequencies when sound is transmitted near the ground, and this would apply to wolf howls, which are typically 150–780 Hz.[309] At transmissions made at 1-m elevation the ground attenuation is greatest at 300–3000 Hz, and the "higher the source, the lower the frequency for peak ground attenuation."[310] Therefore, howling from a high elevation allows a greater proportion of lower frequencies to be transmitted. Wolves stand about a meter tall.

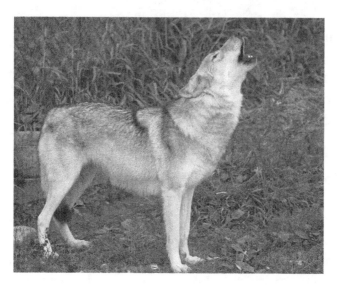

Figure 4.7 A wolf transmits low-frequency sounds farther by pointing its muzzle upward. *Source*: Helen E. Gross|Dreamstime.com.

A wolf howling from a ridge with muzzle pointed upward transmits low-frequency sounds farther than if it stood at sea level. Even at low elevations wolves typically elevate their muzzles while howling (Fig. 4.7).

Considering that peak ground attenuation occurs at higher frequencies the closer to the ground, maximum transmission range near the ground should use neither high (>4 kHz) nor low (<1 kHz) frequencies regardless of habitat type. Low frequencies become less a disadvantage with increased elevation because most low-frequency attenuation is caused by the ground. Sound reception depends partly on existing background noise near the receiver and by the receiver being able to recognize the signal. The degree to which sound is absorbed in the atmosphere depends on temperature, humidity, and frequency. Scattering occurs when an acoustical signal is disrupted (e.g. reflected, refracted, diffracted) by objects or environmental conditions, but atmospheric turbulence is probably the most important factor. Refraction is caused by gradients in air temperature, fluctuating wind speed, and changes in wind direction between sender and receiver.

The more heterogeneous the surroundings (including the atmosphere) the greater the scatter and subsequent attenuation of a propagated signal. The amount of reflected acoustical energy received increases with distance from the source, and as sound is scattered and loses energy it becomes less focused, seeming to arrive from several directions simultaneously.[311] Scattering and attenuation in a deciduous forest are more pronounced in summer than in winter after the leaves (stratified objects) have fallen. Wolves howling inside a dense forest in summer are less likely to be heard by conspecifics than if they howled from high on a ridge, and their location will seem less exact to the receivers. The difficulty is worsened in windy weather.

If howling is a form of long-distance communication, what does it signal? During one study packs of wolves in *Superior National Forest*, Minnesota (hereafter called *SNF*), seldom moved when responding to human howls.[312] Large packs replied to howls more quickly than small packs, as did packs at kill sites or harboring pups at den or rendezvous sites (Chapter 8). In these last two situations the contents of the location seemed more important than the space itself. Lone wolves never replied.

Captive wolves and coyotes and their wild conspecifics can be induced to howl by human mimics.[313] Attempting to make wolves howl by artificial means becomes less effective if they have recently howled.[314] You could call this the "howled-out effect." Dr. Doolittle was surely a fictional character, which makes me wonder why no one has yet asked a basic question: if these sounds truly have adaptive and communicative functions then why do human "howls" elicit howling responses from wild canids? Hunters have long known that wolves can be coaxed within shooting range by howling to them.[315] And why do captive coyotes, eastern coyotes, and wolves howl along with their human companions in plain sight[316] and in response to howling dogs, sirens,[317] fire whistles, or someone playing the trumpet or clarinet?[318] Moreover, they typically wait 40 seconds[319] or so before answering distant human mimics, an indication the response is not simply a howl-jerk reaction. These observations pose serious obstacles to the notion that howls transmit discrete and varied signals or that their use is context-specific instead of straightforward emotion.

If wolf howls have specific significance to other wolves then our own must seem like gibberish. If we "howl" something relevant it can only be accidental. So why would they answer? The most parsimonious explanation – the one having the least speculative baggage – is that their howls are applied over a broad context of nonspecific – and thus nonreferential – communication. If so, then wolf howls and our howled replies are like two tribes shouting at each other across a river each in a language indecipherable to the other. And after the grammar and vocabulary on both sides have been identified and sifted out, human and wolf howls perhaps carry the same two wind-borne emotions, one by the group, the other by its individual members.

I have no evidence to back these ideas, although certain anecdotes are intriguing. Crisler reported that when one of her captive wolves escaped all she needed to do was howl, which coaxed the other wolves into a *chorus-howl* and brought the prodigal running back, anxious to join in. Chorus-howling in some situations might not be a signal at all, but simply the discharge of a pleasing emotion.[320] Also according to Crisler, if a human joins a chorus-howl at a pitch that mimics one of the participating wolves that member of the chorus immediately adjusts its pitch in mid-howl and makes it different.[321] This could explain why the first choruses in a chorus-howl are structured simply, becoming more modulated as the event progresses until toward the end the individual voices "varied so much in frequency that many howls ... could not be measured even in the highest quality sonagrams [*sic*]."[322]

The question naturally arises that even if howling transmits a signal, why should listeners pay attention? Suppose chorus howls convey accurate and explicit "information" about a pack's "intentions" to defend its territory: this is our space, and you better not come over here. Pack A sends such a message stating its "intention" to escalate aggressions if the warning is ignored. Pack B, not to be outdone, howls back a similar message. According to current thinking this threat of potential confrontation is sufficient to keep the groups apart and limit aggression.

Now consider pack C, which comprises only lying wolves of a mutant cowardly type likely to turn tail at the slightest provocation. Nonetheless, pack C howls terrifying threats, causing its neighbors to quake in their wolf skins and remain where they are. After many generations natural selection might gradually favor lying howls over truthful ones, at which time every howling wolf would be a mendacious wolf, making it advantageous for conspecifics to ignore howls altogether. A signal's usefulness vanishes once its interpretant has been lost. According to John Maynard Smith, "this argument was put in more mathematical language, but it simply amounts to saying that you should not believe what an opponent at poker tells you."[323]

Such hypothetical scenes are challenged by those claiming to demonstrate that (1) contesting animals use a range of behaviors corresponding with different levels of aggression, (2) a signal embodies "information" about the signaler's future behavior (i.e. it correlates with the signaler's future response), and (3) "information" is actually transmitted because the signaler signals and the receiver responds (i.e. the recipient's behavior is influenced by the signal).[324]

The second and third have been discussed (Chapter 3). To address (1), we have no evidence of canids practicing deception, but if they do it would pay them to distinguish between the signs, I'm a very large wolf, and I'm going to bite you. The "information" transmitted should be difficult to misinterpret (receiver) and just as difficult to fake (sender). The context must also be appropriate for both parties: piloerection and teeth-bared are of no long-distance use against invisible enemies. Nothing about future intentions is actually signaled, and in many species submissive displays might be better indicators of retreat than threat displays are of attack. "Thus an act may be correlated with an immediately preceding or following act, and yet be a poor guide to whether a contestant will ultimately retreat or attack."[325] Such widespread inconsistency seems illogical if the actual function is to transmit "information" about the signaler's intentions.

Howling to wolves and trying to separate individual voices in their combined reply is difficult because "when a group responded together, their howls were frequently so similar in pitch that recognition of each individual was not possible."[326] This statement is not inconsistent with the above quote from Crisler. To our ears subtle fluctuations in the frequencies of a chorus-howl might not be detectable in the pitch. It seems to me that the capacity and readiness to make such facile adjustments might work against howling as signature vocalization, but this is conjecture.

Wild wolves, unless habituated or socialized (Chapter 9), are shy of humans. They also avoid other packs.[327] If some distance away a pack might respond to human howls by howling in reply, but human howling directed toward a pack nearby is likely to be ignored while the wolves silently retreat.[328] An extraordinary thing can happen in this second situation: human howlers are approached by a curious pack member,[329] usually a single animal, ordinarily the dominant male or female.[330] The animal's motivation is unknown, but one wolf barked,[331] perhaps in alarm, and others howled. The deep pitch of their howls could express aggressive motivation (perhaps signaling large size) consistent with Morton's hypothesis.[332]

Had the humans conducting these experiments shouted or played "Animal" by *Pearl Jam* through a loudspeaker at full volume, would these wolves have approached? Probably not. Did human howls, shamefully lacking in basic wolf lexicon, actually deceive a socially functional adult wolf into suspecting its territory had been invaded by strange conspecifics? Although unproven, the most likely answer is yes. If true then the notion of anything except identity being transmitted and received in howls is questionable.

If wolves mistake a single human's howls for a missing pack member, either of two events should occur: (1) the entire pack approaches expecting a reunion, or (2) the pack howls back only if a member is missing.[333] We have no evidence of either. The investigators just mentioned were approached by single animals seeming to display agonism or alarm, and whether all pack members were accounted for was unknown. They concluded that the wolves regarded them as "strangers," whether other wolves or something else was left unsaid.[334]

As noted, the howls of individual animals are unique, making them potentially recognizable to conspecifics,[335] and wolves can detect the difference between live howls and those previously recorded and played back.[336] However, the capacity to detect auditory differences is one thing; recognizing the voice of a conspecific based on its vocalizations is quite another.

Canid vocalization is fluid, not fixed. Neighborhood dogs sometimes chorus-howl in early morning.[337] Although wolves in nature howl and rarely bark the opposite can be true in captivity, where they can start to bark like dogs, learning to do this in about a week.[338] Other captive wolves behave like their wild counterparts, howling instead of barking.[339] Isolation of confined domestic dogs induces them to bark more; similarly, isolating captive wolves increases their incidence of howling. They howled most when alone, less when someone was nearby and had just left, and least with someone present for at least 15 hours.[340] Both might be affective responses to isolation and removal of social contact. Mech claimed that wolves in the high Arctic howled if disturbed (although not enough to run away), on waking up, and when separated from other pack members; in other words, when aroused.[341] Captive wolves sometimes bark when excited (e.g. at feeding).[342]

5 Space

Philopatry is attachment to place. Wolves and other dogs occupy finite spaces called home ranges and often territories as well to which they are philopatric. Both home range and territory are conceptually straightforward, but often used loosely and sometimes interchangeably. An animal's *home range* is "that area traversed by the individual in its normal activities of food gathering, mating, and caring for young."[1] The boundaries of a home range are often vaguely defined and flexible. The caribou (*Rangifer tarandus*), a circumpolar deer, might migrate 1300 km over the course of a year, the entire distance comprising the home range. Droughts, floods, population fluctuations, human encroachment, intensive predation, excessive self-exploitation of resources, and other factors cause animals to move and establish home ranges elsewhere. Young animals of many species leave the *natal* home range to establish their own. In practical terms, a home range is where an animal spends its life; that is, where it shelters, mates, rears young, interacts with others, eats and drinks, and eventually dies.

A *territory* is the part of a home range that an animal defends, ordinarily against conspecifics but sometimes against other species too.[2] Note that the definition of home range says nothing about it being defended. In birds, a territory is often just the nest and immediate surrounding area, although the home range might be much larger.

5.1   Use of space

Home range and territory are synonyms when applied to wolves residing in the same location all year, the boundaries of one being the boundaries of the other (Fig. 5.1).[3] Wolf territories are usually dynamic, their margins expanding and contracting over the seasons and through the years, permanently fixed only when up against a river, cliff, or some other physical barrier,[4] and although the same trails might be used regularly the routine usually varies.[5] However, routes used by generations of Minnesota wolves were traveled so consistently that trappers could easily predict their movements,[6] evidence that boundaries can also remain stable.[7] Some territories in southwestern Québec had been maintained for 30 years,[8] and Finnish wolves moved through their territories in patterns so regular that "there are hills, eskers and islands on wolf routes that bear names proving them to have been used by wolves from ancient times."[9]

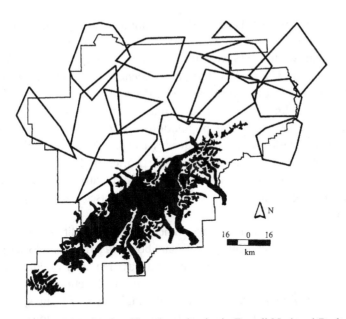

Figure 5.1 Mosaic of wolf pack territories in Denali National Park, Alaska, during winter 1989–1990. Areas in black represent the glaciers surrounding Mt. McKinley.
Source: From *The Wolves of Denali* by L. David Mech *et al*. Copyright 1998 by University of Minnesota Press.

Some wolves occupying SNF, parts of Alaska, and the Canadian Rockies appeared to monitor peripheries of their territories on a regular cycle.[10] Because of substantial differences in altitude and seasonal distribution of game, wolves in the Canadian Rockies sometimes have a summer territory and a winter home range often separated by more than 100 km.[11] Wolves inhabiting the central Canadian Arctic are similarly territorial from late April into late October when denning and rearing pups.[12] These summer territories averaged about 2000 km^2 for males and 1100 km^2 for females. Territories are abandoned in autumn when the pups are old enough to travel. The pack then becomes nomadic through winter, following caribou herds from their calving grounds on the tundra to wintering areas in the boreal forests (Chapter 6), at which time home ranges expand to 63 000 km^2 (males) and 45 000 km^2 (females).[13] Wolves in northwestern Alaska also prey on migratory caribou but do not follow them, and their territories are far smaller, averaging 1000 km^2 in summer and 3400 km^2 in winter.[14] The availability of alternative prey (the moose) might account for this difference.[15] Therefore, wolves that prey mainly on caribou can be migratory themselves, following the herds on their annual treks and territorial only during the breeding season (Chapter 7).[16]

The amount of space defended varies greatly depending on the status of the regional population, the availability of food, and how the food is distributed. A pack of four in northern Wisconsin ranged over about 388 km^2,[17] another pack of four in Michigan used 673 km^2;[18] packs of 2–15 in SFN occupied 80–400 km^2.[19] In the *Bearville Study Area*, Minnesota, winter territories ranged from 78 to

153 km^2.[20] Packs of 20–29 in Denali each used about 1000 km^2;[21] an earlier report gave an estimated range of 80 km wide, or 5024 km^2.[22] Territories of Mexican gray wolves in the southwestern US were thought to be about 7400 km^2.[23] Wolves in Italy use 200–400 km^2;[24] a pack of 10 in the *Nelchina Basin*, Alaska, 13 000 km^2.[25] That of one pack in Yellowstone measured 264 km^2.[26]

Territories of neighboring packs sometimes overlap, large ones especially.[27] They remain exclusive when wolf populations are low and starting to expand, but overlaps occur with increasing frequency as space becomes limited.[28] If the population has peaked (i.e. is at *saturation*) territories are likely to shrink so that more individuals can be accommodated, and large territories are unnecessary if game is plentiful. Mean pack size at saturation increases even if the number of packs remains about the same.[29]

Regardless of its size, with a territory comes the responsibility of monitoring the boundaries against encroachment by both neighbors and strangers. Wolves make the rounds of their territorial boundaries, but not always regularly or consistently in a circuit. While traveling they might turn in the opposite direction[30] or head directly toward the *core area*.[31] The use of space is uneven, more time being spent in some portions (e.g. core areas) than others, in part because the concentration of prey is also likely to be uneven.[32] Territorial boundaries and movements through territories sometimes follow paths of convenience, but not always. A pack in the Nelchina Basin climbed a 2100-m peak all the way to the crest when easier routes were available.[33]

Packs are most nomadic from late autumn through early winter, or starting when the pups are mature enough to follow.[34] They visit outlying areas of their territories, often for the first time in a year.[35] During the period from March through June there is typically a marked reduction in movement during the period of mating, denning, parturition, and rearing of pups (Chapters 7 and 8).[36]

Wolves everywhere use fire lanes, fire breaks, logging roads, highways, stream beds, lake ice, and ski and game trails in preference to traveling through dense forest or deep snow.[37] Wolves on the Sibley Peninsula, Ontario, used the shorelines extensively.[38] At nearby Isle Royale, wolves preferred moving along the lake shore or winter ice, pedestrian and moose trails, open ridges, and hard-crusted snow.[39] Wolves in SNF made extensive winter use of roads, trails, and frozen lakes and streams.[40] Those in *Beltrami Island State Forest*, Minnesota (hereafter *BISF*), favored frozen drainage ditches and traveled extensively on roads even though doing so exposed them more often to humans.[41] Wolves in the Nelchina Basin traveled preferentially on ice-covered rivers and streams.[42] Those in Denali favored highways for travel and to locate Dall's sheep in winter, which often used the highways themselves.[43] Wolves in the Canadian Rockies used roads, foot and game trails, and open areas through forests[44] and those on Vancouver Island, British Columbia, took advantage of areas cleared underneath power lines.[45] A pack in Sweden followed snowmobile tracks.[46] Wolves in Italy made extensive winter use of plowed roads during nocturnal foraging trips into urban areas,[47] those in the American West followed livestock trails, canyons, washes, and highways (presumably all year).[48] Wolves in general often move single file when traveling in deep snow, those behind stepping in the tracks of the ones in front,[49] and a pack in Algonquin Provincial Park, Ontario, walked in a ranger's snowshoe tracks.[50]

Pack size is increased through reproduction and low rates of *dispersal*, or emigration.[51] A wolf population's rate of increase is related to its existing density (i.e. is density-dependent) and rate of dispersal. However, the dispersal rate is density-independent, correlating instead with mean pack size and a measure of the prey's availability, or the prey/predator ratio,[52] and it increases in areas of low wolf densities until stabilizing with prey availability.[53] As a consequence, the number of packs and mean pack size appear to be independent of prey numbers.[54] These relationships render wolves vulnerable to population crashes in times of prey scarcity, as documented in SNF[55] and on Isle Royale.[56] Space restrictions at both locations make them strikingly similar to zoos. On many islands and in all zoos true dispersal is impossible. It could be argued that wolf populations like the present ones in Scandinavia and even SNF are not conceptually different because pressure from civilization limits viable egress, erecting invisible barriers quite unlike moats and fences but no less effective.

Wolves multiply rapidly if undisturbed in the presence of plentiful game,[57] their rate of increase restricted ultimately by competition; in other words, population growth rate, being density-dependent, correlates inversely with the number of wolves.[58] Great Lakes wolves in BISF increased quickly after all US wolves attained federal protection in the early 1970s.[59] The population in SNF rose by 32% a year following a severe winter that made white-tailed deer unusually vulnerable to predation.[60] Wolves in a protected area of Alaska increased by nearly 30% annually over 13 years, similar to the yearly net increase of their principal prey, moose and caribou.[61] This occurred despite illegal poaching within the protected site and legal shooting of wolves that ventured into unprotected areas. The initial 41 gray wolves released into Yellowstone between 1995 and 1997 multiplied to more than 170 within 10 years, or about 300 if contiguous areas outside the park are included.[62]

After a period of intensive aerial hunting ended, wolves in the *Finlayson Lake region* of the Yukon reached pre-reduction density in 5 years, increasing from 29 individuals to 245 within 6 years.[63] The number of packs rose from 14 initially to 23–28, or to the pre-reduction number of 25; mean pack size went from 4.4 to 7.8 and expanded to 9 after 8 years. Populations of unexploited wolves tripled in Russian Karelia in <10 years.[64] These patterns render large populations increasingly susceptible to ecological disturbances. A shortage of white-tailed deer in SNF during the 1970s had a strong effect on the wolf population, which was at saturation. These became manifested as malnutrition (particularly in pups and adolescents), smaller litters (or none at all), greater pup mortality, and increased incidences of trespassing across territorial boundaries. This last increased strife among packs, resulting in more adults being killed.[65]

The history of Isle Royale's wolves is what might be expected when escape is nearly impossible. The original wolves, thought to have crossed a rare ice bridge from Ontario in 1948 or 1949,[66] found an Eden overrun with moose. From 1959 through 1974 the wolf population, which ranged from 17 to 31, divided into a large pack and 2 or 3 small ones.[67] Authorities believed the population had come into balance with its resources of food and space. As time passed, any such apparent equilibrium proved a fantasy. With food plentiful and space still available the new immigrants multiplied, reaching a peak of 50 individuals by 1980. For the founders initial dispersal was unnecessary to find mates, new sources of food, and unoccupied areas to establish territories.

From 1975 to 1980 the Isle Royale population increased annually, with the exception of 1977, and fluctuated from 34 to 50 wolves. The original 2–4 packs split and expanded into vacant areas until there were 5. One of the original groups, which had existed since 1968, was gone by 1979, supplanted by a new one and forced into an area where there were no moose in winter. This group moved east, split, and its smaller components dispersed as best they could, trying to avoid established territories all around. During 1980 to 1982, the wolf population on Isle Royale crashed, plummeting from 50 to 14. One major pack disappeared completely; the rest were greatly diminished. Four breeding females remained. Such an event involving wolves had never before been witnessed.

Territorial boundaries collapsed in 1981 along with the population. It was a period of extensive dispersal, malnutrition, and "conspicuous mortality."[68] One pack used the entire north shore and two others mutually trespassed at will. With the exception of one pack, 1982 saw order established again. From 1982 until 1986, the Harvey Lake pack clung to a swatch of poor habitat, attacked frequently by packs surrounding it. In 1984 a pack to the west killed Harvey Lake's dominant female, and in 1986 an eastern pack usurped the survivors. Now there were again 2 packs.

What had caused the collapse? From December through April Isle Royale wolves depend almost completely on moose. The rest of the year's diet is 80% moose with beavers (*Castor canadensis*) constituting most of the balance. Beavers are not available in winter. Concentrations of both prey declined steadily from 1976 to 1981 before stabilizing at low levels in the early 1980s. North American wolves that rely heavily on moose are adversely affected when the moose population falls below 0.2–0.4 per km^2 (Chapter 6).[69]

Death from malnutrition and intraspecific strife became more common. Not only was dispersal impossible, it had become increasingly difficult to practice mutual avoidance, which wolves do exceptionally well given adequate space. Between 1981 and 1986 researchers found six wolves killed by others. There had been 5 in the previous 21 years. These new ones had been lone wolves (also called *loners*) and members of packs caught while trespassing or intentionally attacked by neighbors. The Harvey Lake pack had been attacked at least four times within its own territory before being displaced, once while feeding on a kill at its core area. In 1982 a group named West Pack II traversed the whole island at 19 km per day, the fastest recorded in 16 years. The apparent motivation was not to find and kill prey, which this pack did more efficiently than most, but to track other wolves.

At its peak of 50 in 1980, Isle Royale had a wolf density of 92 per 1000 km^2, the highest of any known wild population.[70] Compare this, for example, with 2.6 wolves per 1000 km^2 in southcentral Alaska during spring 1982[71] and 38.5 per 1000 km^2 in SNF, a saturated population, in 1968.[72] With game plentiful, wolf territories on Isle Royale shrank in the early 1970s as moose numbers increased and fewer wolves dispersed. A declining moose population over the next 10 years led to the expansion of territories accompanied by heightened strife between packs, trespassing, and a shuffling of large packs into smaller ones with fewer members. Despite all the fluctuations resulting from restricted space and the dynamic two-way push and pull of predator and prey, at no time between 1971 and 1991 did territory size and pack size demonstrate any correlation.[73] By the early 1980s the population had reverted to a near copy of itself 20 years earlier.[74] Following a fleeting spike through the rest of the 1980s, the population plummeted again, to an all-time low of 12 animals in 1991.

5.2   Territorial disputes

Defense of a territory ordinarily involves aggression only against conspecifics. North American wolves, however, do not always honor the distinction. *Intraspecific aggression* (aggression between or among members of the same species) is most common along territorial boundaries or in *buffer zones* between adjacent territories, and the results are often fatal, especially to the dominant animals.[75] During these disputes wolves belonging to a smaller pack might be killed or driven off and their territory usurped.[76] As just mentioned, wolves in small packs can even be killed inside their own territories by trespassing packs,[77] or outside them when they too become trespassers.[78] Lone invaders are chased and sometimes killed,[79] or occasionally permitted by a pack to trail behind at a distance and scavenge the leftovers.[80] In some situations loners might be restricted to poorer habitats (e.g. marshes, swamps) less likely to be visited by packs,[81] or to the peripheries of a pack's territory.[82] Nonetheless, they sometimes compose a substantial part of the population: loners counted for 18% of the wolves observed in southwestern Québec.[83] Domestic dogs are also attacked if they wander across the boundary of a wolf pack's territory.[84] Deaths among wild wolves have occasionally been attributed to "breeding disputes."[85]

Contiguous packs ordinarily avoid each other where territories overlap.[86] During a study of radio-collared wolves in Denali, 22% died annually; of these, at least 52% were killed by wolves occupying adjacent territories, although the number was probably higher (another 39% died of natural causes, some perhaps wolf-related, and at least some of the carcasses were eaten).[87] Sometimes a monitored wolf is killed by others but investigators arrive too late to decipher the circumstances.[88] Intraspecific strife brought on by prey scarcity was the main cause of natural mortality of adult wolves in SNF between 1970 and 1976.[89] Killings caused by intraspecific aggression rose in BISF as the population neared saturation, territories shrank, and dispersal into areas nearby became difficult.[90] As a population nears saturation new packs become difficult to establish. In the presence of adequate prey, interstices between territories are consumed by expansion of adjoining territories rather than establishment of new ones.[91] As the remaining interstices shrink,[92] emigrating wolves are forced to migrate farther.[93] Short-range dispersal is especially difficult where territories overlap.[94]

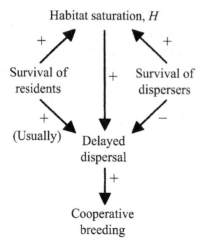

Figure 5.2 Diagrammatic scheme illustrating results of delayed dispersal. Intense competition for territorial space, as measured by habitat saturation, H, favors delayed dispersal. However, this is not determined extrinsically for each population but it is a dynamic outcome of the survivorship of resident and dispersing individuals, which have independent and direct effects on delayed dispersal and might override the effect of habitat saturation. Most important, improved survivorship of dispersers increases H but has a negative effect on delayed dispersal. Increased survivorship of residents usually favors delayed dispersal, although parent–offspring conflicts can sometimes produce the opposite outcome. *Source*: Kokko, H. and J. Ekman. (2002). Delayed dispersal as a route to breeding: territorial inheritance, safe havens, and ecological constraints. *American Naturalist* **160**: 468–484. Copyright by University of Chicago, reprinted with permission.

Habitat saturation, as noted previously, delays dispersal.[95] It also closes genetic distances within a population as dispersing wolves colonize locations near their natal packs[96] and emigrate into packs of close relatives.[97] If saturation is a constraint favoring retention of offspring and cooperative breeding, it is also stochastic, controlled by births, deaths, and dispersals within the population (Fig. 5.2).[98] Competition for space is heightened. One restriction can be extended longevity of the breeding pair, which leaves no possibility of adolescents breeding in the natal territory. In such situations leaving requires balancing two possibilities: low reproductive opportunities elsewhere versus prolonged *survivorship* of the territory holders. Ultimately "saturation is not determined externally by the environment: it is a dynamic outcome of the dispersal decisions of individuals."[99]

5.3   Pack dynamics

Mech defined a wolf pack as "a group of individual wolves traveling, hunting, feeding, and resting together in a loose association, with bonds of attachment among all animals."[100] I define a *pack* as a stable social unit with bonds of attachment, usually composed of related members, that travels, hunts, rears young, and defends a common territory together. This definition is broader by the addition of territorial defense, yet more restricted by requiring the communal rearing of young. At its core is a breeding pair of unrelated individuals, the dominant male and female. Packs in saturated populations, as noted, are more likely to consist of related individuals.[101] In general, territorial boundaries at saturation have more stability if wolves are not exploited and prey remains abundant.[102] Nonetheless, both factors are dynamic,[103] as are packs themselves. Six Denali packs disbanded while being monitored to be replaced by newly formed ones; others formed but did not persist.[104] Small packs of up to three are often transient.[105] The causes of a pack's disintegration can be death of a dominant wolf, failure to produce pups, or inability to establish a territory.[106]

The fluidity of pack membership depends to some extent on season but more often on *recruitment* (births, immigration, return of temporary emigrants), permanent dispersal, and mortality. Pack size varies. Sightings in Siberia of packs numbering >100 are undocumented.[107] The largest pack of gray wolves reliably reported is 36 from southcentral Alaska.[108] Packs in northwestern Alaska averaged 8.5 and ranged from loners to 23.[109] The big pack on Isle Royale averaged about 15, but 22 wolves were seen together on a February day in 1964.[110] Historical winter pack size ranges from 2 to 14 in the Canadian Rockies, with most comprising 4–7 wolves.[111] In the 1930s pack sizes in SFN ranged from 5 to 30, with 5 most common.[112] By the 1970s they comprised 5–20 with 5 being least common.[113] The typical pack size of moose-hunting Yukon wolves was 6–10.[114] The most common pack size for North American wolves is 7 or fewer.[115]

Pack size does not necessarily increase with increasing population,[116] although established packs in unsaturated regions might lose members as wolves emigrate to form new territories.[117] At such locations conflict at territorial boundaries is often more frequent and intense.[118] The mechanisms controlling pack size are unknown, although dimensions of the territory are probably not among them.[119] These factors correlate weakly or not at all, contradicting some earlier studies of some of the same packs in which different technology was used.[120] This general conclusion holds only for unexploited populations.[121]

Mech listed four possibilities that could explain pack size and considered the last two most important: (1) the smallest number to efficiently kill prey, (2) the largest number that could feed to satiation on a single kill, (3) the largest number with which pack members could form social bonds, and (4) the amount of social competition acceptable to pack members.[122]

Possibility (1) is certainly not limiting (Chapter 6). Single wolves can kill adult moose and caribou,[123] and a pack of 2 or 3 on Isle Royale routinely killed moose.[124] During a time when the Isle Royale wolf population was not at saturation and food was plentiful there were more loners and small packs.[125] As to possibility (2), pack size correlates inversely with per-capita food intake (Chapter 6), the idea being that a tipping point indeed exists where not enough kills could be made to feed all members.[126] However, packs can circumvent this problem by splitting temporarily into smaller groups, as they commonly do in summer. Large packs split in winter too, although what sometimes appears to be a split pack can be a group of younger wolves trailing behind.[127] Possibility (3) remains to be tested, (2) but would seem to make it irrelevant. In wild wolves (4) is more or less self-regulating.

A wolf pack takes several forms. The traditional family group consisting of a monogamous pair of adults and one or more litters of their pups[128] is the most common configuration. Even how packs coalesce depends on exigencies of the situation. The release of gray wolves into Yellowstone provides insight into how varied and facile a process this is. Mechanisms accounting for the formation of 29 breeding pairs were documented, excluding 5 pairs established prior to release into the park.[129] Two pairings were recorded when loners met, and 21 new packs formed as dispersing groups (usually siblings) met and joined a group of unrelated wolves. Five such pairs formed when one or more emigrants joined another wandering group. Four pairings occurred when an unrelated pack member took over a breeding position after a dominant wolf died.[130] In one case, a dominant male was usurped by an outsider. Six pairs formed after a dominant male died and was replaced by a wolf from outside the pack, although this never happened after the death of a dominant female.

Among Yellowstone's wolves only males ever left the natal pack and immigrated successfully into other packs as breeders. Females never dispersed into established packs. They either did not mate, became subordinate breeders, dispersed as loners to join a group of males, or dispersed with other relatives when a pack split. Even in saturated populations enough holes can be found in the *social fence* – that common territorial boundary between adjacent packs – to allow outbreeding. Yellowstone researchers, for example, documented instances of a lone dispersing male mating with a subordinate female and occasionally even joining her pack.[131] In any case, a mate and vacant space are difficult to find under saturated conditions.[132]

Pack budding occurs when dispersing wolves form a new territory within part of the natal range.[133] Splitting is often related to food availability (Chapter 6). During *pack splitting* two or more wolves (sometimes siblings or parent–offspring) leave the natal pack, join an unrelated dispersing group, and establish an association in a new territory that includes an unrelated breeding pair.[134] For example, a group of 2–4 split from a pack of 12 in the *Nelchina Basin* and moved 732 km northeast.[135] Like budding, splitting sometimes permits dispersing wolves to stay in the vicinity of their natal packs.[136] A pack of 15 Denali wolves split and after producing pups consisted of 11 and 13 members occupying adjacent territories but no longer associating.[137] Another pack split into groups of 11 and 9.[138] After a pack in Poland's Białowieża Primeval Forest split, their territories overlapped completely.[139] Many splits are temporary, in which case the pack continues to maintain a common territory.[140] A Nelchina Basin pack contained about 10 members but sometimes split into groups of 3 and 7.[141] Another in Canada's *Wood Buffalo National Park* split into two groups that rejoined 10 days later.[142] The big winter pack on Isle Royale in the 1960s occasionally split into two groups of 5 and 10, for example, or 7 and 8, eventually reuniting, although some separations persisted through summer.[143]

5.4   Natural controls on wolf populations

Mammalian populations are limited by intrinsic (behavioral) and extrinsic (outside) mechanisms. The first can be considered social, the second ecological.[144] Only some species of mammals have the capacity to control their own numbers, and the mechanisms are always intrinsic. For our purposes here, *intrinsic mechanisms* are defined as those intricate components of every animal's makeup expressed behaviorally. Three specifically come into play when the population of a species is self-limiting: (1) female territoriality, (2) dispersal of individuals from natal territories, and (3) self-suppression of reproduction before resources become limiting. This last might become more important in saturated populations.[145] Wolves should be governed mainly by intrinsic mechanisms because the dominant female assists her mate in defending the pack's territory, pack members other than the breeding pair typically disperse, and mechanisms for suppressing reproduction are in place to some extent (see below).

In the final analysis, self-regulation of populations should occur only in species in which females compete for space to rear their young or are forced by territorial boundary restrictions to associate with male relatives. Conversely, species in which females are not territorial or have some means of separating lack the capacity to self-regulate. Keep in mind that an animal's territory is a specific location, an actual piece of space within its home range. The size of the space – maybe several square meters for a small rodent, several thousand square kilometers for a pack of wolves – is theoretically irrelevant. Female territoriality still restricts the amount of room available to breed. The defense of territories by females is most common in rodents, rabbits (although not hares), terrestrial carnivorans (including canids), prosimian primates (lemurs, lorises, and tarsiers), and insectivores, and comparatively rare among bats, anthropoid primates, marine mammals, and ungulates.[146]

Depending on species a territory can consume the entire home range or just part of it and contains all the resources its defenders require to survive. Territories, in other words, are about more than food,[147] although as discussed below, food matters most. All species with territorial females produce *altricial offspring*; that is, offspring born with limited mobility (or none at all), blind, often deaf, sometimes naked, unable to move from place to place, and basically helpless. Species whose young are altricial but somewhat mobile, or produce young that are *precocial* at birth (unusually well-developed or advanced),[148] do not have females that defend territories but the males commonly do.

An important determinant in female territoriality rests on altricial young being vulnerable to *infanticide*, although among wild wolves this seems to be a minor problem. With the exception of a few primates, infanticide has not been observed in species with precocial offspring or any in which females are not territorial.[149]

Female territoriality limits population growth by restricting the number of breed-ing females and mitigates the chances of a dominant's offspring being killed by "outsiders," mainly strange females intent on usurping her position in the pack. Not surprisingly, alliances for protection of offspring in group-living animals occur most commonly among females.[150]

Extrinsic mechanisms are ecological factors that limit populations of species unable to control their own reproduction. This would seem to exclude wolves, but all else considered their numbers are controlled ultimately by prey density. Extrinsic mechanisms include anything not part of an animal's internal "self"; in other words, not of intrinsic origin. Examples are weather, predation, disease, and availability of food. Animals can influence none of these except the last, although each impinges on their populations. When extrinsic factors are out of balance a population lacking control over its reproduction can overrun the landscape, eventually outstripping the resources. Ungulates, which constitute the principal prey of North American wolves, are highly vulnerable to extrinsic mechanisms. Wolves are important in controlling ungulate populations,[151] and the same is true in reverse (Chapter 6).

The abundance of wolves where neither they nor the prey are exploited depends on prey availability.[152] A test of this hypothesis was made in two areas of north-eastern British Columbia where wolf numbers were systematically reduced and then left to recover.[153] Prior to wolf reduction the populations of ungulates – caribou, moose, elk, and Dall's sheep (*Ovis dalli*) – were stable or declining, but all increased once the wolves had been killed. After hunting stopped, the wolf population increased rapidly, at least temporarily exceeding the number predicted to come into balance with prey biomass, a result inconsistent with social self-regulation. Rapid recolonization supports the idea that dispersal is the principal mechanism by which wolves adjust to changes in prey density.

Another evolutionary benefit of dispersal is to separate relatives of the opposite sex, thereby lowering the possibility of inbreeding.[154] Nonterritorial animals can usually do this by just walking away. As mentioned, however, emigration in territorial species can be restricted at adjacent boundaries if popu-lations are saturated. We would therefore expect that in species with female territoriality the rate at which juveniles disperse is generally higher at low popula-tion levels, slowing as populations rise. Low population density should enhance dispersal of territorial species,[155] as demonstrated by the higher percentage of emigrants. This applies to wolves, which disperse rapidly in unsaturated regions (Fig. 5.3).[156]

When emigration is unrestricted by territorial conflict the opposite pattern is seen. As noted previously, during the 1990s wolves in the Finlayson Lake region multiplied quickly. Dispersal rates were low and correlated directly with mean pack size, indicating eventual intrapack competition for food.[157] The result was a stabilizing influence on average pack size. Dispersal rate, however, was indepen-dent of both the number of packs and population density.[158] The rate at which this population grew correlated inversely with emigration rate; in other words, the

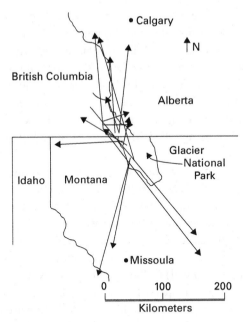

Figure 5.3 Dispersals of <50 km of 14 wolves from the Glacier National Park area, 1985–1997. *Source*: Boyd, D. K. and D. H. Pletscher. (1999). Characteristics of dispersal in a colonizing wolf population in the central Rocky Mountains. *Journal of Wildlife Management* **63**: 1094–1108. This material is reproduced with permission of John Wiley & Sons, Inc.

limiting effect of dispersal on pack size noticeably influenced population growth. In this case a low incidence of emigration from small packs enhanced growth of the population.

Other mechanisms help limit inbreeding. Great Lakes wolf siblings, for example, typically disperse at different times and in different directions,[159] which reduces the likelihood of their meeting later in the same pack and possibly reproducing. Others that disperse in spring might return to the natal pack after being away for several months,[160] in which case siblings that have already left are not potential mates. This is not always the case, however. Three littermates in the Northwest Territories dispersed as a unit during their first autumn and were still together when killed by trappers the following February nearly 300 km (straight-line distance) from the den.[161]

A wolf dispersing from a saturated population must often travel farther and still have difficulty finding vacant space, adequate prey, other lone wolves with which to pair, or a pack amenable to immigration.[162] However, those leaving in low-density areas are believed to travel the farthest.[163] In either case, leaving home is dangerous if it means crossing territorial boundaries of alien wolves. Wolves that disperse or make *forays* away from the natal territory are subject to unfamiliar risk factors.[164] Highways are especially dangerous.[165] Lower survivorship of emigrants has been reported at some locations but not others.[166] Loners, if inexperienced late-stage pups or adolescents, are less likely to survive than dispersing adults.[167]

Nonetheless, pups as young as 15 weeks have been known to disperse, or in mid-August of the birth year.[168] A 10-month-old wolf designated M15, GPS-collared and released in Italy's northern Apennines in March 2004, ranged into the southwestern Alps to the French border before being found dead of unknown causes 11 months later.[169] Wolf M15 also used highway underpasses and drainage culverts, traveling mostly at night and resting during the day. Even becoming road-wise is often no help: a GPS-collared female wolf in Minnesota crossed highways at least 215 times before being killed "illegally," presumably by a hunter or trapper.[170]

Wolves sometimes travel astonishing distances while dispersing and can cover up to 200 km per day.[171] Wolves routinely cross the Finland–Russian border,[172] for example, and those emigrating from Ellesmere Island across the frozen Robeson Channel to Scoresby Sund will have traveled well over 2000 km.[173] The distance dispersed seems mostly unrelated to sex,[174] although female bias has been reported.[175] The current record dispersal is that of a female in *Fennoscandia* (Norway, Sweden, and Finland combined) GPS-collared in Norway 6 December 2002 at the age of 7 months.[176] She dispersed 14 June 2003 and was shot by a reindeer owner in northeastern Finland 1 March 2005. (Reindeer are domesticated and semi-domesticated caribou.) In that time she dispersed 1092 km in a straight-line distance, but traveled a conservatively estimated actual distance of >10 000 km.

Dispersing wolves are obviously not averse to crossing large stretches of ice. The current population in southern Scandinavia immigrated from Finland or Russia, perhaps across the ice-covered Baltic Sea in winter where the 150-km distance between Finland and Sweden is interrupted by the Åland archipelago. Wolves inhabited these islands until 1844, having crossed from mainland Sweden or Finland in winter.[177] They also periodically inhabited Kolguev Island off northwestern Russia in the Barents Sea, crossing 80 km of sea ice from the mainland to hunt reindeer.[178] So too, they were rare inhabitants of Novaya Zemlya, an archipelago in the Barents Sea.[179] The southern end of Novaya Zemlya is separated from Vaygach Island to the south by the 56-km Kara Strait, which evidently froze at some point in the past. Wolves living on islands in the Canadian Arctic must have crossed a minimum distance of 40–50 km; others have recolonized Greenland from Ellesmere Island 30 km away.[180] Wolves were once found on Newfoundland, 25 km from Labrador, and the original colonizers of Isle Royale walked 25 km across frozen Lake Michigan from Ontario's Sibley Peninsula. Wolves recently crossed 160 km of frozen Arctic Ocean from Siberia to colonize remote Wrangel Island.[181]

Most dispersing wolves are offspring leaving their natal packs,[182] usually older pups or adolescents approaching sexual maturity, less commonly adults. Dispersal has been correlated inversely with age in some studies,[183] the reverse in others. About 28% of Denali wolves disperse annually from their natal packs, most commonly in April and May.[184] Half emigrated before age 2 years, another 41% between 2 and 3 years.[185] Dispersing wolves everywhere then find others of the opposite sex and establish territories in vacant areas.[186] The concentration of prey can be a factor too, with more wolves dispersing when prey is scarce.[187] Emigration is not always voluntary, and a wolf is occasionally forced out of its natal pack.[188]

The pace of emigration quickens as adolescents attain sexual maturity.[189] Dispersal in North America ranges from 21 to 35% annually and occurs throughout the year.[190] For example, 28% of tracked wolves emigrated each year in southcentral Alaska of which 40–50% were adolescents and biased slightly toward males.[191] In northeastern Minnesota up to 30% of wolves dispersed monthly, and annual dispersal encompassed pups (10%), adolescents (49%), and adults (17%) with no sex bias.[192] Dispersing wolves from an expanding population in Finland were young adolescents (average age 13.5 months), and the sexes emigrated in equal proportion.[193] A study of wolves in SFN showed numbers of males and females emigrating to be about equal, with 24% adults, 53% adolescents, and 23% pups.[194] One animal stayed in the natal territory until 54 months of age. Of 74 pup wolves radio-collared in SNF, 23% dispersed the first year and 34% the second year, or more than half within the first 2 years.[195] The remaining 32 animals stayed in their natal packs beyond 2 years including two that were still there 7 years later. Four departed after 28–32 months and seven after >3 years.

Dispersal of wolves in BISF occurred throughout the year but was most common just before winter, and adolescents of both sexes rarely stayed with the pack beyond breeding age (about 22 months).[196] The mean age of dispersers in the Finlayson Lake region was 2.9 years, and there was no difference between sexes.[197] Lone Great Lakes wolves generally pair before winter.[198] Annual dispersal from territories was 25% in northwestern Alaska and did not vary between adolescents and adults.[199] Dispersing males averaged 3.4 years of age, females 2.9 years, and only one animal was <1 year.

In Denali, 15% of radio-collared wolves immigrated annually into other packs and another 8% disappeared and could not be monitored because their collars failed.[200] Some of these might have dispersed or died. Immigration into other packs was also high (21%) in an exploited population in southcentral Alaska, and nearly three times as many males as females dispersed.[201] The average estimated age of the males was 30 months and that of females 33 months. Half the dispersing males and 40% of the females were <2 years old. Wolves in southcentral Alaska dispersed from natal territories at all months of the year, but mostly from April through June and October through November.[202] Dispersal distances ranged from 23 to 732 km.[203] Emigrating wolves usually left large packs (average size 7.6 individuals). If accepted into another pack, it was likely to be smaller (average size 2.8). The favored time to leave the natal pack in northwestern Alaska was April through September, and both sexes migrated about the same distance (males 154 km, females 123 km).[204]

Denali wolves immigrating into established packs were predominantly young males, and they entered as subordinates.[205] At least one paired with a pack member and established a budding pack of two. Why immigrants are sometimes tolerated instead of being killed is unknown. A male of 2.5 years from a neighboring pack was accepted into a pack of Yellowstone wolves that had lost its dominant male.[206] Acceptance followed 6 hours of interactions associated with dominance ↔ submission (Chapter 3), play-solicitation (Chapter 9), and courtship (Chapter 7). This wolf subsequently became the new dominant male.

Some wolves disperse from natal packs in February at the start of the breeding season;[207] others leave in late summer and early autumn[208] or throughout the year.[209] Many of these forays are temporary, and dispersers eventually return to their natal packs.[210] Obviously, wolves might or might not disperse permanently the first time.[211] Some break away gradually after temporary forays,[212] presumably returning if conditions elsewhere are less favorable.[213] These excursions can extend from a day or so to several months, and the distance traveled might be a few kilometers or a hundred or more. Wolves in northcentral Minnesota made up to six such forays during which they moved 5–105 km and their time away ranged from 1 to 265 days.[214] As noted by one investigator, "dispersal is not necessarily a 'one decision-one trip' event" but can take place over months or even years.[215]

Dispersal can obviously occur when a population is either declining or expanding.[216] During a steep decline in the SNF population the annual movement out of natal packs was 70% for adolescents and 19% for pups, but 47% and 4% during a time of stability.[217] The transition of adults did not change. Half the nonbreeding wolves of an expanding population in Finland dispersed,[218] a percentage similar to that of an expanding population in the central Rocky Mountains.[219] Success depends ultimately on the abundance of prey, finding a mate, and securing available space.[220]

The third intrinsic mechanism that controls reproduction in wolf packs is suppression of subordinate females by the dominant female to prevent their breeding with her mate. Inbreeding is also controlled by discouraging mating among related members of the pack, principally the dominant male with his subordinate daughters. Such controls are necessary because the second mechanism – dispersal from the natal area – is not always convenient.[221] The maintenance of strict territorial boundaries has a downside: peripheries are likely to be contiguous if the population is saturated. Territories often shrink as packs grudgingly shift to make room for others, and the newer territories are typically smaller.[222] The social fence keeping out the neighbors has two sides because it also prevents your own young from leaving. To repeat, wolf packs in saturated areas are apt to contain more closely related individuals.[223] This increases the potential for inbreeding.

Reproductive suppression is often evident as populations approach saturation.[224] In canids this has been discussed for gray wolves,[225] African wild dogs,[226] and Ethiopian wolves.[227] A form of reproductive suppression in gray wolves begins *in utero*. A small sample of Alaskan animals revealed mature females to shed an average of 7.3 ova during ovulation with an average of only 6.5 being implanted and becoming fetuses.[228] At other times a scarcity of prey can exert an inverse effect on population growth by reducing litter sizes.[229]

How often does infanticide occur in wild wolves and free-ranging dogs? Incest is sometimes evident when related canids of reproductive age are not separated in captivity where normal dispersal is impossible.[230] Infanticide occurs too,[231] probably more often than in nature.[232] The presumed dominant female's fear of her offspring being killed by another female might not be entirely applicable to canids.[233] A breeding female wolf diligently guards young pups for their first 3 weeks and moves quickly toward them when other pack members – including her mate – approach.[234] How much of this behavior has evolved to guard against infanticide by outsiders or even potential competitors inside her own ranks is unknown. It nonetheless appears that females with new pups are at least temporarily dominant over all pack members until pups leave the den.[235] This can be surmised by occasional submissive behavior by dominant males approaching dens where their mates are sequestered with litters.[236]

A dominant female canid is more apt to kill pups of subordinates than they are to kill hers. When food is scarce, a dominant female African hunting dog might kill pups of lesser females born inside her territory.[237] Her drive to monopolize all available resources for her own young perhaps induces her to eliminate their competitors. In this case she commits the infanticide, not a stranger, and not her subordinates. Typically these are older daughters helping rear the current year's offspring. Like gray wolves they guard the den and bring or regurgitate food for the breeding female and her most recent litter (Chapter 8).

A group of captive dingoes demonstrated infanticide. A pair named Curly and Toots and their progeny were allowed to breed over three years.[238] Toots produced litters of five, seven, and four pups during this time, sired by Curly. All her daughters came into estrus at 11 months and became pregnant, but none of their pups survived. During the second year Toots' only daughter, Genevieve, mated with her father and two brothers and gave birth to four pups 10 days after Toots produced her litter. After 2 days Toots moved her pups into Genevieve's den and both females nursed them all. Later Toots and her pups killed and ate Genevieve's offspring, which by that time were only half the size of Toots' (Fig. 5.4).

The next year there were eight mature females, one of which was killed by excited males. Toots transferred Genevieve's pups to her own den where she killed and ate them, and both females nursed Toots' four pups. When Cleopatra produced three pups Toots killed them immediately, then she and several of her adult sons ate them. Afterward, all three lactating females nursed Toots' litter and threatened any adults except Curly that came near the den. One pregnant female was killed during this time, and the other three, all pregnant, were often attacked by Cleopatra (their sister) and Beethoven, one of their brothers. At this point the experiment ended.

5.5 Painting the social fence

Territories are presumably maintained by patrolling. Urine sprayed on objects along the periphery (scent-posts) is thought to serve as a "keep out" sign (Chapter 4).[239] Urine eventually washes away or its odor dissipates, and scent-marking must be

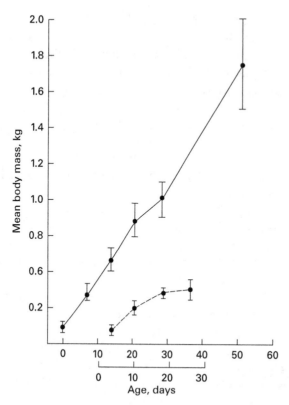

Figure 5.4 Mean growth of two litters of captive dingoes sharing a den. Toots' litter (solid line) born 4 June (1 male, 6 females); Genevieve's litter (dashed line) born 14 June (4 males) killed by Toots 17 July. Error bars are presumably ±SD.
Source: Corbett, L. K. (1988). Social dynamics of a captive dingo pack: population regulation by dominant female infanticide. *Ethology* **78**: 177–198. This material is reproduced with permission of John Wiley & Sons, Inc.

repeated at intervals. This is "painting the social fence."[240] Some have thought that each wolf's urine has a unique and identifiable scent, similar to a personal aftershave or perfume, but this has never been demonstrated.[241] Urine-marking is usually performed only by the dominant male and female.[242] Its frequency increases during adjustments of territorial boundaries or when expressing dominance within a pack.[243]

Raised-leg urination (Chapter 4) is a sign of territory ownership or of staking a new claim to vacant space.[244] Dispersing wolves are said to monitor scent-marks closely, presumably to avoid the property's owners.[245] Observation of urine-marking is the most reliable means of distinguishing a breeding pair from the rest of the pack.[246] Newly formed pairs establishing a territory urine-mark the boundaries extensively.[247] Wolves therefore start urine-marking as they mature, but before individuals are allowed to paint the social fence they must be an established dominant pair or else outside a hierarchy (i.e. newly formed pairs).[248]

How effective is urine-marking? Consider these points: (1) canids can supposedly tell their own urine-marks from those of strangers, (2) urine-marks are deposited around the peripheries of territories, (3) territory owners over-mark the urine-marks of strangers when placed within their boundaries,[249] and (4) urine-marks are believed to deter strangers. We can accept the first three as probably true, but not the fourth. Maybe such marks along territorial boundaries serve as guide posts for residents instead of warnings to stay out.[250] The den site – presumed core area of a wolf pack's territory – has not yet been established when newly formed pairs start to mark territorial boundaries.[251] Modeling urine-marking as a *random walk* shows theoretically that neither a den site nor a neighboring pack is necessary provided: (1) the wolves remain in the vicinity of their urine-marks and (2) receive positive feedback.[252] Other models requiring existing den sites and foreign – as opposed to familiar – urine-marks[253] are not more valid projections of reality.

5.6 Space use by free-ranging dogs

Humankind has historically ignored or persecuted ownerless dogs, and the term *pariah dog* (Fig. 5.5) is both telling and appropriate. A list of offensive behaviors contributing to this universal dislike includes "defecation, biting, barking, street wandering, pack forming, exploring garbage and public copulation."[254] Accordingly, "it could be argued that urban society now needs a toothless, silent, sterile and constipated creature if the real problems of dogs in the cities are to be confronted."[255]

Some key terms now need to be refurbished and expanded beyond the brief mention given in the Preface. The canid literature separates dogs without owners as feral or stray. *Feral dogs* are considered wild animals,[256] usually

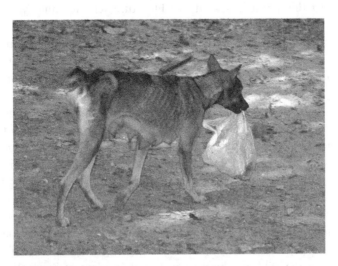

Figure 5.5 "Pariah Carey," a street dog in Siem Reap, Cambodia, carries home her groceries from a curbside pile of trash.
Source: Kent Davis, DatASIA.

aggressive when approached or trapped.[257] They exist independently of humans, generally avoid human contact, and often turn to hunting small animals and eating carrion if garbage is unavailable to scavenge.[258] For the most part they live without human assistance and display no evidence of socialization to humans (Chapter 9).[259] Some are born feral; others escape from their owners and become lost or simply choose not to go home. Like wolves, feral dogs sometimes occupy different resting areas of the home range preferentially according to season and ambient temperature.[260] Note that the feral state is behavioral, not evolutionary, that individuals can become feral within their lifetimes. *Feralization* is therefore a process by which "domestic animals become desocialized from humans, or never become socialized, and consequently behave as untamed or wild, non-domestic animals."[261] The process of becoming feral, in other words, requires developing a fear of humans.[262]

Strays have been defined as ownerless dogs living in urban, suburban, or rural areas that depend indirectly on humans for food or shelter.[263] Some are born ownerless, although many escape, become lost, are abandoned to the streets when a family moves, or turned out simply because no one wants them. In urban locations they subsist mainly on garbage and take shelter in spavined buildings and wrecked cars, in alleys and parks and vacant lots, and under steps and porches. I follow the convention of combining feral and stray dogs into a single category of *free-ranging*, defined as dogs not under immediate human control.[264] In some locations owned dogs are also free-ranging either all or part of the time. They rummage in garbage, mate with other free-ranging dogs, and are distinguished for purposes here only by having homes. Where appropriate I discuss them too. Most free-ranging dogs we see on city streets do not have owners, and they number in the millions.

Comments to this point are what the literature tells us, and we should be skeptical. The categories of owned and unowned free-ranging dogs are obviously fluid and without well-defined borders, a dog sometimes slipping from one into another and back again.[265] In some places dogs are fed occasionally and allowed to sleep on the premises while direct social interaction with the human residents and veterinary care are withheld. In other situations an owned dog can move onto the street and then into the woods, and a pup born free-ranging might be adopted and raised as a pet. Free-ranging pets, as mentioned, rummage through trash and eat garbage even when adequately fed at home.[266] Subsisting on garbage, regardless of ownership status, is not living independently of humans, making a feral garbage-eating dog living in the woods no different from a stray doing the same thing on city streets. Socialization is hardly relevant, considering that urban dogs relying on garbage are seldom socialized to humans either.[267]

Self-sustaining feral dogs of known domestic origin have not been documented in recent times except where they interbreed with dogs that have lived for thousands of years in the wild and become truly independent of humankind. These would include the dingo of Australia, southeast Asia, and New Guinea. What appears to be an ordinary mutt running through a forest in Australia or Thailand might carry the wild heritage of a dingo. In other words, the real basis of feralization requires a genetic component not likely to exist throughout most of the world. In the end, neither feral nor stray is a useful term when applied to dogs.

Availability of resources – food, water, and shelter – substantially influences home range size in free-ranging dogs, the home ranges of owned dogs usually being smaller because these amenities are provided.[268] Home ranges of owned dogs are typically <5 ha,[269] although one of nearly 2 km^2 has been reported.[270] When owned dogs are never restrained, their home ranges tend to exceed those of dogs let loose only occasionally.[271] In addition, large owned dogs range farther than small ones.[272]

Depending on circumstances free-ranging dogs can be up and moving at all times in search of something to eat.[273] The routine might depend on when people eat and discard food.[274] Those in Burdwan, India, were active during the lunch period, a convenient time to cadge handouts.[275] *Crepuscular periods* of dawn and dusk (both called *twilight*) are favored,[276] especially during hot weather,[277] although activity sometimes intensifies after dark[278] and some dogs, for whatever reason (e.g. avoidance of humans), are active only after nightfall.[279] Apparently these varied patterns hold true in urban, suburban, and rural areas. Activity is reduced at midday in hot weather[280] and generally repressed by temperatures >27°C.[281] During cool weather activity might pick up during daylight hours[282] regardless of other weather conditions (e.g. rain, snow), as it always does on cloudy days in all seasons.[283] Severe cold lowers activity regardless of time of day, but least at midday. Australian dingoes are mainly crepuscular,[284] sometimes active at night and least active during the hottest time of day.[285]

A study of urban Baltimore's free-ranging dogs made in the early 1970s showed that 40% of important behaviors – socializing, traveling, mating, foraging, and resting – took place in alleys.[286] Sidewalks, streets, vacant lots, and parks were used much less often. During peak morning hours 68% of dogs were in transit, 38% of them moving through alleys. Although only 11% were observed foraging, 88% were in alleys. The popularity of alleys was attributed to fewer motor vehicles, limited human activity, and high concentrations of garbage. Free-ranging dogs in rural areas maintain similar patterns with daytime activity reduced in hot weather.[287] Like wolves they prefer traveling where access is easiest (e.g. roads, game trails, crop rows, fire lanes).[288] Many are more resourceful and in better condition than their urban counterparts,[289] although urban-dwellers are often in good condition too.[290]

Defense and maintenance of space is strictly a social endeavor. The wolf is territorial, the dog is not or barely so, making the wolf "a landed proprietor, organized for the serious business of earning his way in the world."[291] Territoriality in dogs, when apparent, seems rudimentary and ephemeral. Gathering at the town dump and chasing off another group of dogs expecting to scavenge appears less like territorial defense than gaining temporary priority to a common food source.

I found no reliable evidence that free-ranging dogs[292] or lone wolves defend territories, although both have home ranges. Lone Great Lakes wolves reportedly tolerate each other, even staying in the same vicinity without interacting,[293]

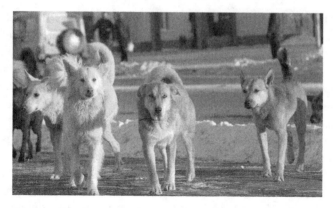

Figure 5.6 Russian street dogs.
Source: Vladimir Sofronov|Dreamstime.com.

behavior similar to that of dogs living on their own. Lone wolves seldom howl.[294] Free-ranging dogs are similarly less vocal than pets inhabiting socialized environments (Chapter 4). A free-ranging owned dog is more likely to bark at a human or another dog from its yard or porch than when wandering the streets several blocks from home. This makes intuitive sense if domestic dogs have true territories and not simply home ranges. If so then territories, if they exist, are small, usually no larger than a porch or part of yard adjacent to a house. Free-ranging owned dogs in Berkeley, California, were never aggressive despite their aloofness toward one another, and wandered through the home ranges of others without reprisal.[295] This is to be expected because home ranges are not defended.

Territoriality was not apparent in free-ranging owned dogs in Newark, New Jersey.[296] Neither agonism nor urine-marking could be correlated with defense of space. Competition for shelter sites was not evident. Free-ranging dogs, whether owned or not owned, often form loosely associated groups that intermittently travel and forage (Fig. 5.6). Typical group size is two to eight.[297] About half the dogs monitored in urban Baltimore were solitary, a fourth in twos, and the rest in groups up to five.[298] Most free-ranging dogs observed in St. Louis, Missouri, were also alone; twos were common, although never two females.[299] Singles and less often twos were the norm in Mexico City and Madras.[300] In St. Louis, early morning groups of up to seven dogs might come together but only for a minute or so, and the longest associations of several dogs were estrous groups comprising a female in heat attended by males (Chapter 7).[301] The more permanent associations were usually not random, some dogs favoring certain companions.[302] Most free-ranging urban dogs studied in Newark were owned, and the majority of these were also solitary.[303] Aggression and other forms of interaction were rare, and the dogs mostly avoided each other. A trio of unowned adults monitored in St. Louis showed both males to urine-mark frequently, the female rarely.[304] During the few times she did, one or both males immediately over-marked her scent.

Of free-ranging owned dogs observed in Berkeley, 82% were solitary, 14% in twos, and <3% were seen in groups of three or four.[305] Group formation was ephemeral and brief, usually occurring when solitary dogs met while traveling.[306] About half of Ethiopian village dogs were alone when observed, two together less common than groups of three or more.[307] Dingoes in northwestern Australia supposedly formed territorial packs, yet 25% were sighted when alone, 21% in twos, and 54% in groups of >3; mean group size was 2.1.[308] Unfamiliar dogs in general are more apt to avoid each other and less likely to form groups when chances arise.[309] Even among dogs that know each other, the trend is toward fleeting associations, and mutual avoidance is often the much stronger tendency.[310] Aggression is seldom a factor in group formation. Just 3 of 243 groups of two or more dogs observed in Newark separated because of aggression.[311] Group formation in urban street dogs does not depend directly on food resources. Garbage is scattered and variable, most available right before collection, least so immediately thereafter, but no variation was discerned in group sizes throughout the weekly collection cycle in Newark.[312] In fact, Newark dogs spent only 9.2% of their time actively foraging, a percentage not significantly different when unowned and free-ranging owned dogs were compared.

Dogs in Queens, New York, thought by their owners to be confined inside fenced yards during the day, were actually free-ranging, able to climb over the fence, duck under it, or in one case lift the gate latch to escape and roam the neighborhood.[313] Those that routinely escaped "lockdown" included two residing inside fenced yards with prominent Beware of Dog signs. These animals, unlike some in other studies, were social when loose and commonly formed transient groups with other free-ranging pets and strays, sometimes traveling briefly in groups up to five.

Urban dogs reportedly defend territories in part by urine-marking during the breeding season.[314] However, that owned domestic dogs respect urine-marks as representing territorial boundaries is unproven, and most seem eager simply to add their own signatures on top.[315] Newark dogs urine-marked by raised-leg urination after agonistic encounters, but the frequency was not different between familiar and unfamiliar dogs, nor between owned dogs and those without owners.[316]

Whether urban free-ranging dogs establish and defend territories is doubtful, and studies claiming they do have not provided supporting data.[317] The general lack of aggression seen in street dogs[318] calls the notion into question, although when aggression occurs at all it is sometimes directed at dogs of other groups.[319] Rural dogs in groups seem more inclined toward aggressive behavior, although still infrequently. Some, like wolf packs, even split temporarily and come together later.[320] Aggression is most likely when competing groups try gaining access to a common food source (i.e. a garbage dump) or when pups were being reared.[321] Even then, defenders of a litter respond to the invaders not by attacking them but by barking and visual displays of dominance (e.g. ears- and tails-erect).[322] Groups of rural dogs threaten other groups and even chase them, but physical contact almost never occurs.[323] In common with wolves, itinerant solitary dogs are sometimes killed (although rarely) by free-ranging groups in residence.[324]

Free-ranging owned dogs are more inclined than strays to be aggressive, the intensity of aggressive behavior correlating inversely with distance from home.[325] Urban dogs, even within their home ranges, usually run when approached.

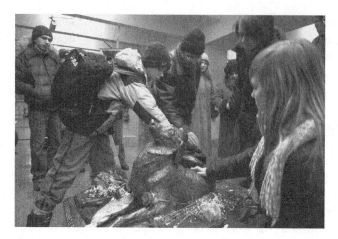

Figure 5.7 Statue honoring Malchik, a street dog that lived at a Moscow subway station. *Source*: Moscow Metro, www.mosmetro.ru.

Ownership has an enormous influence on a dog's social life. The tendency to roam, for example, decreased in 90% of dogs after castration.[326] Putative territorial behavior of owned dogs is restricted to the home area where food is provided.[327] Dogs that share a home naturally socialize more than with other conspecifics. That owned dogs become most aggressive when near home has been seen both as evidence of territoriality and "further indication of our bond with them, i.e., dogs behave as if we were conspecifics to be threatened."[328] It actually demonstrates neither. Even the increased tendency of owned dogs to bark at strangers when near home[329] is not evidence of territorial defense.

Home ranges of unowned free-ranging dogs vary in size depending on availability of food, water, and shelter, but most in urban areas are <10 ha.[330] The more abundant the resources the smaller the home range needs to be. Resources in rural areas, food in particular, are usually scattered and home ranges are larger. Some reported home ranges of rural free-ranging groups of dogs are 72 km^2,[331] 2850 ha,[332] 1872 ha,[333] 444–1050 ha,[334] 0.2–11.1 ha (summer),[335] and 10–25 ha.[336] This last centered around a garbage dump, which represented a concentrated source of food. The size of an urban dog's home range often depends directly on the resident human population: its social status, density, willingness to make food available, and attitudes toward ownerless dogs.[337] Home range size increases for adults of both sexes during breeding and pup rearing.[338]

Malchik, a black stray living in Moscow's Mendeleyevskaya subway station, became a hero after being stabbed to death by a 22-year-old fashion model. A bronze likeness of him was erected at the station's entrance, paid for by his many admirers (Fig. 5.7).[339] Malchik's killer was sentenced to a year of psychiatric treatment. Urban dogs elsewhere travel by foot through their home ranges, but about 20 of the 500 or so inhabiting Moscow's underground stations simply take the subway. They wait patiently on the platform along with the human commuters. When a train stops and the doors open they enter the car, hop onto a seat, and disembark a few stops later.

How urban free-ranging dogs use their home areas to gain resources is illustrated in the following narrative based on Alan M. Beck's fascinating description of the morning routine of Shag and Dobe, two homeless dogs living in Baltimore 40 years ago.[340] Shag was a mongrel but carried a strong component of Old English sheep dog. Dobe was a Doberman. Both were adult males sharing a home range.

The sky is still dark at 4:30 a.m. on 2 September 1970. Beck sits in his parked car outside the Amalgamated Clothing Workers of America (ACWA) building as sunrise creeps closer. At 6:00 he looks in his rearview mirror and sees Shag and Dobe approaching. Beck gets out and follows them at a distance. Neither dog seems concerned about his presence.

Shag and Dobe turn into an alley where they join several other dogs peacefully rummaging through garbage cans, now and then lifting a bag off the top for closer examination. Some of the cans have already been tipped over and the bags ripped apart. Dogs, feral cats, and rats are foraging together in good fellowship, sometimes within a few centimeters of one another, the knee-deep smorgasbord having put aside any evil thoughts of predation. The scene could be easily misinterpreted: mutualism and sharing are barely linked, the first resulting in the second only incidentally during synchronized foraging.[341]

At 6:20 Shag and Dobe move to the alley beside the ACWA building and drink from a puddle underneath the air-conditioner. They lie down to rest on a patch of grass. Dobe gets up and leaves at 6:34 while Shag naps another 5 minutes. Then he stands, stretches, and goes off in Dobe's direction, trotting through several alleys until finding his partner scavenging at an overflowing Dumpster behind an apartment house. They move on together.

At 7:00 and back on Madison Avenue, Shag's friendly greeting of an anus sniff is rebuffed by two small pet dogs just let outside by their owner. Undeterred, he and Dobe continue down Madison and 10 minutes later find a garbage can tipped onto its side. Shag expertly opens a take-out container and scarfs the remains of a spaghetti dinner with bread, then laps up the spilled sauce.

The dogs leave after 3 minutes of scavenging, proceed through more alleys and a playground, and stop at a grassy median to rest. Neither sleeps. Instead they stare at a building across the street where at 7:52 a second-floor window opens and someone whistles. They run over, and a woman drops hot dogs and chopped meat to them. In a survey of the neighborhood, 20% of respondents admitted to feeding strays.

By 8:43 Shag and Dobe are back at home base, the ACWA building. They take another drink of water, crawl into some bushes where the air is cooler, and are asleep by 10:20. In 4.3 hours they have spent 124 minutes resting, 137 minutes on the move, 29 minutes foraging, and only 2 minutes in social contact with other dogs, less time than usual. In evening the pattern is repeated. Their home range, encompassing only 0.26 km^2, contains every comfort and necessity. The dogs were later adopted by different neighborhood owners. Although Shag continued to be released daily onto the streets, he preferred staying near home to roaming. Now warm, secure, and well fed, his home range shrank to 0.52 ha (0.05 km^2).[342]

All things considered, the term home range seems more accurate than territory for the familiar space occupied by free-ranging dogs, and *group*, rather than pack, better defines free-ranging dogs traveling together.[343] To make the case requires revisiting how pack is defined: a stable social unit with bonds of attachment, usually composed of related members, that travels, hunts, rears young, and defends a common territory together. The absence of clear evidence of territoriality is enough by itself to disqualify free-ranging dogs as pack forming. In addition, free-ranging dogs, unlike wolves, do not rear their offspring as a group with both parents and occasionally others participating (Chapter 8), nor are the individuals seen wandering streets and rural areas together likely to be related.

Evidence to refute these statements would most likely come from observing dingoes and dingo-dogs, many of which are truly wild animals with other life-history patterns mirroring those of wolves. In common with lone wolves[344] and coyotes[345] – and unlike most other free-ranging dogs – solitary dingoes wander widely.[346] A male in eastern Victoria traversed 230 km in 9 days and then returned to its natal home range. Another moved 105 km in 87 days, also returning.[347] When on the move a dingo might travel rapidly, examples being 19.2 km in 7.5 hours and 17.2 km in 6.1 hours[348] making use of roads, logging tracks, and fire trails in forested areas.[349] Also like wolves, dingoes often make temporary forays from natal sites before dispersing permanently. Unlike wolves, final dispersal is usually nearby. At one location dispersal distance averaged 20 km, being slightly farther for males than females.[350] More than 75% of 200 dingoes marked or radio-collared in central Australia were later seen, located, or recaptured within 8 km of the original capture site, and 95% were within 20 km.[351] Dispersal is more common at population saturation and low food availability. Lone wolves are sometimes accepted into existing packs. Lone dingoes, in contrast, rarely if ever immigrate into other groups and go out of their way to avoid other dingoes.[352]

The risk to dispersing dingoes is high, as it is for wolves. Most deaths are also human-induced, mostly from automobiles and control activities (trapping and poisoned baits), but at least two mortalities were trespassers killed by resident dingoes, which suggests territorial behavior.[353]

Dingoes and dingo-dogs have been collared and their movements mapped. Philopatry is evident, but territoriality is not. Spaces occupied by the Fortescue River resident dingoes were 44.5–113.2 km^2; as with wolves, there was no correlation with group size.[354] Home ranges were about 2700 ha in northeastern New South Wales,[355] 124 (males) and 45 km^2 (females) in eastern Victoria.[356] As with other canids they expand and contract depending on food supply. Those at Mt. Dare, South Australia, expanded at the end of a drought when resident dingoes were forced to live almost exclusively on grasshoppers.[357]

I mentioned at the start of this chapter that territory and home range are terms used loosely and often interchangeably, and nowhere is this more apparent than in the dingo literature.[358] The Fortescue River investigation redefined the concept of territory without mentioning defense of space,[359] making it no different than home range. Three features characterize areas occupied by dingoes and dingo-dogs, all conforming with how home range is traditionally defined: (1) relative stability over time, (2) area varying inversely with the abundance of resources, and (3) group size unrelated to dimensions of the bounded space.[360] The same characteristics apply to territories with one crucial difference: a territory is defended. Shag and Dobe would have qualified as a "pack" of two except the Baltimore streets and alleys through which they traveled were never proprietary but shared amiably with other free-ranging dogs. Ignoring such an important distinction led the Fortescue River investigation to trip over this fallacy of presumption: "Dingo packs displayed strong site attachment, and their territorial boundaries were quite stable from year to year ... This further corroborates the suggestion that the packs were territorial and validates the concept of long-term or composite territories."[361]

These conclusions validate nothing when territories are conceptually indistinguishable from home ranges. If dingoes are territorial they ought to actively repel intruders. Lone wolves entering occupied spaces are usually chased and often killed. Because fights are not unusual when wolf packs meet at territorial boundaries, interpack strife has been identified as a major cause of adult mortality at several locations: Denali,[362] Isle Royale,[363] different sites in Minnesota,[364] and Yellowstone.[365] Trespassing dingoes, in contrast, are greeted with friendliness when not ignored or avoided, and attacked only rarely.[366]

The dingoes of Australia and New Guinea are free-ranging dogs despite not having been socialized to humans for thousands of years, and like domestic dogs their direct ancestor is the gray wolf. As the wildest of free-ranging dogs, do they form true packs? The reasoning seems to be that because certain individuals are related, occasionally forage together, and occupy a defined space, this makes an association of dingoes a pack and not simply a group with a fluid membership. Existence of a social hierarchy in the Fortescue River dingoes was sought but never verified.[367] One investigator described their social system as resembling that of wolves, and of coyotes to a lesser extent.[368] The reverse seems truer in the case of coyotes, especially if efficiency of hunting large prey increases with group size (Chapter 6).[369]

Dingoes gather on occasion where game is clumped (e.g. water holes during droughts) but mostly forage alone or in twos.[370] Aboriginal myths mention only individuals or pairs, rarely larger groups.[371] N. W. G. Macintosh, who for many years studied dingoes over much of Australia, wrote, "I have never yet seen a dingo pack hunting and I do not believe it ever occurs; indeed, it is rare to see more than 2 dingoes in company in the daytime."[372] Some would consider such statements to reveal fleeting snapshots of dingo societies. According to the long-term Fortescue River project, dingoes ostensibly lived in packs and occupied territories, but were inclined to split into small groups while foraging. Wolves sometimes do this too. Thus sightings of only loners or two or three individuals together is insufficient to refute the pack concept.[373]

Social structure seems unaffected by habitat. Dingo-dogs monitored in eastern Victoria behaved similarly to those in arid regions. They occupied overlapping home ranges (Fig. 5.8), were related, and did not appear to defend territories.[374]

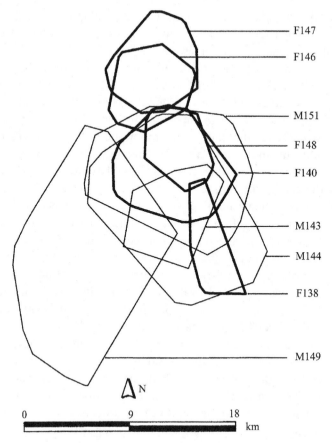

F147

F146

M151

F148

F140

M143

M144

F138

M149

N

0   9   18
                                              km

Figure 5.8 Overlapping home ranges of nine dingo-dogs on the Nunniong Plain, eastern Victoria, Australia.
Source: Reproduced with permission from the *Australian Mammalogy* 32: 23–32 (Robley, A. *et al.*). Copyright Australian Mammal Society 2010. Published by CSIRO Publishing, Collingwood, Victoria, Australia. http://www.publish.csiro.au/nid/256/ paper/AM09030.htm.

In a comparative study of dingoes in wet, mountainous southeastern Australia and the hot, arid central region most dingoes were alone when seen. Of >1000 animals observed, 73% were solitary, 16.2% in twos, 5.1% in threes, and 2.8% in groups of four.[375] Compare this with observations of Alaskan wolves. During sightings of >5000 wolves, 91% were accompanied by at least one other individual.[376] It might be true that dingoes, like other free-ranging dogs, are both solitary and social. Many animals observed alone might be part of a loose group, the members of which are social intermittently. "Thus, it looks as though dingoes, while apparently operating mostly independently, belong to loose but amicably social associations of many animals."[377]

Dispersal rates often seem high compared with wolves, and this has been attributed in part to weaker group cohesiveness.[378] Although most dispersing

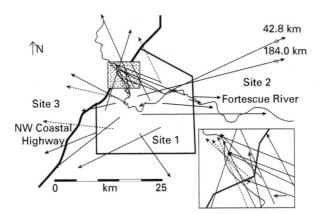

Figure 5.9 Dispersal of individual dingoes (solid arrows) and groups (dashed arrows) all represented as minimum straight-line distances. The NW Coastal Highway is the eastern boundary of Site 3; the gray line denotes the boundaries of Site 1. Inset map is a 300% enlargement of the stippled area.
Source: Reproduced with permission from *Wildlife Research* 19: 585–595 (Thomson, P. C. *et al*.). Copyright 1992 CSIRO Publishing, Collingwood, Victoria, Australia. http://www.publish.csiro.au/nid/144/paper|WR9920585.htm.

dingoes are loners, sometimes a whole group emigrates (Fig. 5.9). Specific individuals travel and associate together, giving the appearance of a pack. As with wolves, some members make forays and eventually disperse, and groups temporarily increase in size with the inclusion of maturing pups. A wolf pack's cohesion is often regulated seasonally, being least cohesive in summer when pups are immobile and members of the pack fan out to forage alone or in small groups. Perhaps dingoes operate like this all year and there is no comparable time, as wolves have, when cohesion tightens, the group becomes nomadic, and prey is almost exclusively large. As I show later (Chapter 6), although dingoes are capable of killing large animals, their diets resemble those of coyotes more than wolves.

Dingoes go out of their way to avoid strangers at watering sites,[379] behavior in keeping with other free-ranging dogs at garbage dumps. How much philopatry affects these trips to obtain needed resources has not been studied. Long-term monitoring at one location showed dingoes to rarely leave the home range,[380] presuming resources are adequate or at least not better somewhere nearby. Yet dingoes gathering at watering sites obviously leave their home ranges unoccupied. Seasonal concentrations of prey might break down home range barriers temporarily, perhaps similar to the situation of tundra wolves mentioned previously that follow caribou herds part of the year.

At Nadgee, southeastern Australia, the average home range was 10 km².[381] Home ranges were not mapped, but doubtfully all had equal access to the beaches and a coastal lake. Dingoes preyed on black swans (*Cygnus atratus*) and Eurasian coots (*Fulica atra*) along the lake shore and patrolled the beaches singly or in twos for seabird carcasses. Birds made up 36.2% of the diet from April to June, but

11.9% during July to September. There can be little doubt that home ranges were abandoned. A year when swans and coots were particularly numerous at the lake coincided with a sharp increase in numbers of dingo tracks. Dingoes congregated around the lake, and one pair even produced a litter. In sum, evidence collected to date favors free-ranging dogs occupying home ranges but not territories.

6   Foraging

By now it should be clear that a pack or group of social canids is a collective stomach in search of food. Wolves and free-ranging dogs feed by hunting and scavenging. As defined here, *hunting* is the act of finding, pursuing, catching, and killing prey, *scavenging* the act of feeding on carcasses or separating edible components from human refuse and other mostly inedible materials. Both terms are covered by *foraging*.

Foraging has the obvious benefit of supplying nutrients from which animals gain energy required for growth, reproduction, respiration, generation of body heat, and all other physiological processes driven and controlled by what we call "life." However, it also has a cost, measured as the energy used to secure food. African wild dogs often chase prey for several kilometers at sustained speeds of 48 kilometers per hour,[1] a tremendous energy expenditure culminating in a burst of strength and effort needed to bring a large ungulate to the ground. Tundra wolves commonly leave the den or rendezvous site (Chapter 8), travel 25–30 km, make a kill, and return with large portions of meat to feed pups and the breeding female all in a matter of hours.[2] Not every hunting trip is successful. If more fail than succeed – that is, if cost exceeds benefit over time – the eventual end is starvation and death. Although wolves can be opportunistic foragers[3] they are primarily hunters of large herbivores. Energetic constraints force them to be. A body mass of 21.5 kg is the point at which carnivorans generally shift from small to large prey,[4] and wolves cross that line. The transition is abrupt: carnivorans smaller than 21.5 kg feed mainly on prey <45% of their own mass, those larger than this select animals >45% of their own mass.

6.1   Wolves as predators

The overall objective of foraging is to elevate energetic benefit above cost and keep it there. The immediate cost is maintaining constant body temperature, which becomes increasingly difficult with declining air temperature. Canids living in cold climates need more food than those inhabiting hot deserts. Their *basal metabolic rates* (*BMRs*) are comparatively higher when adjusted for body mass. They need to hunt regularly and consume lots of food to sustain constant internal temperature (for example, Great Lakes wolves preying on moose in winter averaged a kill every 4.7–5 days).[5] Ambient air temperature and availability of water

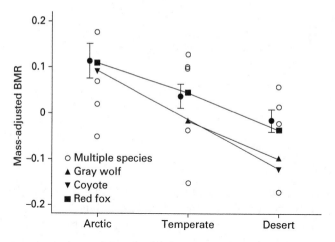

Figure 6.1 Mass-adjusted basal metabolic rate (BMR) among canids adjusted with different climates. Means (±SE) are weighted to account for multiple observations on a single species. See original report for details.
Source: Careau, V., J. Morand-Ferron, and D. Thomas. (2007). Basal metabolic rate of Canidae from hot deserts to cold arctic climates. *Journal of Mammalogy* **88**: 394–400. Copyright 2007 by American Society of Mammalogists, published by Allen Press, Inc.

greatly affect BMR. High air temperature and scarce water favors a low BMR to prevent overheating and conserve water in the tissues. Frigid ambient air requires high BMRs to sustain internal body temperature and prevent hypothermia. Animals living in temperate climatic zones should have BMRs somewhere in between (Fig. 6.1).[6]

One way to keep a favorable cost–benefit balance is by killing large prey animals, which offer bigger packages of potential energy than small animals, and the best way of attaining positive results consistently is by hunting large prey in groups. For individuals scattered across the landscape, gathering each day for a group hunt would be inefficient; a better way is for the hunters to live together. These notions pervade our beliefs about wolves and can be distilled into two simple statements: (1) a big pack is able to kill large game more efficiently than a little pack or individuals hunting alone,[7] and (2) big packs therefore consume more meat per capita than small packs or lone wolves.[8] Both presumptions reinforce the idea that group hunting favors communal living,[9] but neither is true.

In wolf societies a few do most of the work and support the lesser contributors.[10] Packs typically include early adolescents, which by winter are as big as adults[11] and eat as much but can be indifferent or mediocre hunters.[12] Adolescent wolves often have poor success pursuing and killing ungulates in the absence of experienced adults, and in summer they sometimes subsist by scavenging old kills or subduing small prey.[13] However, groups of adolescents (e.g. siblings dispersing together, Chapter 5) that prove inept hunters individually gain efficiency as a group.[14] Adolescents hunting alone in summer have been known to kill adult caribou,[15] but this is after a winter of traveling with the pack.

Loners were once thought to be disadvantaged outcasts forced to scavenge or exist on small game at the peripheries of territories, scratching out a bare existence.[16] Sometimes they are,[17] but healthy wolves are powerful, fearless hunters fully capable of capturing and killing ungulates, and they often hunt best alone or in packs of two or three. Lone wolves and wolves in twos killed more deer in SNF than a pack of five.[18] There the average wolf in winter consumed 345 kg of white-tailed deer meat, or 2.9 kg per wolf per day.[19] Average minimum daily consumption for pack members was 1.63 kg, or near the estimated minimum of 1.7 kg necessary to keep a wild wolf alive.[20] Wolves hunting in pairs each ate about 4.45 kg per day, or 2.6 times the estimated minimum requirement. Isle Royale wolves eat more moose meat than anything else. An adult moose is not only difficult to bring down but dangerous when attacked (see below). Nonetheless, per capita food intake declined with increasing pack size, although variance was larger in the small groups.[21] Each wolf in packs of 6–12 received just 60–70% of that acquired by loners or pairs.[22] In general, consumption rate increases with ungulate density.[23] Where moose are not preyed on their estimated equilibrium density in North America is 2 per km², dropping to about 1.3 per km² with presence of a single species of predator (the wolf).[24] A density of 0.2 moose per km² might be the threshold below which wolves are unable to survive.[25]

Canids are remarkably resistant to starvation. An adult male Scotch collie starved purposely for 117 days lost 63% of its body mass (a decline from 26.3 kg to 9.8 kg when the experiment ended) and recovered in complete health after feeding resumed.[26] Wolves can survive at least 3 weeks without food and quickly regain lost body mass.[27] When food is available they often eat more than seems possible. In fact, the amount of food wolves can consume is staggering. Thirty-four captive wolves, after having been briefly starved, consumed all edible parts of a 670-kg horse within 2 days.[28] Small packs of 2 or 3 in the Finlayson Lake region, Yukon, killed an average of 27 moose every winter, medium-sized packs of 4–9 killed 35, and packs of 10 or more killed 46, in total 10–15% of the population.[29] Wolves in southcentral Alaska existed on a diet of 70% moose by mass, consuming 7.1 kg per wolf per day in winter.[30] Over 3 years in winter (total of 110 days) a 15-member pack on Isle Royale consumed an estimated 9000 kg of moose, or a daily average of 82 kg, equal to 5.5 kg per wolf per day.[31] On the basis of these numbers, an adult white-tailed deer of 67 kg could feed 12 wolves, allowing each animal 5.5 kg assuming everything was eaten including the antlers. This is barely a snack. Nonetheless, both wolf density and pack size correlate directly with density of the prey.[32] Size of the prey is not a factor: a moose can weigh six times more than a white-tailed deer yet pack sizes are basically the same in regions where one or the other is preyed on exclusively.[33]

Do wolves "wolf" their food? A pack of four in the Canadian Rockies ate most of an adult female mule deer (*Odocoileus hemionus*) in 4 hours, and a pack of three killed and ate two mule deer and an elk calf in 5 days.[34] Several times the Isle Royale pack of 15 ate a calf moose within 24 hours, the equivalent of about 9 kg per wolf.[35] In another instance, the pack killed and ate a cow moose that weighed about 270 kg and consumed half the carcass in 1.5 hours, equal to about 9 kg apiece. In earlier years a pack of seven or eight had been seen to eat three-quarters of an adult moose in 2 days, or 16 kg per wolf per day.[36] A wolf of 32 kg, in other words, would have consumed an amount of moose meat equal to its body mass over 48 hours.

Feeding on a new kill is selective initially. The first parts of a caribou eaten are the viscera (exclusive of stomach contents), soft parts of the neck, and the ribs.[37] Nearly everything else, including heavy muscle tissue, hooves, long bones, skin, and skull are often consumed too until all that remains is some hair and stomach contents. The moose-eating wolves of Isle Royale seem to prefer the nose, heart, throat, shoulder, upper hind leg and pelvic region, and abdominal areas.[38] They too leave little, often returning to a carcass until nothing is left except the long bones, skull, parts of the spinal column, mandible, teeth, and some hair.

Carcasses are revisited[39] or not abandoned: a pack of five in southwestern Québec stayed near a moose carcass for 7 days.[40] Time on a large moose is 1.3–3.1 days,[41] and still the wolves often return to clean up any scraps. This pattern is true for other large ungulate kills such as bison: 2.5 days on the initial kill before moving on, then revisiting once or twice for 2.3 days each time.[42] Small packs sometimes stay on large kills longer than large packs,[43] but this is not a trend.[44] A pack might stay several days near a kill, feeding intermittently on the carcass until nothing useful remains and their collective hunger prompts them to move along and kill again.[45]

Wolves have superior endurance, able to trot at 8 km per hour continuously for 190 km[46] and travel many kilometers without pause, even in deep snow.[47] Those on Isle Royale might travel 100 km between kills. During one month the largest Isle Royale pack traversed 446 km of winter terrain averaging 50 km per day of actual traveling and usually moving at a trot.[48] Wolves in the Nelchina Basin made daily treks of 10–72 km and averaged 39 km.[49] A pack of 10 occupied a territory of 13 000 km^2 through which it moved continuously, averaging 25 km per day, and once 142 km over 4 days during March and April,[50] killing about every 1.7 days. Tundra wolves in Finland crossing on hard-crusted snow were reported to travel 200 km in a day.[51]

Wolves are not always on the move. Gray wolves at *Gates of the Arctic National Park and Preserve* (hereafter *Gates of the Arctic*) observed in November and March budgeted time as follows: resting or sleeping (48.8%), walking (32.1%), feeding (9.8%), behaving socially (6.8%), and running (2.5%).[52] Packs in BISF in winter spent their time traveling (28%), sleeping (34%), resting (31%), and feeding (6%).[53] Wolves on Isle Royale were resting or sleeping almost half the time.[54]

Kill rate represents the number of kills by a wolf pack divided by number of wolves in the pack divided by some unit of time (e.g. days of observation).[55] Both kill rate and wolf density correlate strongly with density of the prey.[56] The *functional response* describes how kill rate varies with prey abundance; the *numerical response* summarizes changes in predator abundance with prey density.[57] These factors potentially regulate (as opposed to simply limiting) prey numbers.[58]

The functional response is important because it embodies two key features: prey death rate (i.e. kill rate) and rate at which the number of predators increases.[59]

A strictly prey-dependent functional response (the traditional model) depends only on prey abundance and assumes predators encounter prey randomly[60] instead of having to search for food, then afterward share or compete for it.[61] This is doubtfully realistic except in some carnivoran Eden. A more practical situation assumes the functional response to depend on the ratio of prey/predator abundance.[62] Models of this type evaluate mechanisms controlling prey–predator systems using a bottom-up approach; prey-dependent models examine these same mechanisms from the top down.[63] Ratio-dependent models predict the proportional increase of both prey and predator; prey-dependent models predict just the benefits derived by the predator from an increase in prey abundance.[64] Stated differently, the rate at which the predator population grows depends on the prey/predator ratio, and so should the functional response.[65] Taken in sum, it seems sensible to compute kill rate for each pack separately.[66] The only data set large and tight enough to test thoroughly comes from Isle Royale where careful records of moose–wolf interactions have been kept since 1959. There, satiation by wolves is a prominent feature of the functional response, becoming asymptotic as kill rate approaches maximum.[67]

Pack size has a strong negative effect on kill rate.[68] That of wolves on moose and caribou in the Yukon correlated inversely with size of the pack,[69] and the same was true in Alaska.[70] Yukon wolves in small packs of 2 or 3 killed moose at nearly twice the rate of medium-sized packs (4–9), which in turn had a kill rate 40% greater than large packs (10–20).[71] In fact, pack size was the only factor affecting the kill rate.[72] Large packs, on average, killed moose more often than did small packs, although the small packs often matched them. Packs were small when the population was first expanding, and the efficiency at which they killed was unexpectedly high. Kill rate in this population was unrelated to territory size (Chapter 5), the distance traveled daily (presumably in search of prey), moose/wolf ratio, number of packs in the vicinity, snow depth, or moose density. In times of deep snow, moose are more vulnerable to predation.[73] The critical snow depth (>90 cm) was seldom reached while observations were in progress.[74] These and other data show that optimal pack size for hunting large ungulates is two wolves,[75] not several.[76] Sometimes large packs usurp the kills of smaller ones,[77] in which case numbers matter.

Distance traveled is evidently unrelated to numbers of moose or the moose/wolf ratio, indicating that "competition for prey resources did not influence prey search rates of wolves."[78] These findings are generally true of other locations, including Gates of the Arctic. Its wolves prey mostly on caribou, the abundance of which did not affect the kill rate.[79] Nonetheless, prey must still be found, and travel distance affects kill rate. In summer, the movements of wolves in the central Canadian Arctic are restricted by immobile pups, forcing them to search large areas of tundra for caribou.[80]

Search distance depends on many factors including terrain, season, weather conditions, distribution of the prey according to its social organization (e.g. scattered, clumped), and so forth.[81] Large packs are known to split temporarily when hunting, and this probably raises the daily per capita food intake of members.[82] A pack in the Nelchina Basin split on occasion, regrouping later. Pack splitting also occurs among wolves at Gates of the Arctic[83] and in northwestern Alaska.[84] Wolves in Algonquin Provincial Park sometimes separated into smaller groups in winter to hunt white-tailed deer.[85] If ungulates are abundant even large packs might stay intact. A pack numbering up to 20 in the Nelchina Basin was never seen trespassing into spaces occupied by neighboring wolves and rarely split even temporarily, presumably because moose were numerous inside its own territory.[86]

The age and physical condition of an ungulate affects its susceptibility to predation.[87] When ungulates are plentiful wolves tend to select young of the year and old adults, which are weaker, more vulnerable, and less dangerous than prime-age adults.[88] In Mech's Isle Royale survey calves were only 15% of the winter moose population but accounted for 36% of winter kills; otherwise, no moose killed was young and healthy.[89] Most were 8–15 years old, and 39% showed signs of debilitating maladies such as jaw necrosis, bone deformities, and heavy loads of tapeworm cysts in the lungs.[90] Although few moose and caribou killed by Yukon wolves had evidence of starvation, adults of prime age were in the minority.[91] The high predation on calf moose (31% the of moose killed) was nonetheless unrelated to the number available, probably because yearling moose were also common. The summer diet of wolves in northwestern Alaska was 51% caribou and 42% moose.[92] The caribou were mostly in good condition; the condition of the moose was marginal. Wolves on the Kenai Peninsula also preferred calf moose.[93] Half killed in winter were malnourished, and 35% of adults killed throughout the year had been debilitated by age, arthritis, malnutrition, or severe periodontitis.[94] Wolves in the Nelchina Basin killed calf moose preferentially to adults by a ratio of six,[95] and calves were also hunted selectively in the Yukon.[96] Wolves in the Canadian Rockies, however, preyed equally on adult and calf elk.[97]

Prey diversity among predatory carnivorans such as canids increases with body size.[98] From late summer into autumn Denali wolves of all ages spend considerable time individually hunting mice.[99] Small prey organisms having scattered distributions are exploited more efficiently by lone hunters.[100] As Murie pointed out, a large number of mice would be required to satisfy a 45-kg wolf. After feeding his pet wolf Wags on dried salmon and table scraps, Murie tossed her 19 mice and 2 shrews, which she swallowed whole and without any sign of satiation.[101] A small prey animal offers a much reduced package of nutrients, and wolves often lose weight over the summer. A healthy adult male live-trapped during both summer and winter on the Kenai Peninsula was 37.2 kg in summer and 49.9 kg in winter.[102]

A pack of four in Oneida County, Wisconsin, preyed almost exclusively on white-tailed deer throughout the year. Deer composed at least 93% of the annual diet (presumably by mass), the balance consisting of rabbits, hares, and rodents;[103] the prey in northcentral Minnesota was as much as 98% white-tailed deer by mass.[104] The annual diet of wolves in the Canadian Rockies was 80% ungulates and 18% rodents (including beavers). There, packs split or become more loosely knit beginning in late spring as the snow melts and opens up the range. The result is a seasonal shift in the composition of prey. Wolves often hunt alone or in twos, and the summer diet contains 69% ungulates and 32% rodents (including beavers) compared with winter (85% ungulates, 14% rodents).[105] In Denali wolves the annual diet was 69% ungulates, 27% rodents.[106] Denali wolves also hunted alone, in twos, or in groups, depending on season and prey availability.[107] They hunted ungulates preferentially, but ate more Alaskan marmots (*Marmota broweri*), other ground squirrels, and mice in summer after the caribou left. Marmots can be 8 kg.[108]

The evolutionary place of wolves and dogs is with the carnivorans, but unlike cats they are not obligate eaters of meat. The summer diet of wolves in SNF consisted of small animals (e.g. grouse, mice and voles, marmots, snakes, insects) and vegetation, and in winter shifted to white-tailed deer and snowshoe hares (*Lepus americanus*) almost exclusively.[109] Summer scats of Great Lakes wolves in BISF contained remnants of several species of rodents ranging in size from mice to woodchucks (*Marmota monax*), striped skunks (*Mephitis mephitis*), various birds and bird eggs, insects, even bits of black bears and wolves, although white-tailed deer and moose (and beavers to a lesser extent) were the principal prey.[110]

Lone wolves kill adult moose and elk,[111] and even adult bison.[112] A bull musk ox is about 272 kg.[113] A lone male wolf was seen to kill one over the course of little more than an hour.[114] An adult wolf hunting alone can kill a mature white-tailed deer.[115] Caribou bulls are about 165 kg, cows 95 kg, September calves 54 kg.[116] Lone wolves have no trouble chasing down and killing a running adult by attacking it on the shoulder, flank, or neck.[117] This observation contrasts with those made on Alaska's Brooks Range when the landscape was free of snow. Both adults and calves easily outran pursuing wolves, and most pursuits were unsuccessful even when caribou were taken by surprise.[118] In Denali, 2-week-old calves kept up with cows when chased by wolves.[119] Wolves in Russia attacked red deer (*Cervus elaphus*) at distances of 10–200 m and gave up when the prey was not captured quickly.[120] Many of the kills involved straggling animals that were sick or injured, one of which was chased and killed by a lone sled dog despite its being smaller and slower than a wolf.

An old report cited anecdotal evidence of wolves preying on Indian and Eskimo dogs in the Northwest Territories.[121] Wolves on the outskirts of Fairbanks, Alaska, killed and occasionally ate owned dogs (whether free-ranging or chained outside was not stated).[122] Wolves in Minnesota and Wisconsin have been known to kill owned dogs[123] and cats,[124] deliberately seeking them out as prey and eating them.[125] Most confirmed attacks occurred in the owners' yards. A wolf attacked a dog near its doorstep and did not retreat until beaten with a shovel. When dogs were chained outside wolves killed and carried them off, severing their collars in the process. Portuguese[126] and Italian[127] wolves occasionally kill dogs or prey on them,[128] including hunting dogs.[129] Wolves elsewhere on the Iberian peninsula capture and eat domestic dogs and cats.[130] In Latvia, dogs make up 22% of domestic animals attacked by wolves.[131] Free-ranging dogs in Spain are much less common in areas occupied by wolves.[132] Dogs are the most frequent domestic prey of wolves in Poland's Carpathian Mountains, and predation on pets and livestock occurs most often where dens and rendezvous sites (Chapter 8) are near pastures and residences.[133] Wolves following sleds or sled tracks was once common at some locations. A lone wolf on Ellesmere Island reportedly followed a sled track for more than 300 km.[134] Whether it considered the dogs potential food is unknown. Wolves on Ellesmere Island in the early 1950s were attracted to dogs at a summer field station and on one occasion attacked them.[135] In the Voronezh and Belgorod regions of western Russia in the 1970s domestic dogs were the favored prey of presumed wolfdogs,[136] and Russian wolves have been known to prey regularly on dogs.[137] Iranian wolves preyed mostly on livestock (sheep and goats) and reportedly killed and ate dogs that chased them too far from the shepherds and other dogs.[138] Wolves in Finland killed both domestic cats and dogs, devouring them completely.[139]

Wolf predation on dogs appears to have been common at one time in the American West and in the North American Arctic and subarctic.[140] A Montana wolf killed 15 dogs over 2 years, and a North Dakota wolf named Badlands Billy "killed 15 dogs in a single encounter while they were pursuing him along a narrow mountain trail."[141] In contrast, a group of free-ranging dogs in interior Alaska occasionally interacted with red foxes, coyotes, and wolves,[142] and some wolves famous for killing livestock were seen playing with dogs and courting them.[143] Alaskan wolves scavenged the carcasses of red foxes and other wolves, although they rarely preyed on foxes.[144] Wolves that have been socialized to humans are seldom aggressive toward dogs (Chapter 9).

Packs ordinarily kill one ungulate during a hunt, but if prey is plentiful they might kill more than one.[145] The killing of wild ungulates in excess of their immediate needs is unusual for wolves, but when these *surplus killing* events occur they are carried out with swift efficiency. Wolves in Canada's Northwest Territories killed 34 calf caribou within a few minutes and fed on just half the carcasses;[146] wolves in the Keewatin district of central Canada killed caribou in excess of their needs and ate only the tongues and unborn calves.[147] Two wolves in Sweden killed at least 40 reindeer in 2 weeks, 8 in one night,[148] and a pack of 2–4 wolves in the Nelchina Basin killed 7 adult caribou.[149] Multiple kills of both caribou and moose were reported from northwestern Alaska,[150] of caribou at Gates of the Arctic,[151] and of domestic sheep in the Caucasus.[152] Some observations of mayhem include an element of the fantastic: "Dmitriev-Mamonov reports that he has seen a wolf jump over a high fence with a medium-sized ram between its jaws and then cover over a mile."[153] Surplus killing seems more likely when the distribution of prey animals is clumped or otherwise rendered vulnerable (e.g. many newborn calves, deep snow, stormy weather).

The same conditions make livestock more susceptible to wolf predation. Wolves prefer wild ungulates over domestic livestock, and increased livestock predation often signals a decline in natural prey abundance.[154] At certain places and times the effect has been devastating. Wolves in Russia were not hunted for several years after World War I when the economy was in shambles. Wolf populations rose quickly, and in 1924 and 1925 about a million cattle were supposedly killed.[155] Numerous US reports, especially in the late nineteenth and early twentieth centuries, described the uncontrolled slaughter of cattle and sheep, but many accounts were exaggerations presented to lawmakers as a rationale for wolf eradication.[156] Ernest Thompson Seton, for example, claimed that two wolves in New Mexico killed 250 sheep in one night and did not take a bite from any of them.[157] This certainly fits the definition of surplus killing, but Seton's account, like many others, was unconfirmed. Some wolves became famous cattle and sheep marauders. They were given nicknames and achieved fleeting fame as outlaws until trapped, poisoned, or shot by government officials or bounty hunters. Lots of them were old or maimed by traps[158] and might have experienced difficulty capturing wild ungulates. Livestock, and sheep in particular, are comparatively easy to kill, and in 1997 a lone wolf in Montana did kill 28 sheep during a summer night.[159] Another Montana wolf introduced from Canada killed 41 sheep in a single week. It was trapped and moved to a different region but returned and killed another 15 sheep, not feeding on any of them. The occasional slaughter of 200–300 sheep has been reported in Italy.[160] Surplus killing seems to have no function other than discharging the hunting urge.

The principal reason wolves move from place to place is to find food on a more or less regular basis. Wolves tend to hunt nearer the centers of their territories, avoiding potential conflict with neighboring packs at the peripheries.[161] Daily movements vary with prey availability, season, and nature of the landscape. In summer, breeding female wolves in BISF hunted more often in daylight than at night, when they stayed with their pups, although they still managed to visit most of their territories.[162] Dominant males were less likely to be found near core areas, and most subordinates traveled with them a third of the time. Subordinates often began a series of solitary movements as summer progressed, visiting peripheries of the territory and spending little time at rendezvous sites. Packs that had not produced pups showed no seasonal differences in use of territories. If tundra wolves lose their litters or fail to produce them "the pack resumes its usual nomadic movement pattern within its territory."[163]

Air temperature can affect activity. Wolves in Poland were less active when the temperature exceeded 20°C.[164] Summer movements of wolves collared and tracked by radio telemetry in southern Ontario varied by individual and were independent of weather conditions. At dusk the pack scattered to hunt individually. A female spent most daylight hours with her pups at one of three rendezvous sites, often with other pack members.[165] A young female, in contrast, was active throughout the day, once traveling 2 km in 2 hours. These wolves preyed extensively on beavers during summer and autumn, which were abundant, making more extensive ranging unnecessary.

The diel movements of wolves are therefore driven by foraging opportunities. Some individuals are more nocturnal than others,[166] but all can be active in daylight as well.[167] The wolves of Vancouver Island were more active at night,[168] and movements of southern Ontario wolves in summer were mostly nocturnal.[169] Wolves in the high Arctic hunted day and night in summer,[170] although even at midnight the illumination is bright enough to see prey. In summer the wolves

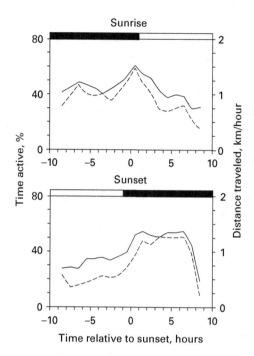

Figure 6.2 Patterns of mean active time and distance traveled by 11 wolves relative to sunrise and sunset in the Białowieża Primeval Forest, Poland, 1994–1999. Black bars indicate night with overlap into dawn, clear bars depict day with overlap into dusk.
Source: Theuerkauf, J., W. Jędrzejewski, K. Schmidt, H. Okarma, I. Ruczyński, and S. Śnieżko *et al.* (2003). Daily patterns and duration of wolf activity in the Białowieża Forest, Poland. *Journal of Mammalogy* **84**: 243–253. Copyright 2003 by American Society of Mammalogists, published by Allen Press, Inc.

monitored by Murie in Denali began hunting at dusk (occasionally late afternoon) and rested during the day.[171] Those in the Białowieża Primeval Forest, Poland, were active both day and night with peak activity at dawn and dusk (Fig. 6.2), a pattern based mainly on behavior of the prey.[172] Foraging by Minnesota wolves was also crepuscular in summer, presumably because prey animals (mainly beavers) were most active at dawn and dusk.[173] Foraging can be dictated by human activity, as it is in free-ranging dogs (see below). Wolves near human habitations avoid persecution by being nocturnal, like some living east of Rome.[174] These wolves learned to approach livestock pens without being detected by dogs and knew where garbage was likely to be found. At dawn, before the populace awoke, they retreated silently to hidden resting areas.

Wolves see well.[175] Crisler considered them to be sight-hunters, describing how a tame wolf raised its head and ran straight for a caribou herd; a husky that often accompanied it "followed the zigzag scent trail."[176] Vision permits quicker, more directional responses in open landscapes, becoming at times superseded by olfaction in dim light and wooded or mountainous habitats. Wolves apparently do track prey by scent and are thought to distinguish old ungulate tracks from new

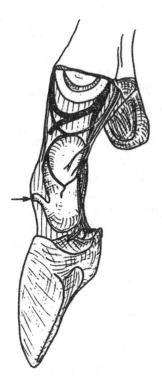

Figure 6.3 Schematic drawing of the forefoot interdigital pocket of a Japanese serow (*Capricornis crispus*). Arrow indicates the opening of the duct.
Source: Atoji, Y., Y. Suzuki, and M. Sugimura. (1988). Lectin histochemistry of the interdigital gland in the Japanese serow (*Capricornis crispus*) in winter. *Journal of Anatomy* **161**: 159–170. This material is reproduced with permission of John Wiley & Sons, Inc.

ones, although at times they seem incapable or indifferent.[177] Wolves in Sweden followed the 4-day-old tracks of three moose for 2 km.[178] These tracks had been made in snow, and whether the wolves used scent or sight is unknown.

Ungulates leave odorants produced by glands in the legs and feet and augmented by urine as they move across a landscape. Although canids doubtfully possess "interdigital glands" (Chapter 4), somewhat analogous structures are common in ungulates. However, theirs are not glands per se, but reservoirs holding glandular exudates. They form dorsal pockets of skin between the primary digits of the feet, enlarged by *sebaceous glands* and a few apocrine glands (Fig. 6.3).[179] I therefore call them *interdigital pockets*. Some of the compounds collecting there are believed to be emollients for lubrication[180] and antimicrobials functioning to prevent foot infections.[181] "The movement of lifting, gathering, sagging and interspacing of hoofs mechanically discharges the gland [*sic*]."[182] Traces of scent are probably left with every step.[183] Numerous volatile compounds have been isolated from the interdigital pockets of white-tailed deer, black-tailed deer (*Odocoileus hemionus*), moose, reindeer, fallow deer (*Dama dama*), roe deer (*Capreolus capreolus*), and Japanese serow (*Capricornis crispus*).[184] Still unknown are how long these odorants persist and which are detectable by wolves. American Indian dogs in the seventeenth century reportedly followed moose by scent,[185] but whether the tracks were used is unknown.

Deer also have tarsal and metatarsal glands on their legs. Tarsal glands, like interdigital pockets, produce antimicrobial substances.[186] When a deer lies down, the metatarsal gland on one side is in contact with the ground[187] and leaves a scent. White-tailed and black-tailed deer of all ages urinate on their tarsal glands then rub their legs together, the urine and glandular secretions mixing to form odorants that are carried on the body,[188] spill onto the ground,[189] and atomize in the surrounding air. Volatile components produce scents believed to function in individual recognition,[190] but might also leave scent trails useful to wolves. Substances from these glands have been thought to signal alarm to conspecifics or warn of a dominant buck nearby.[191] Urine alone releases common volatile compounds into the environment that provide information about an individual's sex and state of maturity.[192]

6.2   Competitors of wolves

Quickly consuming an ungulate is one way of not losing it to scavengers – mainly ravens – which steal large proportions of kills at some locations[193] but not at others.[194] Ravens are predators of small animals in addition to scavengers of wolf kills.[195] The loss is most severe when a large prey animal is killed and the pack is small[196] because a carcass then takes longer to consume.[197] Ravens often follow wolves[198] or are attracted by their vocalizing or the howling of human mimics.[199] They "announce" a new kill by circling above it and calling,[200] landing to feed on blood-stained snow while waiting for the wolves to become satiated[201] or feeding along with the wolves on blood trailed in the snow if the prey is wounded but still mobile.[202] Ravens in the Finlayson Lake region stole an estimated 50% of edible meat from small packs (2 or 3), 25% from medium packs (4–9), and 11% from packs of 10 or more.[203] Although wolves occasionally drive ravens away from a kill, the effect is short-lived.

Other scavengers are tolerated less well. Finland's wolves compete for reindeer with wolverines (*Gulo gulo*), and a resurgence in the wolf population caused wolverines to abandon many parts of their former ranges.[204] Wolves kill coyotes if they become too bold or aggressive near kill sites,[205] as do cougars,[206] and some wolves seem to simply dislike coyotes. A male wolf in Montana was known for killing leg-trapped coyotes.[207] In 1920 a hunter caught and shot the wolf after placing leg-traps around a trapped coyote that was still alive. The coyote was still too tempting. Its own leg caught, the wolf dragged itself to the coyote and killed it. The release of gray wolves into Yellowstone resulted in a surfeit of carrion but precipitated an annual winter decline in the coyote population of 25–33%, most of the loss attributed directly to wolves.[208] In nearby *Grand Teton National Park*, Wyoming, competition from wolves has also exerted a negative effect on the coyote population.[209]

A wolf-killed ungulate offers coyotes a scavenging banquet, although taking advantage of it must be balanced against the risk of getting injured or killed.[210] As a result, coyotes become more vigilant and spend less time resting when scavenging kills.[211] Coyotes sometimes contest wolves for ungulate carcasses and occasionally succeed if they have superior numbers.[212] Wolves ordinarily feed at will, forcing coyotes to wait. In such instances the coyotes approach only after the wolves are satiated and move off to a rest site nearby within sight of the carcass. A dominant male wolf can usually retain full control over a kill and keep coyotes at a distance.

Whether coyotes succeed in feeding at all therefore depends on the number of wolves and their state of hunger, the number of coyotes, and whether the kill is new or old. Wolves at a fresh kill feed preferentially on the internal organs and muscle tissue. The active consumption rate (feeding rate averaged over a feeding bout, or single "sitting" at a kill) increases as these parts are consumed, but food intake declines as they disappear leaving greater proportions of skin and bone.[213] Each bite extends the sequence of diminishing returns until the remains have less value than the energy required to kill again. At this point the wolves abandon them to coyotes, ravens, and other scavengers.

In the Nelchina Basin, 13% of kills (mostly moose) were contested by brown bears (*Ursus arctos*).[214] A wolf is no match for a bear, although a wolf pack can often harass and threaten a bear enough to keep it away from the kill. Sometimes a bear makes a kill but is chased away by wolves. Two adults and two adolescent wolves were described attacking an adult brown bear in possession of an adult moose carcass. The bear was not driven off but harassed in a way that individual wolves could feed briefly and intermittently.[215] Bears themselves are potential wolf food. Wolves in the Nelchina Basin killed an adolescent bear and consumed most of it, caching what was left. Finnish wolves have also reportedly killed and eaten bears.[216]

6.3   Wolves hunting and scavenging

Preparation to hunt together involves several activities, the first being to awaken the participants from their naps.[217] Sometimes the play of younger wolves arouses the dominant pair. This activity includes chases, games of keep-away with a bone or stick, ambushing, and so forth. At other times one of the pair awakens first and then wakes its mate. Often this is the female. During one series of observations she then urged the male to become active and go foraging. The male was reluctant and seemed to need prodding. Occasionally an adolescent serves as an alarm clock. When both parents are awake the group-ceremony commences (Fig. 3.11). Pack members assemble nose-to-nose and tail-wag excitedly. As described earlier (Chapter 3), they crowd around the dominant male, displaying low-intensity active submission (e.g. nose-pushing, face-pawing, licking-up).[218] Group-ceremonies often culminate in a chorus-howl before the hunters depart.[219]

Or do not depart, because the dominant male might lie down again. The female could then start out alone, her mate following a short distance before lying down again. The two then howl.[220] A female without pups reversed this procedure, sleeping through her mate's 48 impatient howls.

Wolves often stalk large prey on open landscapes, moving slowly and keeping their bodies close to the ground.[221] If detected they might lie down and even sleep while the potential prey continues to graze.[222] When threatened, musk oxen gather together tightly and form a defensive circle facing out. They behave this way whether confronting wolves or dogs.[223] If the calves stay inside the circle or between the adults they are nearly invulnerable. The wolves' deceptive disinterest might encourage adult musk oxen to become sufficiently calm for their vigilance to diminish and individuals to separate. If the wolves attack before the defensive circle forms they can induce the musk oxen to flee, offering a chance to attack the calves,[224] which are slower, more naïve, and less dangerous than adults.[225]

Ungulates on open ground seem circumspect in the presence of canid predators, often grazing calmly within sight. Their predators show no interest until ready to hunt, often napping or interacting with each other as if no other animals existed.[226] Wolves seldom appear to stalk caribou because they are easily approached, often within a few hundred meters, and instead of moving away the caribou continue grazing until chased.[227] Sometimes in the middle of a pursuit a wolf might stop and watch, at which time the caribou also stop until the chase commences.

Wolves are particularly wary of adult moose, and any animal that stands its ground, even if badly wounded, is apt to survive.[228] Sometimes a pack temporarily abandons a wounded moose only to return later after it weakens. Mech, having watched a lone Great Lakes wolf harassing a wounded bull, concluded that "an individual was observed seriously attempting this indicates that at least the wolf thought it might succeed."[229] And sometimes it does. The breeding male of a radio-collared pack in Denali was observed killing a moose by himself, but the process took 36 hours.[230]

Wolves quickly give up if a chase of any ungulate seems futile[231] or the prey fights back. Isle Royale wolves managed to kill <8% of moose chased or brought to bay.[232] Wolves on the Kenai Peninsula had similar experiences.[233] Of 38 observed encounters, 6 moose became aggressive and were left alone, 14 ran before making a stand and driving off their pursuers, 8 escaped by running, and only 2 were killed. Wolves chased every moose that ran. A similar pattern was seen in wolves hunting red deer in Russia.[234] If a deer ran it was chased, if it stood its ground the wolves usually withdrew. Wolves in Sweden typically chased reindeer farther than they chased moose, although members of both species frequently escaped.[235]

Murie was among the first reliable witnesses to document group hunting by wolves. In this case the prey were caribou and Dall's sheep in Denali.[236] In observations of wolves hunting musk oxen on Ellesmere Island, 3 of 21 chases observed by Mech resulted in kills.[237] Mech also gave an accounting of his Isle Royale studies.[238] Of 120 moose detected, 24 stood their ground and fought, and the wolves gave eventually gave up. Another 96 fled, 43 of which escaped. The wolves caught up with 53, 12 of which turned, fought, and escaped. Of 41 that continued to flee 34 outran or outlasted the wolves and got away, 7 were killed, and one escaped an attack after being wounded.

When snow is deep in an intermittently open landscape Great Lakes wolves often pursue a moose in single file.[239] Those in front attack the rump, flanks, or legs and hang on.[240] When the moose has been slowed sufficiently by their combined weight another wolf tries to grab its nose and pull down the head. If this can be accomplished, the rest of the pack piles on until the prey falls and is killed. Sometimes a moose fights off its attackers before collapsing, in which case the pack surrounds it, licking the bloody snow and seeming to assess its strength with half-hearted lunges. If the moose shows no signs of succumbing the pack might abandon it or return later to finish it off or feed on the carcass if the victim has died of its wounds. Sometimes a couple of pack members remain with a wounded moose until the rest return.

Grabbing the nose is a common technique when the prey is large and especially dangerous. On Ellesmere Island the first wolf to reach a running musk ox tries to grab its nose and hold tightly while a second leaps for an ear.[241] Wolves are occasionally trampled during this process. In the seventeenth century, Indians on the Gaspe Peninsula, Québec, used dogs to pursue and attack moose, the first dog grabbing the nose and holding on while the rest attacked from all sides. Their job was keeping the victim busy until hunters could arrive to kill it with arrows.[242]

Wolves in the Canadian Rockies also pursue ungulates single file on open landscapes, but in forested areas where visibility is limited they line up abreast: "When game is jumped the wolves are often in a position to outflank the animals and to effect speedy capture."[243] Whether this reflects "strategy" remains to be determined, and I hesitate to use the term with its implication of intentionality. The Crislers were convinced the wolves they observed on the Brooks Range used "strategy" and "tactics" to hunt caribou.[244]

A hunting sequence can indeed appear strategic and actually culminate in cooperation despite each participant responding to different signals and patterns of reinforcement. Running prey stimulates the chase response of wolves.[245] Picture two wolves resting on the tundra, one watching caribou in the distance (Wolf A), the other (Wolf B) gazing in another direction. The caribou sense the wolves' presence, but feeling no immediate threat they continue to feed, except for one animal that runs. To Wolf A the sight of running prey is a primary signal (S_1, Chapter 3) triggering a predictable primary response (R_1), which is to pursue a running ungulate. The sudden sight of Wolf A running at full speed serves as a secondary signal (S_2) to Wolf B, triggering a primary response in it too. Because this is a familiar pattern repeated and learned through reinforcement, Wolf B knows from experience that Wolf A's behavior indicates the potential of a food reward.[246]

Chases across open landscapes sometimes single out a wounded or sick animal or one especially frightened that might be easy prey,[247] a hunting method also used by African wild dogs.[248] Like wild dogs, a wolf might enter a fleeing herd (caribou in this case) and run with it, focused on a single animal.[249] Wolves and African wild dogs preferentially pursue an ungulate that runs when the rest of the herd remains stationary, and at times an entire herd is put to flight putatively to "identify" a slow or weak individual.[250] Wolves pursue caribou herds supposedly to isolate the calf with least endurance.[251] Murie described a scene in which a wolf chased a caribou herd at full speed, actually moving into the herd, which split into three groups.[252] The wolf ignored the running animals to either side, intent on a calf far ahead. Eventually it weakened, slowed, and was captured.

Observational evidence indicates that wolves can identify vulnerable animals from among many, explaining how the young, slow, old, and debilitated are singled out and killed selectively in disproportionate numbers.[253] This hypothesis was tested using borzois (Russian wolfhounds) to choose, chase, and kill saigas (*Saiga tatarica*), a species of antelope native to the Eurasian steppe. "One hundred percent of the animals caught by borzois turned out to be the carriers of various pathologies of the inner organs and of the skeleton–muscular system."[254] Only 30% of saigas shot by hunters were debilitated.

Murie examined 221 skulls of Dall's sheep that died between 1937 and 1941, most killed by wolves.[255] Only 4% had been prime-age animals (2–8 years) without evident signs of disease, confirming an early hypothesis that of wolf-killed ungulates "the majority ... are of old, diseased or crippled animals."[256] This observation has since been verified at other locations with several species of prey. In Yellowstone, human hunters and wolves both prey on elk. Adult female elk selected by wolves averaged 13.9 years, significantly older than the average prime-age females of 6.5 years killed by hunters.[257] Wolves killed comparatively more calves, but calves have lower fitness than adults because there is no guarantee they will survive to reproduce. However, prime-age females are pregnant during the winter hunting season, and killing one of them removes two elk from the population.

Hunting large ungulates even in a pack is risky. Examination of Alaskan wolf skeletons revealed many healed and healing fractures.[258] A male with broken ribs and legs was found alive after having been trampled by a moose;[259] another was alive but also crippled.[260] Skulls had compression fractures, particularly of the nasal and frontal bones, indicative of heavy blows, perhaps from moose hooves. Wolf carcasses with rib fractures inflicted by moose have been found on Isle Royale,[261] and an adult male was thought to have been killed by a moose in SNF.[262] A wolf carcass found in Algonquin Provincial Park showed evidence of having been killed by a white-tailed deer.[263] Two wolf carcasses found on northern Ellesmere Island had been gored by musk oxen,[264] and a wolf with a hind leg so badly injured by a moose that it could barely crawl was shot in the Northwest Territories.[265] An adult female wolf in the Nelchina Basin was seen pursued by a cow moose. The wolf stopped and hid in brush, but the cow ran to the area and trampled the wolf, which then ran off with a limp.[266]

About 9% of the annual natural mortality of southcentral Alaskan wolves resulted from moose injuries.[267] Wolves in the high Arctic, where they pursue

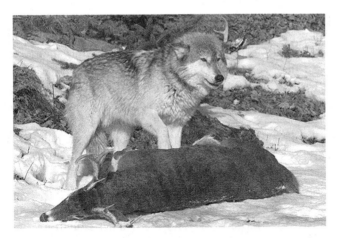

Figure 6.4 Wolf in submissive posture at a new kill being approached by a dominant. Notice the tongue-flick, ears-back, tail-low, and raised front leg poised to face-paw.
Source: © Outdoorsman|Dreamstime.com.

musk oxen, have been seen limping or wounded, and remains of others have been found with broken jaws and ribs.[268] A radio-collared dominant male in Minnesota was found with three fractured ribs that had healed and evidence of having been kicked in the head by a deer; two other wolves were killed by moose, and still another had been impaled by a deer's antlers.[269] In BISF, where the moose experience high natural mortality, most of those eaten are scavenged carcasses.[270]

When the prey is large all pack members gather around and feed simultaneously, and no social hierarchy is apparent;[271] at other times, they growl and snarl.[272] Actual aggression is rare, but order is maintained at the discretion of the dominant pair (Fig. 6.4). After kills, the members of a wolf pack in the Nelchina Basin fed together without animosity.[273] The breeding pair might dominate its older offspring after a kill. Older siblings are dominant over pups, which are fed preferentially by the parents and occasionally even by their older siblings (Chapter 8).[274] The dominant pair controls small kills and might feed first, excluding subordinates that sometimes approach them behaving submissively.[275] A subordinate comes at a crawling crouch, tail-low, head-low, ears-folded, giving the submissive-grin. When close enough it raises its head and face-paws the dominant wolf, sometimes flopping over on its back and lying upside-down in passive submission. The dominant male might ignore these gestures or give a bored snap of his jaws. He might pin-down a subordinate not already supine.

Wolves are eminently adaptable: a Minnesota wolf was seen feeding on a floating moose carcass while treading water.[276] Wolves in Finland swim to islands in lakes where sheep are pastured;[277] others in Canada's Keewatin district commonly chased caribou onto lake ice where the footing was poor and killed them.[278] As mentioned, wolves also forage on vegetable matter when game is scarce, and in the Canadian Rockies they turn to berries, grasses, and sedges.[279] Wolves in BISF and SNF eat fruit (e.g. blueberries, raspberries, strawberries) in summer,[280] and at SNF during August and September fruit composed up to a third of the diet.[281] Fruit remains appeared most often in scats near rendezvous sites (Chapter 8)[282] and might indicate that most of it is eaten by pups. According to a Russian writer, "in the stomach of wolves I have often found wild pears – in one wolf the entire stomach was filled, all swallowed whole, the wolf not even bothering to bite into them."[283]

Wolves occasionally kill and eat fellow pack members caught in traps and scavenge the carcasses of others.[284] This is thought to be a consequence of prey scarcity, although limited cannibalism has been reported when populations are at or near saturation and game is adequate.[285] Territorial invasion is an invitation to suicide. A pack in SNF killed and ate a lone wolf that crossed its boundary,[286] and another in the Nelchina Basin killed and ate a loner caught 18 km inside its protected space.[287] A dominant male on Isle Royale that had been limping badly was thought to have been killed and eaten by subordinate males of the same pack.[288] In Algonquin Provincial Park wolves ate one of their members after it and the white-tailed buck it had been attacking severely wounded each other.[289] They also ate the deer. Undocumented reports of murder, cannibalism, or both are part of the wolf's legend.[290]

Where wolves have been restricted by civilization they tend to become nocturnal and scavenge garbage dumps instead of hunting.[291] Garbage is also used as supplementary food in North America[292] and elsewhere. Packs inhabiting a populated area near urban Rome where large game is absent split on occasion to forage on small animals or garbage.[293] In fact, scavenging at a garbage dump is a universal habit of wolves living in close contact with humans.[294] It represents a clumped food source easily exploited by one or many, although competition can arise from other species. Israeli wolves scavenging at garbage dumps, carcass dumps, and feeding stations competed with griffon vultures (*Gyps fulvus*) and striped hyaenas (*Hyaena hyaena*).[295] Usually the wolves gave way to the hyaenas but chased the vultures. Where garbage is the food source there can be no predator; every visitor is a scavenger. Wolves elsewhere in Europe and Asia (e.g. Russia, Italy, Iberian peninsula, Finland) have been reported scavenging at dumps and livestock burial sites.[296]

Wolves cache leftover food, often within easy access of a den if the breeding female is still confined there with young pups, but sometimes several kilometers away.[297] Alternatively, a nonbreeding wolf might selfishly cache food where other pack members are not likely to find it,[298] although the existence of selfish caching among wolves has not been tested. Like scrounging (see below), food cached selfishly by adolescents suggests that their delayed dispersal is not necessarily offset by cooperation and inclusive fitness gains (Chapter 8).[299] Regardless of motive, a cache by any hoarding animal represents fat reserves minus the negative phy-siological cost of carrying fat.[300] During the caching process the wolf excavates a hole, places the meat in it, and covers it using its nose.[301] Parts of the same carcass can be cached in several locations, and the wolf might return to it over many months.[302] Most of the meat regurgitated to feed pups is carried by the breeding pair (Chapter 8), and probably most of the caching is done by them as well.[303]

The caching of food by wolves and dogs is curious behavior. If the purpose is to hide it from other scavengers, why bother? Mammals that both hunt and scavenge also have keen senses of smell. Bears cache too, but are less thorough and fastidious than wolves.[304] The superior eyesight of ravens enables them to distinguish even minimal disturbances in the landscape. They also reveal behavioral evidence of excellent odor detection and in laboratory experiments readily locate food buried in gravel.[305]

6.4   Prey selection by wolves

Some early observers thought wolves killed nonselectively as opportunity arose.[306] Today we know they often choose certain species of ungulates over others, and preferences appear to be regional. In making these choices wolves seem insensitive to the *dangerous prey hypothesis*, which posits that predators avoid animals that might injure them in favor of those less dangerous.[307] Consequently, wolves would leave moose alone if white-tailed deer were present in sufficient numbers.[308] According to recent investigations, prey selection and prey shifting is more likely based on habitat bias and learning.

Wolves in the Yukon preferred moose to caribou despite moose being larger, more dangerous, and more difficult to kill.[309] Conversely, Gates of the Arctic wolves hunted caribou preferentially even when moose were more common,[310] and Denali wolves also chose caribou over moose.[311] Therefore, danger and vulnerability might not be consistent factors in prey selection. For example, although elk are about half the size of bison, have thinner skin, and run when attacked instead of standing their ground, that Yellowstone wolves choose elk over bison is not evidence of selection based on any known factor.[312] Instead, observational data conform to probabilities assigned by humans based on presumed ease of capture by wolves.[313] This is quite a conceptual leap, and the next is accepting that innate calculations by wolves somehow fit the same pattern.

If two or more ungulate species are present the diet of resident wolves might shift with changes in relative prey abundance, perhaps differences in prey vulnerability, species preferences, and other factors.[314] In such multi-ungulate systems prey switching occurs if a favored prey species declines. When elk became scarce in the area of *Glacier National Park*, Montana, the wolves switched to white-tailed deer.[315] Yellowstone wolves prefer elk and switched to killing bison only when elk became rare relative to bison.[316] The dietary proportion shifted from predominantly elk when abundant (relative to bison) to bison when elk became scarce (relative to bison) (Fig. 6.5), but the shift was abrupt only after elk became rare (relative to bison). Wolves at Gates of Alaska hunted caribou preferentially even when moose were twice as prevalent, and there was no evidence of prey switching.[317] A pack of three wolves in Sweden preyed mainly on moose toward the end

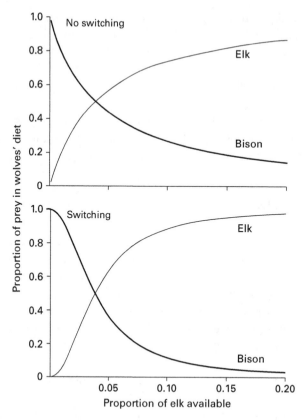

Figure 6.5 Model showing proportion of prey (elk or bison) in the diet of wolves in Yellowstone National Park depending on the proportion of elk available for no prey switching (*top*) or prey switching (*bottom*).
Source: Garrott *et al*. (2007).

of winter, replacing reindeer as their principal food source.[318] The Lapps had rounded up reindeer from the area twice in February 1978, reducing the number available. Nonetheless, 100–200 reindeer remained compared with 20–30 moose.

Reluctance to switch prey seems based on learned behavior, and the underlying mechanism linking behavioral ecology with population genetics would then be *habitat-biased dispersal*.[319] In other words, natal habitat predetermines the ultimate locations of dispersal: wolves born into a forested moose-hunting life will seek a similar habitat and the same prey when dispersing. According to this hypothesis, prey selection and habitat selection are inseparable, and ecological factors explain most of the genetic variation seen in tundra and taiga wolves, the boundary of tundra wolves into the taiga being coincident with the southern range of the caribou migration.[320] Wolves inhabiting coastal British Columbia show marked genetic differences from inland wolves, which are more similar to other North American gray wolves. Geographical barriers are not an issue, yet little intermingling occurs. The perceived reason is because "dispersing grey wolves select habitats similar to their own in which they were reared, and that this differenti-ation is maintained largely through behavioural mechanisms."[321] Early ontogen-etic imprinting on the natal habitat and later prey specialization could account for any seeming reluctance to change either lifestyle or prey choice.

The high dispersal capacity of wolves lessens the importance of geographic barriers to gene flow and suggests how other factors are more influential. Relentless persecu-tion and subsequent habitat fragmentation in western Europe culminated in genetic drift and random fixation of regional genotypes.[322] Today we see a discontinuous mosaic of unique mtDNA haplotypes (Chapter 1).[323] At some locations in North America distinct genetic clusters point to restricted gene flow despite the availability of uninterrupted long-range dispersal, suggesting a contributing factor overriding the wolf's extraordinary ability to move across vast landscapes. Genetic distance between populations correlates directly with latitude and habitat variables as assessed using microsatellite analysis.[324] How wolves come to occupy different habitats depends on the distribution of large prey (e.g. deer and moose in wooded areas, caribou on open landscapes). As shown, in multiple-prey systems certain ungulates are killed prefe-rentially to others. Selectivity stimulates a positive functional response to an increase in the numbers of favored prey. This in turn correlates directly with the local wolf population's genetic structure.[325] If consistently true then wolf dispersal is ultimately habitat-biased,[326] and an emigrant is not simply seeking an empty space in which to relocate but a space just like home.

As with most ecological models the exceptions are puzzling. In the mid-1980s "wolf dispersal into Greenland [took] place *from* terrain supporting caribou ... *into* a vast region devoid of this food source."[327] Wolves can subsist on small game if ungulates are rare or unavailable. Why they would choose to do this has not been explained. Remnants of Arctic hares (*Lepus arcticus*) were the most prevalent components in scats of Ellesmere Island wolves in the mid-1950s, with musk oxen remains constituting just 20%.[328] From the late 1960s into the 1980s, scats from Greenland were dominated by remnants of Arctic hares, lemmings (*Dicrostonyx* spp.), and ptarmigans (*Lagopus mutus*) despite the availability of musk oxen. Wolves also hunted seals (I assume ringed seals, *Phoca hispida*) along Greenland's fjords and on the Queen Elizabeth Islands.[329] At other places in the region they scavenged seal carcasses, in one instance digging through 50 cm of dense snow and 38 cm of sea ice to retrieve an adult ringed seal that had died underneath the ice.[330] They also dug up seal carcasses cached by Inuit hunters and ventured onto the sea ice to stalk seals. Wolves on northern Ellesmere Island were seen lying near a breathing hole waiting for a seal to surface and emerge from the water. Wolves in Russia reportedly killed Caspian seals (*P. caspica*), mainly pups.[331]

Packs split and sometimes an entire pack abandons its territory and moves elsewhere. Prey switching is then inevitable if the habitat is sufficiently different, and appropriate adjustments are made.[332] Previous assumptions about diet achieve finer resolution as new techniques are applied (e.g. stable isotope analy-sis).[333] In addition, suddenly abundant resources can be targeted and traditional prey abandoned temporarily. This is true in coastal British Columbia where autumn salmon become the principal food and not just a supplementary source.[334] Mule deer remains appear in 90–95% of wolf scats in spring and summer, but in autumn 40–70% of scats contain remnants of salmon. At other locations in Europe and North America the usual ecological constraints are in play: number of ungulate species available and their spatial distributions, availability of alternative prey, changes in prey density and migratory pattern, and so forth.[335] Evidently there are no rules governing what wolves eat and how they go about acquiring it, just regional patterns.

Wolves on the Alaska Peninsula patrol the coastline of Bristol Bay seeking carcasses of marine mammals that have washed ashore.[336] These are known to include the walrus (*Odobenus rosmarus*), beluga whale (*Delphinapterus leucas*), harbor seal (*Phoca vitulina*), spotted seal (*P. largha*), sea otter (*Enhydra lutris*), and even an occasional gray whale (*Eschrichtius robustus*). In winter when the bay freezes the wolves travel up to 6 km offshore to hunt sea otters trapped above the ice. These hunts are risky: in one case a pack of 7 apparently drowned when the ice broke apart during a sudden increase in wind and air temperature. Early in the twentieth century wolves were seen on drifting sea ice off Alaska's coast.[337]

Spectacular evidence of prey-based habitat bias has been found in North America. Some wolf packs in northwestern Alaska abandon their territories to follow migrating caribou herds in winter when moose numbers are inadequate to sustain them.[338] In one case packs moved 64–272 km to the caribou winter range from October through February and returned to occupy their territories starting in March.[339] Wolves in parts of western Canada also migrate south to caribou wintering areas.[340] These annual treks can exceed 1000 km.[341] Caribou herds in Alaska, Yukon, and Northwest Territories follow the same pattern.[342] November through March is spent in the boreal forest at the southern end of the range, and the northward spring migration starts in March and April with females reaching calving grounds on the tundra to give birth in early June. Males delay northward movement, but appear on the tundra by June and stay through August. Caribou arrive back at the tree line in September, entering the forest in October.

Migratory behavior by Canada's subarctic wolves was proposed by Capt. J. C. Critchell-Bullock in the mid-1920s.[343] He saw wolves not only traveling with the caribou but appearing to anticipate their movements by occasionally preceding them along the migration route. In addition, he reported seeing foxes trailing along for the leftovers.

The result in both Canada and Alaska has been the evolution of two separate populations of wolves, one comprising pale-colored tundra wolves following caribou on their annual north–south migrations, the other consisting of darker animals that are territorial all year and hunt elk, moose, deer, and nonmigratory caribou.[344] Considering the rapidity and ease with which wolves traverse all types of terrain, the natal habitat and its accompanying ecological components (e.g. type of prey) appear to restrict dispersal more than geography or distance.[345]

Finland's wolves might follow the seasonal movements of semi-domestic reindeer,[346] and Algonquin wolves in eastern Canada make short migrations of up to

62 km to winter "deer yards" outside the boundaries of Algonquin Provincial Park.[347] In years when white-tailed deer congregate at these locations packs might split, some wolves remaining behind in their territories while others make forays to the yards, often staying from late December into March. The deer yards are neutral spaces with no packs claiming ownership, and this evidently quells aggression. At times when few deer remain inside the park the wolves trespass regularly into each other's spaces to make kills or feed on remains of kills abandoned by other trespassers.

6.5   The dilemma of cooperative hunting

Craig Packer and Lore Ruttan assessed the evolution of cooperative hunting using game theory, and much of what I say here is based on their models.[348] When we think about wolves we picture individuals bound by social ties hunting and feeding as a unit. In other words, we think of a pack as the additive or synergistic expression of its parts. Was cooperative hunting therefore the evolutionary force driving wolf sociality? Probably not. Were it so, then hunting in a pack should increase each member's food intake, and this is not what happens. In fact, wolves in pursuit of the same ungulate might not even be cooperating.

Encountering (and presumably pursuing) the prey is an event independent of each pack member's ultimate participation in the capture. Not all invest the same effort during a group hunt. Prey animals vary in size, strength, condition, speed, and experience, affecting a group predator's willingness to participate and allowing some to withhold cooperation. When the prey animal selected is large a pack member can conserve energy and avoid injury by not taking part in the kill, yet benefit afterward by freeloading at the feast. These *scroungers* need to be present at the kill to obtain food, and running with the pack during the pursuit phase of a hunt can present an illusion of cooperation. Scroungers usually go unpunished because familiar pack mates are easier to exploit than strangers.[349] Of the pack of 15 on Isle Royale, only 5 or 6 actually took part in the final chase, attack, and killing of moose while the other members dropped far behind.[350]

Scroungers by definition rely on companions to kill for them and hunt only when necessary. Adolescent wolves often scrounge, as do debilitated ones.[351] The tendency to scrounge correlates directly with pack size[352] because the cost/benefit ratio (measured as per capita food intake) rises with each member added. Those wolves that actually do cooperate with others (*cooperators*) can coexist with scroungers only by preying on single large animals like moose; that is, prey large enough to feed themselves with enough left for scroungers. Prey small enough to be eaten by a cooperator before scroungers catch up does not qualify. Scrounging is tolerated among individuals of similar social standing when food comes in large packages because each bite taken by the owner diminishes the personal value of the remains while increasing their value to others waiting to eat.[353] Those waiting become increasingly more willing to contest ownership of the leftovers. If cost exceeds benefit it pays the owner to share.

When a wolf pack pursues a single prey animal each individual potentially contributes to the kill. Additional participants make the effort more profitable, but raise the probability of success only in situations in which an individual hunter's probable success is already low. As discussed previously, a group's food intake diminishes when individuals can hunt the same prey efficiently, and an experienced adult wolf can apparently kill any large ungulate it encounters.

If living in groups offers no advantages in terms of hunting efficiency and food intake, why do it? Hamilton's models of altruism (Chapter 8) imply an inverse relationship between degree of relatedness and group size (i.e. increasing degrees of relatedness cause the dissolution of social behavior, not its enhancement).[354] Variance in per-capita food consumption seems lower in larger groups of wolves,[355] although whether this affects fitness is unknown. Even if beneficial it must be offset to some extent by the lower per capita intake. The shorter kill interval described as typical of larger packs[356] appears to be a necessity, not an advantage.

Other possibilities might be better care of the young[357] and enhanced protection of kills from other predators and scavengers.[358] Wolves perhaps improve their fitness by staying with the natal pack on attaining sexual maturity. In doing so they delay reproduction[359] and transfer responsibility of regular food procurement to their parents. On dispersal they depart well-fed and probably better hunters.[360] Emigration benefits both the emigrants and those left behind because dispersal is an important mechanism of adjusting to the food supply.[361] Not only are there fewer mouths to feed, but a reduction in pack size increases the kill rate, thereby making more food available per capita. Although as discussed previously wolf density at the population level is prey-dependent,[362] the fact that pack size and number of packs both seem unaffected by prey availability is evidence of the loose relationship between dispersal and prey numbers (Chapter 5).[363]

When the wolf population on Isle Royale declined abruptly in the 1980s (Chapter 5), the average pack size declined concomitantly and the number of loners rose.[364] If prey is scarce and wolf numbers high, wolves might disperse to avoid intrapack conflict and to search out new food sources.[365] If the balance is reversed (low wolf numbers, high prey density), wolves might disperse, seeking unoccupied spaces in which to reproduce.[366] The social organization of wolves on Isle Royale between 1988 and 1991 fit better with the second hypothesis: low wolf density, packs mostly small, high proportion of loners, high numbers of moose.[367] Nonetheless, the expected population increase had not occurred by 1991. To those who studied this population and its interaction with moose over many years, the point was "to know who was gaining on whom and for how long,"[368] and the answer has never been obvious.

6.6   Foraging by free-ranging dogs

Free-ranging dogs everywhere,[369] including the dingoes of Asia and Australia,[370] probably occupy similar ecological spaces as scavengers and predators. The typical diet seems composed of small game, road kills and other carrion, garbage, and vegetable matter,[371] items that can be procured without joining forces with other dogs. Coyotes, putative red wolves, and free-ranging dogs in Arkansas had diets similar to this.[372] Garbage strewn through urban settings represents a dispersed food source best exploited by solitary scavenging.[373] Urban free-ranging dogs also prey on rats and cats.[374] Three dogs in St. Louis were seen chasing squirrels in a park on 61 occasions, all pursuits unsuccessful.[375]

Free-ranging dogs scavenge anything they find; in some countries this includes human feces[376] and human body parts.[377] Nearly any organic matter regardless of condition or origin is potentially food, and even dog carcasses are treated as carrion.[378] Scats of free-ranging dogs in rural Alabama contained traces of grass, leaves, persimmons (*Diospyros virginiana*), cottontail rabbits (*Sylvilagus floridanus*), mice (*Peromyscus* sp.), insects, garbage, and gopher tortoises (*Gopherus polyphemus*).[379] Dogs in Alaska's interior, when not scavenging at garbage dumps, appeared to hunt snowshoe hares cooperatively. To accomplish this the group spread out, flushed a hare, and then converged at the capture site.[380]

Free-ranging dogs observed in Illinois occasionally killed white-tailed deer fawns, but whether individually or in groups is unknown.[381] Neither these dogs nor those studied in Alabama attacked adult deer or livestock of any age.[382] Of 24 white-tailed deer in Arkansas[383] known with certainty to have been killed by dogs, only 2 were shown to be healthy on necropsy.

Murie cited an incident in which two large huskies in Alaska attacked a cow moose and her calf but were driven off.[384] Free-ranging dogs in Zimbabwe are inefficient predators of large game, especially small dogs of 14–15 kg traveling in groups through regions where alternative food is abundant.[385] Most wild animals killed were <50 kg, mainly domestic goats. However, one unusually large dog of 22.5 kg managed to kill three wild ungulates by itself.

Free-ranging dogs have been accused of killing livestock in the American Midwest,[386] and unsupervised owned dogs in North America are sometimes guilty of livestock predation.[387] The same is true in Italy, where owned dogs caused more damage to livestock than those without owners,[388] although a group of these did kill some foals and sheep.[389] Free-ranging dogs in the Voronezhskaya Oblast of Russia reportedly attacked deer, and others in the same area fed on carrion and garbage and were known to kill sheep.[390] Wolves were considered the lesser nuisance. Dogs brought to the Americas by early Europeans reverted to the wild at some locations (e.g. the island of Hispaniola) and soon became serious predators of livestock.[391]

Wild canids said to be wolfdogs preyed heavily on roe deer in the southern Ural Mountains in the 1970s.[392] Unlike wolves, they traveled in large groups in summer, sometimes pursuing deer for up to 4 km and (unlike wolves) vocalizing during the chase. Also during this same time other admixtures in the vicinities of Voronezh and Belgorod were scavengers but also bold predators of domestic livestock, often active during the day, digging dens near urban areas and occupying abandoned buildings.[393] Wolves that reappeared in recent years displaced these animals and free-ranging domestic dogs occupying woodlands.[394]

In areas of Israel where wolves have disappeared, dogs have replaced them in some instances, mostly pariah × Alsatian crosses.[395] They subsist mostly by scavenging garbage but also by killing sheep and goats, activities often blamed on wolves. Three Israeli dogs reportedly killed 70 goats in a single night.[396] Like wolves, after such a slaughter the dogs might not feed on the carcasses. Occasionally a killing is not surplus but simply strange when it serves no gastronomic purpose. Three dogs were observed to attack and kill an adult coyote and then immediately abandon the carcass.[397]

Free-ranging dogs in rural and suburban southeastern Brazil ate animal and vegetable matter and garbage.[398] The animals consumed were mostly invertebrates (57%) followed by mammals (25%), birds (17%) and reptiles (1%). Consumption of mammals ranged from 17–25 kg annually for each individual. Principal prey animals consumed by mass were the South American coati (*Nasua nasua*) and nutria (*Myocastor coypus*). Other mammalian prey consisted of the lesser grison (*Galictis cuja*), white-eared opossum (*Didelphis albiventris*), Brazilian porcupine (*Coendou prehensilis*), and nine-banded armadillo (*Dasypus novemcinctus*). Rats and mice predominated numerically (45%).

A group of dogs that traveled together showed mutual tolerance when scavenging at a garbage dump in Alaska, occasionally approaching each other and feeding side by side.[399] This is similar to the behavior of urban street dogs (Chapter 5). A group in Alabama traveled 8.2 km in 24 hours while foraging,[400] a pattern not unlike wolves. And similar to wolves, free-ranging dogs cache food in times of surplus.[401] What titillates the palate of a Dumpster-diving dog? Fried liver with onions tops the list, followed by baked chicken.[402] Fresh foods are preferred to gamey fare, and liver ranks highest among raw meats.

Owned dogs rely on us for food, and during their domestication humankind seems to have selected for scrounging, perhaps unwittingly. Consider that when a trait arises that benefits other members of a group, selection favors *not* possessing it, but only within groups.[403] By permitting some members to shoulder partial costs of traits advantageous to group living, scroungers parasitize the beneficial acts of other members. Between-group selection, in contrast, promotes traits favoring other members. Tolerated scrounging explains why household dogs and subordinate wolves in a pack receive food regardless of what the givers might prefer.[404]

When it comes to foraging we know more about Australian dingoes than all other free-ranging dogs combined. Dingoes are usually on the move,[405] often when the expected prey is moving too, but climate is a contributing factor. Dingoes in temperate Victoria were active at all times.[406] Those in northeastern New South Wales were alert both day and night with 70% of the rest periods of one small group of adolescents averaging <30 min,[407] but they became most active during crepuscular periods and least so at midday.[408] In arid regions activity is sometimes limited to cooler times when loss of body water can be minimized, and in hot, arid central Australia some dingoes hunt at night.[409] Dingoes in the arid northwest of Western Australia hunted two species of large kangaroos, the euro

(*Macropus robustus*) and red kangaroo (*M. rufus*), both having peak activities at dawn and dusk.[410] Dingoes in the arid Nullarbor, Western Australia, hunted these species at night too.[411] Many animals in the Australian wet tropics are nocturnal. Dingoes there hunted at night, primarily along edges of the rainforest where dense vegetation opens onto pastures and roadsides.[412]

At an average adult body mass of 15 kg[413] the dingo is Australia's biggest and most widely distributed carnivore.[414] Its largest natural prey is the red kangaroo, adult males of which can be 89 kg, adult females 36 kg.[415] Although the diet is varied and coyote-like everywhere, mammals compose most of the prey,[416] in some regions accounting for 96% of food items.[417] At Nadgee, southeastern Australia, dingoes favored such medium-sized prey as the European rabbit (*Oryctolagus cuniculus*), long-nosed potoroo (*Potorous tridactylus*), two species of bandicoot (*Isoodon obesulus*, *Perameles nasuta*), and brush-tailed and ring-tailed (*Pseudocheirus peregrinus*) opossums. Large prey consisted of the eastern gray kangaroo (*Macropus giganteus*), red-necked wallaby (*Macropus rufogriseus*), swamp wallaby (*Wallabia bicolor*), and common wombat (*Vombatus ursinus*). These last two species, at 17 and 26 kg, respectively, were the most frequent prey.

A dingo requires about 7% of its body mass in food per day, the equivalent of a 1-kg rabbit,[418] the principal prey in many locations,[419] but dingoes gorge when opportunity permits. A New Zealand fur seal (*Arctocephalus forsteri*) that washed up dead at Nadgee in September 1975 lay untouched for 5 days until found by three dingoes, which consumed it over another 5 days.[420] Adult male New Zealand fur seals can reach 160 kg, and this one was described as "large." Assuming that it was only 140 kg, that just 40% of the carcass was edible[421] and the dingoes were each 15 kg, the total amount eaten would have been 18.6 kg per dingo, or 6.2 kg per day, equal to 41% of each dingo's body mass. Dingoes at the same location were sometimes left cow legs of 20 kg. The meat was routinely consumed in a night by two or three individuals.

The diets of dingoes and dingo-dogs are probably the same.[422] The variety of items consumed is extensive,[423] easily matching the coyote's extensive menu (Chapter 1). Food consumed ranges from fruits and insects to cattle,[424] and in arid regions of Australia it includes 26 species of animals, although 12 species composed 97% of the diet by frequency at one location.[425] Dingoes in coastal southeastern Australia scavenge along beaches for carcasses of shearwaters (*Puffinus tenuirostris*, *P. pacificus*), little penguins (*Eudyptula minor*), and marine mammals.

Predation can involve a form of prey-shifting, predatory opportunism, and scavenging (Fig. 6.6).[426] Dingoes in northwestern Australia favored two species of kangaroos, switching to cattle carrion when their populations declined and continuing to hunt kangaroos even with fresh cattle carrion in plentiful supply.[427] Cattle are relatively abundant during times of both rain and drought; red kangaroos, birds, and lizards are relatively scarce. Following a heavy rainy period (flush times) rodent populations exploded, and dingoes concentrated on rodents for a year. Rabbits surged next, and dingoes hunted them intensively for the next 3 years. Rodents, rabbits, birds, and lizards were the preferred prey, but as

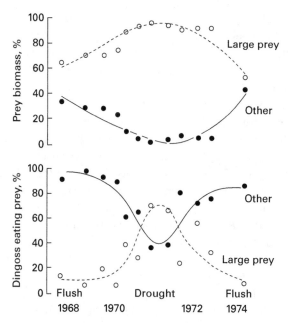

Figure 6.6 Model depicting alternation of dingo predation depending on flush (rainy) or drought conditions relative to body size of prey. Large prey represent kangaroos and cattle. With permission from Springer Science + Business Media: Corbett, L. K. and A. E. Newsome. (1987). The feeding ecology of the dingo. III. Dietary relationships with widely fluctuating prey populations in arid Australia: an hypothesis of alternation of predation. *Oecologia* **74**: 215–227.

drought once again encroached the larger mammals (mainly red kangaroos) were killed more often, as were cattle, although most of the beef consumed was scavenged from carcasses. Kangaroos and cattle carcasses offer more convenient packages of nutrients at such times than the scarcer small animals. Rabbits were the exception regardless of relative density, constituting more than half the diet during both droughts and flush times.

In the Simpson Desert during a 2-year flush period, rodents dominated the diets of letter-winged kites (*Elanus scriptus*), red foxes, feral domestic cats, and dingoes.[428] The expected dietary overlap occurred. The abundance of dingoes increased but did not show a significant positive correlation with rodent abundance. Although rodents composed a measurably higher proportion of the diet (70%), dingoes also consumed rabbits, cattle, kangaroos, reptiles, and invertebrates. This should not be surprising considering that dingoes are larger than foxes and cats; as mentioned before, larger foraging generalists should be expected to have broader diets.[429] Dietary patterns in arid regions can be summarized as: (1) preferred sources sought at all times but more available during flush times (rabbits, rodents) or droughts (cattle carrion), (2) animals killed inversely with their absolute abundance and never common (red kangaroos), and (3) prey killed infrequently whether large (cattle) or small (birds, lizards).[430]

At Kosciusko in temperate southeastern Australia, wombats made up 51.3% of the prey. Their abundance at four locations was similar yet unrelated to frequency in the diet of resident dingoes. However, dietary frequencies for the wombat, kangaroo, and feral horse correlated significantly regardless of their estimated populations. "Thus, the presence of one prey in abundance appears to have induced heavy predation upon scarcer prey."[431] Swamp wallabies were preferred over other kangaroos by dingoes in northeastern New South Wales, which killed them disproportionately to their numbers instead of switching to more abundant red-necked wallabies and eastern gray kangaroos.[432] Remnants of medium-sized and large marsupials composed 89.3% of dietary items in the stomachs of dingoes in southeastern Australia of which two (swamp wallaby, red-necked wallaby) formed the bulk (>50% of items recovered).[433] Parts of sheep (4.8%), cattle (2.4%), feral pigs (4.0%), and European rabbits (7.8%) were also present.

The fact that foraging dingoes will eat any animal matter, dead or alive, has ample documentation,[434] but labeling them simply as opportunists based on variety of items consumed is inaccurate. We know that in some parts of Western Australia dingoes are important predators of large kangaroos;[435] at other locations they subsist principally on rabbits.[436] Often these are choices. Opportunism implies not just consuming items as encountered but a lack of preference.[437] Dingoes are sometimes preferential hunters of large prey species, kangaroos and wombats in particular.[438] Their reluctance to switch from a scarce but favored prey, as just discussed, is supporting evidence. Dingoes in northeastern New South Wales fed on, at minimum, members of 35 animal groups or species yet 5 species composed 76% of the diet.[439] Such results are not unusual.[440] Cattle carrion, regardless of its condition, is not among the dingo's preferred foods and is often not exploited in proportion to availability.[441] In times of food scarcity items ignored previously are not rejected, even desiccated cow hides now months old and mummified in the desert air.[442] Therefore, changes over time in the contents of scats "may not reflect a change in the relative proportion of these species observed."[443] In other words, stomach or scat content analysis might indicate need and not preference.

Claims that large kangaroos and healthy adult cattle are safe from lone dingoes and can be killed only by groups[444] might be true in the case of cattle, which are larger and stronger than a kangaroo. The dingo's bite force is weak compared with the wolf's and correlates inversely with jaw gape, the effective optimal angle being small (25–35°).[445] This might explain why carcasses of large mammals found at dingo kills can appear nearly intact. Small female and juvenile red kangaroos necropsied after a sequence of surplus killing (see below) showed no apparent signs of having been injured except for occasional blood-tinged fur at the throat, and even that was slight. A hind leg was generally attacked first, followed by bites to the thorax and neck. Leg wounds were not deep. However, extensive bite marks were found elsewhere on the skinned carcasses. The victims had not been torn apart as if by powerful jaws, but literally bitten to death.[446]

Like wolves, dingoes are inefficient hunters if percentage capture success is the criterion. Of 272 observations of dingoes chasing kangaroos in the Fortescue

River region just 25 (9.2%) resulted in a capture and kill.[447] Dingoes in groups were slightly more successful than loners, but groups of three and larger were no more efficient at pursuing and killing kangaroos than dingoes in twos.[448] Dingoes in southeastern Australia killed swamp wallabies when hunting alone and in twos.[449] Solitary dingoes in the Nullarbor chased and captured euros and red kangaroos both day and night.[450] Only 10 daytime chases were witnessed, all by solitary dingoes, of which two were successful. As with wolves an increase in group size beyond two evidently does not improve capture efficiency.[451]

Dingoes hunting rabbits fare no better. Rabbits, which are the primary prey of Nullarbor dingoes, were hunted more successfully alone than in groups.[452] Whether digging a rabbit out of its burrow or chasing it on open ground, advantage went to the prey: the success rate was 9.7% for digging and 12.9% for chasing. Whether prey was large or small, "on the Nullarbor the presence of groups of dingoes was evidently not strictly related to improved hunting efficiency."[453]

I found surprisingly few field descriptions of dingoes hunting. One is an anecdotal report of a group attacking kangaroos,[454] another an undated narrative by A. Y. Hassell from the early 1860s. Mrs. Hassell wrote about seeing two dingoes chasing a large kangaroo and described the kill.[455] Sightings of several dingoes feeding together on a large carcass is not evidence of group hunting, nor does the number present simultaneously have special significance. Dingoes in the Nullarbor killed kangaroos alone and shared the kill, but only two at a time were seen feeding together, and it was estimated that no more than three in total ever fed on the same carcass.[456] In the Fortescue River region the proportion of observations of dingoes hunting large prey rose with the number present up to five, but a measure of hunting efficiency by group size was not presented.[457] More individuals were observed feeding on large mammals (average group size 3.3) than pursuing them (average group size 2.8), tentative evidence that not all had participated in the chase.

Dingoes might alter their group sizes depending on prey availability, moving in groups of up to 10 in arid regions, but confirming evidence is slim. Habitat probably has little effect on overall social structure. Of 1000 combined dingo sightings in arid central Australia and the wet mountainous landscape of southeastern Australia, 73% were alone, 16.2% were in twos, 5.2% in threes, 2.4% in fours, and two groups each comprising five, six, and seven.[458]

Like wolves, dingoes seldom kill livestock if other suitable prey is available,[459] but similar to individual wolves in the American West that were labeled legendary killers of livestock certain dingoes at one time achieved similar status.[460] As mentioned, dingoes attack adult cattle infrequently, preying almost exclusively on calves when cattle are attacked at all, and capture attempts seldom succeed if calves are protected by adults. Sheep, in contrast, are easily killed even by solitary dingoes.

Dingoes sometimes kill kangaroos and sheep in excess of their needs.[461] Five dingoes killed 83 red kangaroos at a watering point in *Sturt National Park*, northwestern New South Wales, in 7 weeks.[462] Eighty of these included a few smaller females but most were juveniles, and parts of only half those killed had been eaten. Males, which are much larger than females, typically ignored dingoes even when approached within a few meters.

Two dingoes killed six molting black swans in shallow water, eating four and leaving the remaining two carcasses.[463] Twenty dingoes released on Townshend Island, North Queensland, in late 1993 and early 1994 to get rid of goats that were damaging the ecosystem did the job.[464] By March 1997, only four goats from an original population of about 2500 could be located. Most of those killed initially had not been eaten. Dingoes have also been known to kill sheep and leave the carcasses[465] or begin to eat the victims while they were still alive.[466] Dingoes have also killed cattle (usually calves at watering sites) without eating them.

Red foxes and feral domestic cats prey heavily on small native reptiles, birds, and mammals in Australia.[467] Dingoes, if not persecuted, prey on both foxes and cats or frighten them away,[468] eventually displacing them just as wolves kill and displace coyotes in North American ecosystems.[469] Where dingoes are abundant small animals flourish[470] but kangaroo numbers decline.[471] Where dingoes are absent foxes multiply, negatively affecting the species richness and diversity of small mammals.[472] Overall, the dingo regulates a top-down *trophic cascade* that benefits native mammals including some threatened by extinction.[473] Where dingoes have been excluded by the *dingo fence* red foxes were more abundant, rabbits and dusky hopping-mice (*Notomys fuscus*) less so, indicating that dingoes reduce the incidence of fox predation on these two species by limiting the number of foxes.[474]

7   Courtship and conception

Members of the genus *Canis* have reproductive cycles with several unusual features:[1] monogamy, parental care, monestrus, extended proestrus and diestrus stages, a copulatory lock, incorporation of offspring into the social group, social suppression that keeps subordinates from breeding, obligate pseudopregnancy in subordinate females, and helping behavior by group members including males. I define and discuss these concepts here and in the next chapter, demonstrating how their intricate patterns of timing affect societies of wolves and free-ranging dogs.

Aspects of the reproductive cycles themselves differ in degree but not kind. Most changes are endocrinological and therefore invisible, yet they profoundly affect social behaviors and interactions. To ignore their details in favor of strictly observational information puts aside the biological basis of reproductive behavior, revealing only a partial glimpse of its integrated functions. In addition to the expected differences between wolves and dogs are large individual variations in endocrinological profiles throughout the reproductive cycle,[2] and these are routinely evident even in littermates. I start with an explanation of how the endocrinological factors cycle, stitching in brief mention of the external displays we recognize as courtship. Aspects of courtship in owned dogs, wolves, and free-ranging dogs are then discussed specifically.

7.1   The reproductive cycle – part 1

Wolves breed annually,[3] the time of mating and parturition varying slightly by latitude[4] but occurring between late January and early April.[5] Those in the Canadian Rockies mate in March and early April, the young being born in May and June.[6] Wolves of Denali[7] and southcentral Alaska[8] mate early in March and give birth throughout May.[9] Most Alaskan wolves mate during the first two weeks of March with a range of mid-February through early April,[10] although a captive colony at Barrow mated in March and April, the pups being born in May and June.[11] Wolves at BISF and Isle Royale mate from early February to early March.[12] Pups are born in Minnesota and Ontario during April and early May,[13] including in captive colonies.[14] Red wolves formerly living in Texas and Louisiana mated in January and February and gave birth in March and April.[15] Captive eastern coyotes in New Hampshire were born in April and early May.[16]

Israeli wolves mate in winter and parturition is early to mid-April;[17] Polish wolves breed in February and March.[18] Those in Finland mate in February and March, and pups are presumably born in May except at the highest latitudes. There mating occurs in April and birth is in June.[19] Central Russian wolves mate from mid-February to early March depending on location, with unconfirmed claims that estrus in the Caucasus starts late in December.[20] Litters of Russian wolves were purportedly born from mid-April into the second half of June, again depending on location,[21] and captive wolves in London gave birth mostly in May.[22]

Puberty[23] is ordinarily attained at 22 months,[24] or around 2 years,[25] although some wolves do not mature until 4 years old[26] and in captivity even older pups can breed.[27] Arbitrary but useful divisions are: *pup wolf* (<1 year old), *adolescent (yearling) wolf* (1–2 years), *adult wolf* (>2 years).[28] Wolves and dogs are unusual by being *monestrus*;[29] that is, undergoing only one estrus during a reproductive cycle.[30] The female cycle is traditionally broken into arbitrary stages for discussion. The problem with dividing a closed circle is deciding when a "stage" ends and another begins. Not surprisingly, various authors have described the timing differently. Here I assume wolves and dogs to progress through four stages distinguished loosely by social behavior, physical signs, and endocrinology. They are proestrus, estrus, diestrus, and anestrus. Proestrus and estrus are associated with courtship and discussed here; diestrus and anestrus are covered in Chapter 8.

Both sexes go through *gonadal recrudescence*. In males this results in enlargement of the testes followed by *spermatogenesis* (sperm production) timed to coincide with estrus.[31] Male domestic dogs (including dingoes and dingo-dogs) produce viable sperm continuously with no variation in seasonal sexual response,[32] although testosterone concentrations can fluctuate wildly.[33]

The female cycle is more complex. *Proestrus* (also called the *follicular phase*) in members of the genus *Canis* can be said to represent the reproductive cycle's first stage. Day 1 is marked by a bloody vaginal discharge in combination with a swollen vulva.[34] The vulva is warm to the touch; hence the term "in heat".[35] Proestrus in dogs can extend 3–17 days[36] but 7–9 days are typical;[37] in wolves it lasts about 15 days.[38] Proestrus is longer in female wolves than it is in dogs, with reports ranging from 16 to 45 days.[39] Proestrus in coyotes is much longer, 56–84 days,[40] that of coydogs (28–42 days) intermediate between wolves and coyotes.[41] Proestrus is accompanied by subtle changes in the behavior of both male and female wolves beginning in late autumn or early winter brought on by increasing concentrations of *estrogen*.[42] Reciprocal interest is clearly not in step at first, and one wolf's initiation of courtship is rebuffed or met with apathy by its mate.[43] Male aggression increases and can be especially pronounced in captive groups.[44] A female dog becomes restless, excited, sometimes aggressive toward the male, and drinks frequently; she urinates more often.[45] Only part of the bladder's contents are released with each urination. Scent-marking increases during proestrus,[46] and a free-ranging female in heat is thought to lay down an "odor trail" helping males to find her.[47]

Excretory constituents are also important as olfactory attractants in canid courtship, and the same substances that repel herbivores (Chapter 4) often serve as attractants among canids. Considering how important scent-marking is thought to be, surprisingly little effort has been made to isolate and identify the chemical compounds involved and test their effects on canid behavior. For example, Δ^3-isopentenyl methyl sulfide from red fox urine induces scent-marking by wild red foxes on fresh snow during the breeding season.[48] This substance has also been isolated from wolf urine[49] and is associated with mustelids.[50]

Studies of captive Great Lakes wolves found differences in urine composition according to sex of the animals, hormone status (intact adult males and females, neutered adult males), and season.[51] Subsequent treatment of neutered males and females by administering testosterone, estradiol, and progesterone reduced concentrations of certain volatile compounds typical of castration and increased others characteristic of intact adults, tentative evidence that urinary compounds in scent-marks might be used to communicate sexual identity.[52]

Injection of proestrous females with progesterone induced enhanced male interest in cotton balls swabbed with vaginal discharge.[53] Intact male dogs can distinguish the urine of a female in heat from one that is not,[54] and "estrous urine" is a demonstrated attractant.[55] Sexually experienced male dogs spend more time sniffing the urine of proestrous females than the urine of females not coming into heat.[56] Whatever it is a male dog detects, the possibility of a pheromone is unlikely unless such compounds can be sensed by the main olfactory system (Chapter 4). Dog pheromones have not been shown to exist, and compounds purported to serve this function are not specific just to dogs.

During courtship males also sniff and lick the anogenital regions of females in the proestrous stage. These behaviors suggest that specific odor detection might be important in courtship, but again no "pheromone" has yet been isolated. Whatever attractants a female might exude, the life of an "odor trail" is apparently brief. The urine of a female in heat stored 24 hours in a loosely capped clear glass bottle at room temperature lost its olfactory attractiveness to males, becoming comparable to fresh anestrous urine.[57] The same trend is seen in estrous urine of female rats.[58] This could be a disadvantage. On the other hand, rapid volatility could "facilitate the accuracy with which receptivity is signified."[59]

Urinary excretion of estrogen is concordant with plasma concentration, peaking during proestrus and during the last third of pregnancy.[60] Benzaldehyde is one compound appearing in the urine of proestrous female wolves during estrogen secretion.[61] Whether it or other substances induces the sniffing and licking behavior of males is unknown. Some major components isolated from the urine of female dogs in heat are methyl propyl sulfide, methyl butyl sulfide, and acetone; minor constituents include trimethylamine and five disulfides thought to be associated with estrus.[62] Of possible sex attractants, one of the most promising does not appear in urine. In 1979, methyl p-hydroxybenzoate was separated from the vaginal secretions of estrous dogs.[63] Applying the natural substance or its synthetic equivalent to the vulvas of anestrous and spayed females induced males to display courtship behavior and attempted mountings. Later investigators were unable to replicate the results, demonstrating that methyl *p*-hydroxybenzoate was no more attractive to male dogs than saltwater controls.[64] These last tests should be repeated before the results are considered valid.

The major constituent of urine from captive female coyotes collected in winter and spring was methyl 3-methylbut-3-enyl sulfide.[65] Its concentration fluctuated sharply even over a few days and showed no correlation with state of estrus. This compound was previously identified as a minor constituent of dog urine.[66] Conversely, methyl propyl sulfide and methyl butyl sulfide, major components of dog urine, were present in trace amounts in the urine of coyotes. If these or similar substances are found eventually to vary with hormonal cycles and even prove to be sex attractants they can be disqualified immediately as "pheromones" because: (1) they are common urinary constituents of carnivorans, and (2) they also serve as repellants to herbivores.[67]

Wolves and dogs demonstrate the same visible signs when proestrus begins (bloody vaginal discharge, swollen vulva). The dominant female of a wolf pack and all subordinate females past puberty probably come into estrus,[68] but usually only the dominant animal mates. When a captive female wolf was brought artificially into proestrus in summer, male dogs attempted to mate with her but male wolves, being reproductively out of phase, showed no interest.[69] Eastern coyote × dog crosses mated earlier in the year (November and December instead of February), and both sexes were seasonal breeders, not inheriting the domestic dog's reproductive pattern.[70] Coyote × dog offspring also mated earlier, and neither first- nor second-generation admixtures were in condition to breed synchronously with coyotes.[71]

In wolves and dogs the plasma concentrations of *follicle-stimulating hormone* (*FSH*) and *luteinizing hormone* (*LH*) are low through most of proestrus, kept in check by estrogen,[72] and rising in tandem just before the onset of estrus.[73] Their roles are crucial and often overlooked in discussions of canid reproduction. The pattern by which FSH and LH are secreted, in combination with changes in morphology and secretion by the ovaries, dictate species-specific nuances of the female reproductive cycle.[74] Estrogen spikes from baseline concentrations to peak values late in proestrus; *progesterone*, which is produced by the ovaries, remains low until rising gradually with the surge in LH.[75] Progesterone is apparently required to stimulate complete behavioral estrus (see below) including receptivity to males.[76]

Ovarian follicles (*follicles*) start forming early in proestrus. Their estrogen secretion is regulated by LH, which must be sufficiently elevated to stimulate follicular development.[77] Follicles begin developing into *corpora lutea* during late proestrus, the process continuing into estrus.[78] *Estradiol* (a form of estrogen commonly measured) produced by the developing follicles rises from baseline concentrations, spikes during the last 2 days of proestrus, and falls before the onset of estrus.[79] Progesterone concentrations, which had been low and nearly unvaried at the start of proestrus, rise gradually toward the end,[80] higher levels persisting into diestrus (Chapter 8). The ovarian follicles therefore produce

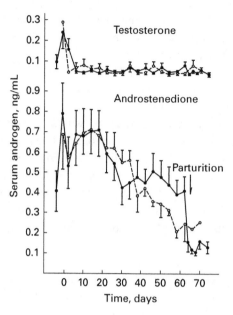

Figure 7.1 Mean (±SEM) serum concentrations of testosterone in three nonpregnant and six pregnant beagles (*top*) and of androstenedione in four nonpregnant and eight pregnant beagles (*bottom*) all aligned to the day of the preovulatory peak in LH. Nonpregnant dogs are indicated by open circles and dashed lines, pregnant dogs by closed circles and solid lines. Day of peak LH was determined by LH assay or else estimated as 65 days prior to parturition. Results from 10 days prepartum forth are also aligned to a parturition on day 65. *Source*: Concannon, P. W. and V. D. Castracane. (1985). Serum androstenedione and testosterone concentrations during pregnancy and nonpregnant cycles in dogs. *Biology of Reproduction* **33**: 1078–1083. Copyright by The Society for the Study of Reproduction, Inc. Reprinted with permission.

progesterone and not just estrogen prior to *luteinization*.[81] However, normal follicular development can proceed in early proestrus only if the progesterone concentration is low. The change in progesterone alters the female's behavior, causing her to accept mating just as proestrus terminates.[82] The length of proestrus and estrus in both dogs and wolves varies considerably among individuals.[83]

As mentioned, FSH and LH are initially held back by estrogen, but both rise sharply at the end of proestrus just after estrogen spikes and progesterone increases.[84] The exact timing varies, but in dogs the surges of LH and FSH usually occur 1 day before or 3 days after behavioral estrus when mating is observed.[85] The *androgens* (male hormones) *androstenedione* and *testosterone* also participate, both increasing in proestrus females. Testosterone peaks nearly in synchrony with LH[86] and declines through the remainder of proestrus.[87] Androstenedione continues rising through estrus and early diestrus before diminishing by about day 40 in both pregnant and nonpregnant females.[88] Its concentration at all times predominates that of testosterone (Fig. 7.1), which starting from day 6 after the LH surge stays at baseline levels.[89] Levels of androstenedione in both nonpregnant and pregnant dogs are elevated and variable near the LH peak, decline through diestrus, and drop abruptly just before parturition (Chapter 8). The origin and function of androgenic hormones in female wolves and dogs are unknown, but they might be produced by the *ovary* and associated with release of LH or the female's behavior at the time of estrus.[90]

Estrus, the second stage in the female dog reproductive cycle, lasts 3–21 days,[91] but like proestrus averages about 9 days.[92] A synonym is *ovulatory phase* when spontaneous *ovulation* takes place.[93] Estrus in wolves lasts 7–9 days[94] and 10 days in coyotes.[95] Some investigators incorporate elements of late proestrus (i.e. a late follicular phase when ovarian follicles are being formed) into this stage, others some features of early luteinization. Regardless of where the reproductive cycle is arbitrarily broken, estrus always includes ovulation and is recognized behaviorally when the female first becomes receptive to mating.[96]

Receptivity results from a decline in plasma estrogen and simultaneous rise in progesterone.[97] The bloody vaginal discharge diminishes and becomes watery,[98] and the vulva softens 1–2 days after the LH surge facilitating penetration by the male.[99] These visible signs, although useful, are unreliable correlates of ovulation,[100] as is measuring the plasma LH surge, which can occur anytime in the final 72 hours of proestrus to the first 120 hours of estrus.[101] For practical purposes ovulation commences 2 days following the increase in plasma progesterone above 1–2 ng/mL in both dogs and wolves[102] and 2 days following the LH spike in dogs.[103]

Follicles are typically present in both ovaries.[104] Although LH and FSH often peak at the onset of behavioral estrus (see below), peaks can also occur 2 days before and 3 days after. Occasionally a graph of LH has two peaks (i.e. is bifurcated). Estrogen secretion in all but the youngest follicles is controlled by LH.[105] The LH surge, which precedes ovulation by about 2 days or so,[106] lasts about 36 hours,[107] quickly follows the spike in estrogen (Fig. 7.2),[108] and is probably triggered by the abrupt decline of estrogen and concomitant rise in progesterone.[109] The spike in FSH that accompanies LH lasts about 110 hours, or three times longer than the LH surge.[110]

The progesterone concentration starts a steep rise 3 days or so after LH peaks (Fig. 7.3),[111] attaining maximum concentration 10 days following the spike in LH and staying high for up to 30 days, or well into diestrus (Chapter 8).[112] The follicles rupture about the same time,[113] and ovulation takes place 1–3 days following the onset of estrus, or within 2 days after the simultaneous surges of LH and FSH when their concentrations drop to baseline levels and remain there.[114] Testosterone concentrations diminish as estrus proceeds, attenuating to baseline levels; androstenedione rises midway through estrus following progesterone's trend.

The 1–3 day spike in LH induces luteinization of the mature ovarian follicles resulting in ovulation and progesterone-producing corpora lutea.[115] Serial ovulations then commence starting about 2 days after LH peaks. Ordinarily the LH surges within 1 day of the shift from proestrus to estrus as assessed by behavior, although observation alone is unreliable and mating can occur from 3 days before the surge to 5 days after.[116]

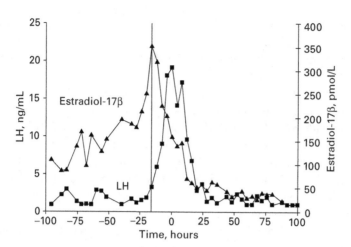

Figure 7.2 Plasma concentrations of LH and estradiol-17β from 100 h before and after the preovulatory surge in LH in a female beagle of 5 years. Note how the preovulatory surges of the two hormones coincide.
Source: de Gier, J., H. S. Kooistra, S. C. Djajadiningrat-Laanen, S. J. Dieleman, and A. C. Okkens. (2006). Temporal relations between plasma concentrations of luteinizing hormone, follicle-stimulating hormone, estradiol-17β, progesterone, prolactin, and α-melanocyte-stimulating hormone during the follicular, ovulatory, and early luteal phase in the bitch. *Theriogenology* **65**: 1346–1359. Copyright by Society of Theriogenology. Reprinted with permission of Elsevier.

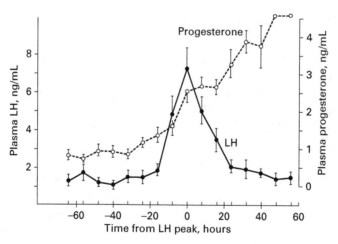

Figure 7.3 Mean (±SEM) plasma concentrations of LH and progesterone obtained from six beagles three times daily during proestrus and estrus.
Source: Concannon, P. W. (1993). Biology of gonadotropin secretion in adult and prepubertal female dogs. *Journal of Reproduction and Fertility* (Suppl.) **47**: 3–27.

Ovulation in members of the genus *Canis* is spontaneous, not induced.[117] The *oocytes* released during ovulation are immature[118] and fertilization is delayed until they mature, probably 2–3 days after release, or 4–5 days past the LH surge.[119] Uncleaved *ova* persist up to 3 days after ovulation, or to day 6 of estrus.[120] The average timing of mating is 1 day following the peak in LH and 1 day prior to ovulation.[121] If the LH peak is considered to be day 0 and ovulation day 2, fertilization is probably restricted to 3 days (days 4–7), which is 2–5 days after ovulation,[122] or during mid- to late estrus.[123]

Multiple fathers of a litter can best be explained by the time needed to complete *meiosis* and not the extended period of ovulation.[124] The dog's oocytes can remain viable at least 7 days;[125] *spermatozoa* reach the oviduct within 25 seconds of ejaculation where they are delayed 8–10 days by elevated estrogen.[126] As progesterone becomes dominant the embryos are transferred to the *uterus*. Long-lived sperm and ova make the exact timing of fertilization difficult to ascertain.

Endocrinological (i.e. "fertile") estrus is timed by the fall in plasma estrogen and accompanying rise of progesterone in association with the LH surge and ends 7–9 days after LH peaks.[127] Matings outside this range are seldom fertile.[128] *Endocrinological estrus* is what I mean by estrus unless behavioral estrus is stated explicitly. The day LH peaks is thus a reasonable measure for the start of endocrinological estrus.[129]

Behavioral estrus, which is stimulated by estrogen, starts when the female assumes the breeding stance with vulva displayed and tail turned to the side and lets the male mount her;[130] it ends when she refuses to be mounted for 2[131] or 3[132] consecutive days. Behavioral signs of estrus are not always timed perfectly with the LH surge and subsequent ovulation. *That fertility and behavior are not necessarily coincident makes behavioral estrus an unreliable indicator of ovulation.*[133] Vaginal smears are probably the easiest and most consistent indicators of how development proceeds.[134] Ovulation usually occurs within 3 days of the start of behavioral estrus[135] and is over in <24 hours.[136] The shift in behavior from restlessness to passivity results from decreasing estrogen concentrations after LH peaks and the simultaneous rise of progesterone.

The wolf's reproductive cycle is known less well than the domestic dog's. Certainly the courtship signals and reproductive physiologies of wolves and dogs are similar enough to permit interbreeding. Whereas dogs attain sexual and functional maturity at 5–12 months, wolves in nature postpone mating until nearly twice this age, although older female pup wolves have been known to reproduce in captivity.[137] As mentioned, gonadal recrudescence is seasonal in wolves. Initiation of the female reproductive cycle identified by the swollen vulva, bloody vaginal discharge, and changes in estrogen and progesterone concentrations is concordant with the male's enlarging testes and rising levels of testosterone and LH.[138]

It was once thought that the reproductive cycle of female domestic dogs lasts 6 months.[139] It actually lasts 7–8, occurs at variable intervals of 5–10 months,[140] and can commence at any time of year.[141] Variation by breed is apparent, but not by size of the animal.[142] The interval between periods of heat is 8.5 months in the dachshund, for example, and 7.5 months in the Labrador and Pekinese. Although the domestic dog can breed in any month[143] there might be a faint seasonal bias held over from its wolfish ancestry. Records of 3754 dogs from the American

Kennel Club Stud Book Register from 1942 to 1943 showed the greatest number of matings occurred in March,[144] and a British survey of commercial dog breeders confirmed that most mating took place from February to May.[145]

7.2   Courtship in owned dogs

The term *courtship* conjures images of ritual preceding a mating act. Any notion that free-ranging domestic dogs court one another seems odd at first, the casual observer's impression being one of unsupervised group sex. How an estrous female interacts with her suitors, and they with her, reveals a surprising repertoire of subtle behaviors.[146] Male dogs are mainly promiscuous, but the female of an *estrous group* (a female in heat being followed by one or more males attempting to mate with her) demonstrates selectivity.

Most of what we know about dog mating behavior has been derived from a series of studies by Frank A. Beach and Burney J. Le Boeuf conducted in the 1960s and early 1970s at the University of California, Berkeley. Theirs were the first experiments designed specifically to tease apart and describe the nuances of relevant patterned behavior. It had long been suspected – but never demonstrated experimentally – that females in estrus mate preferentially with certain males. *Female choice* is common in social mammals living in the wild where its effects have important evolutionary consequences.

Beach and Le Boeuf made their observations using purebred beagles. The first of the Berkeley experiments I describe involved five males and four females conducted through two estrous cycles of the females.[147] The dogs knew each other, having been acquired as pups and raised together in a large outdoor enclosure. A test consisted of releasing an estrous female into the enclosure after removing all the dogs and later letting a male join her. Early trials in which the male was released first and allowed to acclimate to the surroundings had the unintended consequence of leaving the female insufficient adjustment time. Beach and Le Boeuf wrote, "for example, some males mounted ... within 1 or 2 sec after she had literally been tossed through the doorway."[148] So much for beagle foreplay.

When the order of introduction was reversed came evidence of what I shall call courtship. The male approached and sniffed and licked the female's vulva. If she liked the male she allowed this, and then permitted him to mount. Sexual intercourse in dogs commences when the mounted male begins a series of pelvic thrusts, guiding the penis toward the vagina. The glans penis is inserted between the labia majora, gaining partial intromission. The male thrusts deeper and more rapidly, depressing his tail, forcing his pelvis against the female. Her tail has meanwhile been turned to the side. Full tumescence is not attained until the bulbus glandis at the base of the penis swells. The bulbus at full distension fits so tightly into the vulva that its circumference becomes greater than the vaginal opening. The result is a *copulatory lock*, or *tie*, in which withdrawal is difficult or impossible. Once a lock is established the male lifts a hind leg over the female's back and the two stand on four legs facing away from each other. They stay like this until ejaculation is finished and the erection subsides. Copulatory locks in domestic dogs generally last 15–45 min.[149]

One of my recollections of elementary school in rural West Virginia is of the class looking out a window into the school yard late one fine spring afternoon where a pair of stray dogs had locked in *flagrante delicto*. That was during the late 1940s when children's eyes were to be shielded from such spectacles. Instead of pulling down the blind and redirecting our attention, the teacher went outside, fetched a bucket of water from the well pump, and doused the dogs. It was how you took charge of nature in those days.

The dogs, of course, wanted desperately to break the tie and run away, but this was now impossible. The male turned without unlocking and remounted the female, and the two hopped around on six legs yelping and quivering as another bucket of water splashed over them, then another. Our teacher finally gave up and returned, stamping off the mud and wondering aloud how God could permit such filth in the world. She seemed puzzled why the dogs, in not disengaging, had lowered this torment onto her shoulders. We spent the time remaining with chairs turned away from the windows. No matter. The dogs were still locked when classes ended a few minutes later, offering a full opportunity to gather round and watch.

A female in Beach and Le Boeuf's experiments could – and often did – reject a male released into her company, the first observational evidence of female mate selection in domestic dogs. If after 5 minutes together the female refused to let the male mount she was unlikely to do so after 30 minutes or longer. In rejecting a persistent male, an estrous female can simply avoid him by stepping away when he tries to mount. She can also whirl around to face him, buck him off, fall over on her side, roll onto her back, or sit down.[150] Failing this she can threaten him by growling, snarling, snapping, or barking. A final option is outright attack: biting, chasing, even pursuing the male until he loses interest. If the female has tried to reject the male but he still manages to achieve intromission, her behavior from then on is cooperative.

The females in these experiments allowed certain males to court them and rejected others, evidence of female choice. Here a sociological commentary is useful. Peggy had no use for Ken while never rejecting Broadus or Eddie. She also liked John despite his difficulty achieving penetration. Broadus possessed star qualities, being rarely rejected by two of the females and never by the other three. Only Kate found Clark likable, but then Kate liked all the males. Despite his popularity with Peggy, Eddie could never light Blanche's fire. Blanche proved the most discriminating. These tendencies carried over from one estrus to the next. Spot, for example, always reacted negatively toward Clark and Ken, and Blanch consistently rejected Clark, Ken, and Eddie while occasionally accepting Broadus or John.

In some cases what appeared to be avoidance was the female trying to reposition herself underneath a male ineffectually humping her side or leg. At other times a female became overly excited, unable to stand quietly while being mounted. As mentioned, females typically cooperate after a male has mounted, and if a male mounts and fails to achieve intromission the female's reaction is still positive. Now disengaged, she investigates his penis, prances back and forth in front of him, and often turns the tables and mounts him, clasping him in the usual male's foreleg grasp just in front of his hips and commencing to thrust. Some behaviorists have called this behavior *solicitation*,[151] although I stick by courtship, a less slutty term.

Some females showed preferences by "teasing" a preferred male,[152] ending the male's investigation of her vulva or attempts to mount by running away. If the male chased her she stopped and stood still, allowing herself to be examined. If the male declined to follow she returned to him and initiated courtship.

Popularity does not necessarily depend on performance, although it might sometimes appear so. Broadus, for example, was rejected the least and attained the highest percentage of copulatory locks, making him most popular and also the best performer. Eddie placed third and Clark fourth in these measures. John, second in popularity to Broadus, ranked last in locks achieved per mount. Success means making the most of opportunity. Ken, the male rejected most often, nonetheless scored second in percentage of locks. Although the females liked John and allowed his frequent mounting, a conspicuous failure to penetrate rendered him unable to lock. Ken's mounts were fewer than John's, but given the chance he locked often. Clark was least popular and the poorest performer. After the usual rejection he simply lost interest.

Beach further assessed female choice in a later series of experiments using different beagles (six males, four females) under the same conditions as before.[153] This time some of the male dogs were littermates, although tests of kin discrimination were not done. Once again the females demonstrated clear preferences for certain males. Judy was the most accepting, Kathy least so. Littermates Don and Juan were the males accepted most often; Cecil and Joe, another pair of littermates, were accepted the least. Lolita liked Cecil best; least acceptable were her brothers Cassius and Amigo. Judy liked Don best and Cassius least, although Joan preferred Cassius most and liked Joe least. Kathy never rejected Cassius, Don, and Juan while remaining less receptive to Cecil and Joe.

Among the more interesting findings: social preferences when in anestrus was unrelated to female choice during estrus. These same dogs had been used in tests of social preferences and formed specific bonds with other dogs, preferring their company to that of others. Joan had liked Cassius the least among the males in those experiments, but moved him to the top of her list when in estrus. Lolita demonstrated a similar preference for another male, and the patterns of Judy and Kathy, although less pronounced, showed clear distinctions in their preference for male company during anestrus compared with estrus. A lady beagle's best friend in social situations is not necessarily her first choice during that magic moment. Some discrepancy can be traced to the male's behavior, which changes noticeably in the company of an estrous female. Beach wrote: "Males differ with respect to the intensity, duration and variety of their precopulatory activities and this may contribute to the female's sexual preferences."[154]

Also interesting was that competitive dominance between an anestrous female and a male had no detectable effect on female choice during mating. In these tests one dog was released into the communal area and given a bone. After it assumed possession the experimenters released a second dog. Ninety seconds later the dog with the bone was assessed as more "dominant," although this procedure is questionably a true test of dominance (Chapter 3). Of the females, Lolita dominated most often (was least subordinate) when placed with the males individually, but during estrus fell somewhere in the middle, being neither most nor least accepting of males while being courted. Kathy, the most likely to reject a male when in estrus, proved the most subordinate female in dominance tests. When in anestrus Joan dominated Don and was subordinate to Cassius, although in estrus she accepted them equally. Kathy was dominated socially by Amigo and Cassius, but accepted Cassius every time when in heat and rejected Amigo more than half the time.

Using sexually experienced beagles from the first group, Le Boeuf continued work on mate selection, but included extensive monitoring of the males and females in anestrus.[155] The setup to test interactions included a post to which a dog could be chained. The post was at the center of a circle measuring 3.7 m in diameter, its circumference outlined in gypsum dust for easy visibility. From an observation shed, Le Boeuf recorded how a "tethered" dog interacted with a "roving" dog released into the area for 5 minutes. The area outside the circle was large, and the "rover" had the option of not entering the circle to interact with the dog that was tethered. Pairs of dogs (male–female, female–female) were tested in multiple combinations of "tethered" and "roving" when a female was in estrus and when she was not. Pairs of males were also observed.

A roving male visited a female inside the circle on 93% of days the female was in estrus and 79% of days she was anestrus. Roving females visited tethered males more often when in estrus (76%) than anestrus (28%). Overall, males visited females more often than vice versa. Kate was the most gregarious female, almost always visiting tethered males and spending the most time with them regardless of her reproductive condition.

Three females visited some males more often than others and stayed longest. Peggy visited Broadus and Eddie every day she was in estrus and spent the majority of her allotted 5 minutes with them inside the circle. Her visits and time spent with John were somewhat less, and with Clark and Ken substantially less. Similarly, Blanche and Spot visited more often when in estrus and spent more time with Broadus and John than with Clark, Ken, and Eddie. In some cases females spent no more time with specific males when in estrus than when not.

Uncooperative behavior of females in estrus was described earlier and consists of avoidance, threat, attack, or sometimes a combination of these. Female choice was clearly evident in these later experiments. The roving Peggy allowed a tethered Broadus and Eddie to mount her numerous times, Clark only toward the end of her cycle, and Ken not at all. Whether tethered or roving, Peggy courted Broadus and Eddie often, Clark rarely, and Ken never. A quarter of Clark's attempts to mount Peggy and three-quarters of Ken's were rejected outright with threats and attacks, although she rarely acted this way with Broadus, Eddie, and John. Blanche and Spot also had favorite suitors, not always the same ones. Blanche, for example, seemed repelled by Eddie, one of Peggy's favorite paramours, and Kate liked them all.

The single factor preventing these results from becoming a beagle soap opera is the absence of any male–male interaction. In real life the lovely brunette with the doting husband suddenly comes face to face with the meter man, whose blue eyes seem depthless. Even though the meter is located outside of the house he asks to come inside, and she admits him. What this situation presents is female mate choice plunged suddenly into a heady brew of male–male competition. In none of the experiments just described was an estrous female released into a full company of males, a dog-on-dog test of evolutionary fitness. The results were obtained in laboratory conditions. Comparable studies using free-ranging dogs have not been done, although the few observational reports reveal fascinating nuances of both female choice and male–male competition (see below).

Estrous females visited tethered anestrous females as often as they visited males, but spent twice as much time with males. In contrast, anestrous females visited other anestrous females more frequently than they visited those in estrus. Females in either condition visited each other less often. Females sometimes mounted each other. Sometimes the female in estrus courted her anestrous companion. Females showed no preferences for other females. Roving anestrous females visited least often and spent the least amount of time when paired with other groups.

Overall, roving males visited tethered males about as often as females visited each other, but males spent twice as much time together. However, those visiting others were the least visited themselves when it came their turn to be tethered. Clark, for example, so unpopular with the females, visited every male when he roved, yet they entered the circle with him tethered only 40% of the time. Eddie, who seldom visited other males, was almost always visited by them.

Signs of aggression could have accounted for some of these differences. The males, despite knowing each other, displayed aggressive behavior, usually the roving male toward the tethered one. During these incidents the aggressor approached stiff-legged, growling, tail-wagging or tail-high and arched over his back in a display of dominance. Sometimes the other dog mirrored his behavior. The two stood still, touching noses or walking side by side. Usually both stood down and investigated each other's genitals. If one dog was subordinate he retreated and cringed, sometimes rolling onto his back in sudden passive submission. The other dog then straddled him in the stand-over pose, growling. No male attempted to mount another.

Visitations by roving dogs seemed to depend on dominant ↔ subordinate relationships. Clark and John were the most aggressive, never retreating from these encounters. A male seldom entered the circle if the dog to which he was subordinate had been tethered there. In sum, Clark and John visited the other three males 93% of the time but were visited in turn 32% of the time. Clark and John displayed mutual aggression when visiting each other, neither ever gaining dominance. Eddie declined every opportunity to visit Broadus, but Broadus visited Eddie in every test. Both became aggressive when meeting inside the circle, with Eddie usually backing down. Other paired males seemed on friendly terms. Neither Clark nor Eddie displayed aggression when paired, nor did John with Broadus.

Having nibbled around the edges of female mate selection, is there such a thing as male choice in domestic dogs? Certain experimental hurdles make the question difficult to test, and any conclusions at this time are equivocal.[156] Perhaps the most serious difficulty is making certain the females are "equally" in estrus at the time of testing. The onset, rise, and decline of estrus follows a bell curve extending over a period varying from a few days to 3 weeks. No two dogs are alike, and some have shorter or longer estrous cycles than others. How much of this wax and wane a male can detect is unknown, but whether or not he is rejected depends a great deal on where a female is in her cycle when a male arrives at the scene.

Le Boeuf's experiments offer insight, if only a glimpse. When roving, John rarely visited females regardless of their reproductive condition, spending about as much time with estrus females as Broadus spent with those in anestrus. This was not aversive behavior because the females seldom threatened or attacked him. Broadus, who was rarely rejected, spent more time than the other males in the company of tethered females. When in heat they allowed him to mount sooner and more frequently, rejected him least, and courted him often. Clark and Ken were rejected regularly and to about the same extent by Blanche and Spot. Ken, however, persisted even when rejected repeatedly. Clark, in contrast, slunk away after a few brief threats. Other factors being equal, perhaps male "choice" embodies nothing more than stamina and persistence. This seems to be true of free-ranging dogs.

7.3   Courtship in free-ranging dogs

Although dogs can breed before 1 year, a convenient breakdown of age categories is: *pup dog* (birth to 4 months), *adolescent dog* (4 months to 1 year), *adult dog* (>1 year).[157] As already discussed, owned female dogs do not have a seasonal breeding pattern[158] and usually more than one annual reproductive period. Some free-ranging dogs have a single annual cycle similar to wild canids,[159] but others reportedly have more than one, in which case litters are born in May or June and November or December.[160] Street dogs in Katwa, India, evidently have a single mating period from August through October with parturition peaking in December and January.[161] Free-ranging dogs in West Bengal, India, have one annual cycle[162] and the same might be true elsewhere (e.g. Mexico, Australia).[163]

Male dogs do not show seasonal changes in scent-marking, perhaps because spermatogenesis is continuous.[164] Some dogs reportedly pair off while the female is in heat, but the bond is only temporary and the female almost always raises her pups alone.[165] A male dog, having mated, seldom demonstrates permanent attachment to the female, thereby relinquishing any possibility of a familial role. A free-ranging female in heat is quickly surrounded by suitors, and how their interactions sort out can give the mistaken impression of a male dominance hierarchy.[166]

One conjecture has dogs discarding monogamy as a result of domestication. Living near humans provides ample opportunities to scavenge, and the dependence of one dog on another, or weaned pups on their parents, is no longer necessary. As a researcher put it, "in an artificial environment of unlimited human care, promiscuity works."[167] The validity of this hypothesis has yet to be tested, and any such experiment would be prolonged. One way might be to release dogs onto an isolated island with large game and return at 10-year intervals to monitor any tendency toward reversion to monogamy and true pack behavior.

An estrous group, as mentioned, consists of an estrous female accompanied by males attempting to mate with her. Some will be familiar, known to the female by having been littermates but more commonly unrelated dogs with home ranges overlapping hers. Others are likely to be strangers having temporarily abandoned their familiar routes for an opportunity to mate. In the fervor of the moment brief fights break out among the males, along with growling, snarling, and other aggressive displays. Sometimes the female attacks one of the males if he becomes too persistent. Her aggression toward strangers and friends is similar, and she tends to turn on them only if bitten or annoyed by unwanted attention. Over her estrous period a female might mate with several males, each contributing genetic material to the future litter.

Some females mate indiscriminately but most, like owned dogs, seldom mate with strangers and allow only certain males – in some instances only one male – to mount while being courted by several.[168] Strange dogs are consequently shoved to the periphery, their breeding opportunities much reduced. Female strays, like owned females, also show clear mating preferences. An estrous group might form for 2 hours or so each day during which the familiar males persist twice as long as strangers and involve them in proportionately more fights.[169]

A female in heat fails to attract all males in the vicinity. Many, both familiar and unfamiliar, simply continue making the rounds through their home ranges, although strangers are most likely to behave this way.[170] Even familiar males that had mated previously with the female sometimes decline to pursue her during a subsequent estrus.

Any so-called dominance hierarchy among males of an estrous group is fleeting, lasting in sum a few hours over several days, during which time males of all perceived ranks arrive and depart. I say so-called because in clearly defined hierarchies the dominant male usually breeds while his subordinates stand around hoping he becomes distracted and provides them a furtive chance with the female. In the lives of free-ranging dogs, female choice means that a handsome prince who vanquishes most rivals can still lose the lady to his gnomic groom. Large, aggressive males are not necessarily preferred choices.[171] The smallest and most timid often have breeding opportunities, which suggests that large size and aggressiveness have limited selective advantage if these qualities fail to exclude other males from breeding. Confusion and chaos also factor in. Among strays in Bhabanibera, India, only 10% of mountings resulted in locks, and successful copulations correlated inversely with the number of courting males.[172] Up to 10 males courted estrous females, and copulations were unsuccessful when more than three males were present.[173]

In a study of the breeding behavior of street dogs in Newark, New Jersey, rank was assessed in descending order according to the number of fights initiated by males of an estrous group against potential rivals.[174] Estrous groups usually formed early in the day, and most had dispersed by late morning. The observations involved two females that over a summer and winter of the following year were part of eight estrous groups. The perceived dominance rank-order proved independent of body size, meaning that big males held no advantage over small ones. Mating success (achievement of intromission followed by a copulatory lock) was then assessed by observing 106 mounting attempts. Only six were by strange males, none successful. Success by familiar males showed no positive correlation with number of attempts. During a single day of observation, one of two successful copulations involved the male of lowest perceived rank. Familiar males appeared to be more dominant and clearly more successful than strangers, and even those of higher rank usually left the group after having mated. An aggressive male is able to get closer to the female, and by briefly excluding rivals can mount more often. However, proximity and persistence alone offer no ultimate advantages.

The notion of a true male dominance hierarchy in estrous groups of free-ranging dogs rings false because it appears to offer no selective advantage. Certainly, the fittest dog in any such group leaves its progeny behind, but in this case the top dog is no more likely to breed than an underdog and therefore is no more fit despite being the better fighter. Furthermore, instead of preventing others from mating with the female, a successful male then leaves the field to his rivals, granting them equal opportunity to impregnate her. In addition, any perceived dominance ranking is based on an arbitrary system of measurement. Attaining the position of top dog, whatever its advantages, undoubtedly involves more than the inclination to start fights. In animals as diverse as insects and primates, aggression and rank are often no measure of reproductive success.[175]

In summary, both the extent of a male's familiarity with the estrous female and female choice – not rank in any dominance hierarchy or body size relative to the other males – are the important factors influencing mating success in dogs. Although estrous groups are without social order, sexual selection could be a remnant of a monogamous wolfish ancestry.[176]

The dingo's reproductive cycle incorporates features of both the wolf and domestic dog.[177] Where dingoes admix with dogs, the pattern becomes more dog-like. In common with wolves, the breeding season commences later with increasing latitude (Table 7.1). Dingoes at southern temperate latitudes breed in June; those in arid central Australia begin mating in April and May (austral autumn), although droughts can postpone the process for up to 2 months or halt

Table 7.1. Months when dingo litters are born in Asia and Australia. Blank months indicate no data or incomplete data. *Source*: Corbett (1995: 41, table 3.5). Material reprinted from Laurie Corbett, *The Dingo in Australia and Asia*. Used by permission of the publisher, Cornell University Press, and by JB Books, Marleston, South Australia.

		Oct	Nov	Dec	Jan	Feb	Mar	Apr	May	Jun	Jul	Aug	Sep
Asia													
Bangladesh	25°N	◄	◄	◄	◄								◄
Myanmar	21°N	◄	◄	◄	◄								
Laos	18°N	◄	◄	◄							◄		◄
Thailand	14°N	◄	◄	◄	◄	◄	◄				◄	◄	◄
Philippines	10°N	◄	◄	◄	◄	◄							
Sulawesi	0°	◄		◄	◄	◄	◄	◄	◄	◄	◄	◄	◄
Australia													
North	13°S				◄				◄	◄	◄	◄	◄
West	21°S					◄			◄	◄	◄	◄	
Central	24°S								◄	◄	◄	◄	◄
Southeast	37°S		◄	◄	◄	◄	◄	◄	◄	◄	◄	◄	◄

it completely. Relentless crossing with dogs has made the dingo's reproductive cycle more difficult to predict. Dates in which breeding occurs at a given location can vary widely. The fact that breeding by dingoes in Victoria's highlands occurs over 7 months has been attributed to interbreeding with dogs,[178] which have no specific season.

Males reach *sexual maturity* at 1–3 years. In temperate locations they assume the physiological and behavioral characteristics of domestic dogs, capable and motivated to mate anytime. Males in arid regions undergo cyclical gonadal regression and recrudescence and breed annually. Despite seasonal regression, the testes produce spermatozoa all year, just far fewer when out of phase, and hormonal changes probably account for the lack of motivation at this time. Captive dingoes in central Australia ignored proestrous domestic dogs when out of phase but mated with them during their own breeding season. Dingoes taken to Canberra in the temperate southeast assumed the local pattern of no seasonal cycling and the continuous capacity to breed.

Females attain reproductive age at about 2 years and typically experience a single annual cycle. External signs of proestrus are the same as in the wolf and domestic dog (bloody vaginal discharge, swollen vulva), and cellular changes in the vagina follow the same pattern. Proestrus and estrus are also similar and perhaps slightly longer (10–12 days).[179] Proestrous bleeding can last 2–3 weeks.[180] An undocumented observation of captive animals claimed tumescence of the vulva and bleeding to continue 40–50 days prior to mating.[181] Duration of proestrus in wild populations might be closer to that of the wolf's. Generally only the dominant animal in a group reproduces while subordinates go through pseudopregnancy (Chapter 8). Dingo-dog backcrosses become increasingly dog-like, with females experiencing more than one annual estrus.

Dingoes at London Zoo went through annual reproductive cycles in boreal autumn but with widely disparate dates of mating (15 October and 20 December).[182] Males and females urine-marked more frequently in the mating season, and males followed the females closely. Proestrous females were followed by males attempting to lick and mount them. Aggression among males increased, sometimes requiring them to be separated. Behavioral estrus lasted only 3–4 days, during which females courted males and presented themselves to be mounted with tails turned to the side. At least one female showed evidence of mate preference. Dingoes from New Guinea housed apart from the Australian dingoes mated in mid-September.

7.4   Courtship in wolves

Two wolves compose a pack, a social group of two. A lone wolf deciding to pair with another loner "is essentially identical to a group of one choosing not to repel a joiner."[183] Although this is a different arrangement than seen in free-ranging dogs, in neither case is dominance ↔ submission a likely selection factor during initial mate choice.

There are no estrous groups in wolf packs dominated by a monogamous breeding pair. During aerial surveys of wild wolves in February the dominant male and female could be told from other pack members by their propinquity, the male staying at the female's side or following her closely.[184] Mated wolves sleep closer together during the breeding season than at other times of year.[185] Captive wolves behave similarly, the male keeping in nearly constant haptic contact with his mate.[186]

Pairs of breeding wolves often urine-mark intensively, one animal over-marking where the other has just urinated. Dilution of estrous urine from female dogs with male dog urine decreases its attractiveness to males;[187] over-marking by wolves serves the presumed function of masking the female's reproductive status and discouraging male competition.[188] Over-marking has been proposed as an important element in pair bonding,[189] although if pair bonding is indeed the endgame, this hypothesis lies fallow without a testable mechanism. In this case compounds in urine could serve to physiologically "prime" both animals as they approach reproductive readiness. Subsequently, frequent mutual sniffing of scent-marks then reinforces and synchronizes reproductive timing.[190]

Surgery-induced anosmia resulted in decreased urine-marking by an adult female and was associated with her failure to pair-bond.[191] Anosmia of females seemed to have no adverse effects on mating, maternal behavior, or hormonal profiles. Inexperienced anosmic males did not court females and failed to respond to female courtship cues despite having testosterone concentrations and testis sizes the same as fully intact males. An experienced anosmic male did mate successfully. Thus olfactory "priming" of naïve males by urinary and vaginal odors of proestrous females might be necessary to induce courtship. Experienced males appear capable of circumventing olfactory signals and relying instead on visual, auditory, or tactile cues.

Almost everything known about courtship in wolves comes from watching them in captivity. Like dogs, wolves[192] and eastern coyotes[193] show mate preferences. Literature on the behavior of wolves in confinement paints their societies as disturbed and incomplete, offering only partial insight into courtship and pair-bond formation. This is especially true when mature animals are matched haphazardly and thrown together with little regard for factors other than pup production.[194] Wild wolves form pairs at all times of the year,[195] not just during the reproductive phase. Monogamous attachments probably derive from friendship and familiarity strengthened by traveling and foraging together and eventually establishing a territory (Chapter 5). Pair formation is not limited to the female's estrous period as it sometimes is in dogs, but rather a prelude to a lifelong relationship based on shared responsibilities.

Zimen's observations of the captive group he monitored (Chapter 9) are relevant here. Finsterau, the dominant female, came into heat in mid-February, although for months previously she had been "pressing against Wölfchen [the dominant male] and whimpering, rolling on her back in front of him, and pulling his coat."[196] Despite her being in estrus (as shown by vaginal bleeding), Wölfchen showed no interest. Näschen, another male, assumed Wölfchen's courtship role and he and Finsterau eventually mated.[197]

During their courtship, Näschen followed Finsterau everywhere, licking her coat and genitals and staying in nearly constant physical contact. Finsterau approached Näschen sideways and then from the front and turned her tail aside to be mounted. Afterward each wolf licked its own genitals. Then, "Finsterau dashed excitedly at Näschen, jumped up at him, whimpered, and rolled on her back in front of him exactly like a wolf showing friendly submission."[198] The others were not passive bystanders. They "also began running about, and they all ran around one another in friendly, excited fashion." After the mating season Wölfchen remained dominant, but Näschen and Finsterau formed a permanent bond and were seldom apart. Wölfchen often stayed with them, and "these three animals now formed the inner circle of the pack around which the other members revolved."[199]

Social animals can attain sexual maturity but not demonstrate *functional maturity* by participating directly in reproduction, a situation heightened when same-sex competitors render any attempt to breed dangerous or otherwise not worthwhile. Many wolves that fail to reproduce are therefore physiologically capable but repressed socially from doing so.[200] Subordinate females allowed to reproduce are obviously fertile and not physiologically suppressed.[201] A young adult wolf in the wild can circumvent the problem by deferring functional maturity and staying in its natal pack instead of immigrating. By waiting until its perceived fitness "is higher than that of other individuals that attempt to reproduce at the same age and under the same conditions," it disperses to find a mate.[202]

The intense agonism and attendant displays of dominance ↔ submission reported in captive wolves are largely artifacts of confinement and the subsequent inability to disperse (Chapter 9). Sexual competition among captive wolves can prevent subordinate females from breeding. The situation is often reversed simply by placing these animals in packs having different social compositions,[203] thereby simulating a sort of *faux* dispersal. Captive wolves aggressively interrupt each other's attempts at courtship and sometimes continue to direct aggression at animals that are copulating and locked. Such behavior is uncommon in the wild, perhaps evidence that tensions are discharged harmlessly when space is not restricted. Monitoring of wolves in Yellowstone showed slightly increased aggression during the mating season but no overall increase in agonistic behavior compared with other times of the year.[204]

Social activity, including courtship, intensifies with the onset of the breeding season. Large size and even being the dominant wolf in a pack does not guarantee breeding.[205] In a pack of wild Russian wolves the breeding male over four consecutive years was small, lame, and "not a fierce competitor."[206] In an extended family observed by Murie at Denali there were two breeding pairs, but the dominant male had no mate.[207]

In captive wolves, the younger males begin following the females even before they become receptive, attempting to sniff and lick their reproductive parts and making clumsy attempts to mount them.[208] Usually they are rebuffed but not deterred. The drive is intense: unpaired wild wolves have been seen following female foxes.[209] Once the females come fully into heat the older males begin to court them. Instead of trying to immediately mount a female, a male prances around her, placing his forelegs on the ground and keeping his hindquarters elevated. He wags his tail, nips the female's ears, face, and back, and attempts to mount her sideways. If the female accepts him she turns her tail to the side, and he mounts. Reciprocal courtship is common. The female approaches the male submissively and backs up to his head, tail turned to the side.[210]

In two captive groups in Minnesota all female adults, adolescents, and three of five older pups reached proestrus.[211] Males that courted most received the most courtship in return from females. These males had the highest *testosterone responses*.[212] They were the most aggressive toward other males, received the least aggression in return, and scent-marked most often. Only females that actually produced pups actively scent-marked. Subordinate males in the presence of dominant males did not scent-mark. The sexual behavior expressed by subordinate males showed no relationship to aggression, either emitted by them or received from dominant males. It did, however, correlate directly with female courtship and testosterone response. Males with the highest testosterone responses directed the most aggression at those with the lowest responses. They also expressed more sexual behavior toward females.

All females that ovulated courted the males. Among captive wolves in estrus males were courted more often by subordinate females than by dominant females.[213] Not all estrous females were equally attractive to males as measured by sexual attention received (i.e. male courtship). However, receipt of sexual attention did not correlate positively with the frequency and intensity with which she courted a male, but with duration of her vaginal discharge. Female courtship, on the other hand, correlated inversely with discharge duration. Males of low status were courted more often by low-status females. These males were more attracted to high-status females, which courted them less. In sum, no evidence has been found that social interaction suppresses the reproductive cycles of wolves. Nearly all eligible pack members in the two captive groups where high stress can be expected went through normal physiological cycles during the reproductive phase, becoming sexually mature at the appointed time with only the dominant animals attaining functional maturity. Biology has few unbreakable rules, and in some captive groups the parent of a litter might be a subordinate wolf of either sex.[214]

How do wild wolves avoid inbreeding? The high level of *heterozygosity* characteristic of healthy wolf packs is attributable entirely to active choices wolves make to breed with unrelated partners. This has been shown with striking clarity in the Yellowstone packs, where "inbreeding avoidance is nearly absolute despite the high probability of within-pack inbreeding opportunities and extensive inter-pack kinship ties between adjacent packs."[215] The same occurred at Algonquin Provincial Park after the killing of wolves in areas surrounding the park became prohibited.[216] Both situations are temporary with inbreeding inevitable unless unrelated animals are recruited or imported. At least for now, the Yellowstone wolves continue to show vibrant genetic diversity.[217]

What accounts for *inbreeding avoidance*? The obvious explanations of familiarity and kin recognition (Chapter 8) fail as explanations at a mechanistic level. One possibility is activity by the *major histocompatibility complex (MHC)*, a polymorphic complex of genes that helps initiate the immune response; that is, the discrimination of self from not-self, thus making possible the recognition of infectious disease organisms. It also forms a remarkable link with the olfactory systems.[218] In this context MHC genes are not pheromones but ubiquitous components of the vertebrate immune system. Together with bacterial activity they influence body odor and subsequently mate choice based on odor attractiveness, serving as olfactory "signatures." Most studies have involved mice and humans, and mouse data suggest that dissimilar odors attract most strongly.[219] The reasoning is that odors smelling "not like me" are likely "not related to me." Metaphorically, this means that what a mouse smells on another mouse is degree of relatedness predicated ultimately on genotype. Mating with a mouse that smells completely different might offer some assurance of outbreeding, and the same pattern could also be at work among Yellowstone's wolf packs.

A mouse detects chemical signals through its MOS and VNS (Chapter 3). That some MHC genes activate VRs indicates a vomeronasal organ function in detection of sex attractants. However, the MOS also participates, and it detects not just volatile organic aerosols as once thought but nonvolatile compounds too.[220] *Like the VNO, the MOE requires direct physical contact with the source of scent before nonvolatile odorants associated with social recognition signals can be detected.*[221] This finding has astonishing implications. It offers a testable model for linking odorant properties with specific neuroreceptors and thus assessing important facets of social behavior based on something more substantial than observation and conjecture. As mentioned, interpreting behavior from observation alone remains speculative until validated biologically.

The canid VNO is less functional than thought previously, suggesting that pheromones (however defined) doubtfully play the dominant role once assumed, although in rodents the VNO and MOE act in concert. As mentioned, the requirement of direct odorant contact for both rodents and canids remains, in the latter case mediated almost entirely through the MOS, and this potentially explains why a male dog or wolf sniffs and licks estrous urine, sniffs and licks the female's proestrous vulva. It also offers an explanation of female choice at a molecular level by posing testable hypotheses of how the female of an estrous group makes selections of certain male dogs and rejects others. What we have assumed to be choices based on familiarity could have an alternative explanation: the males selected are those that to the female smell most different from herself. Consider this: "*When peptide/MHC complexes are released into the extracellular space and appear in urine and other bodily secretions ... any information contained in their chemical complexity becomes a property of the entire individual*."[222] This includes not just sexual attractiveness and availability, but degree of relatedness. At least in terms of smell, opposites attract.

Incest, like admixing, occurs if mates are scarce or unavailable,[223] but its occurrence in undisturbed populations is unusual.[224] Where it has been studied in the wild (e.g. Alaska, Michigan, Minnesota, Yellowstone) the suppression of incest is facilitated by: (1) active avoidance of breeding with related pack members, (2) dispersal from the natal pack, (3) pack splitting, and (4) frequent turnover of breeders and recruitment of replacements because the tenure of breeding-age wolves (about 4 years) is shorter than the typical lifespan of a pack.[225] A claim that the earlier maturation of females (Chapter 8) is a factor inhibiting breeding among littermates[226] has not been validated.

Inbreeding is pronounced in some European populations.[227] In Scandinavia, for example, a population of wolves that included 28 breeding pairs in 2002 had been founded in about 1980 by three immigrants from Finland.[228] Inbreeding was unavoidable.[229] *Inbreeding depression* followed, eventually reducing average litter size by 1.15 pups. The arrival of a lone male in 1993 added genetic diversity but was insufficient to eliminate the effect.[230] In an unusual situation three female littermates of a Finnish pack stayed after the dominant female was shot, two of which mated with their father, the other with their brother.[231] To date, no inbreeding depression has been seen in Mexican and red wolf captive breeding programs despite the small number of founders.[232]

A few carnivorans are not susceptible to inbreeding depression, and for these dispersal has little evolutionary benefit.[233] Canids are among those affected. Consequences are reduced recruitment of young wolves and subsequent population decline,[234] and congenital defects.[235] Severe and prolonged inbreeding of wolves in Swedish zoos culminated in inbreeding depression manifested as a reduction in the average weight of pups, shorter lifespan, smaller litter size, and sharply increased heredity blindness.[236]

The introduction of wolves into Yellowstone starting in 1995 continues to be an interesting experiment on inbreeding avoidance. No wolves had lived there for 70 years.[237] With game plentiful and exploitation outlawed, opportunities arose to watch and measure in accelerated motion all nuances of wolf society. Most observations until then had been of established packs. Unless viewed over several years this can be like describing a complex machine without any notion of how its parts have been assembled. Pack formation and splitting in Yellowstone could be monitored from the start. Data from known genealogies would reveal how wolves dispersed, avoided inbreeding, defended territories, and hunted ungulates.

Establishment of a new pack commences with a breeding pair, the fundamental unit of wolf societies.[238] The newly released wolves in Yellowstone formed seven packs initially, four of which maintained the same core group of individuals at least through the first 10 years.[239] Some of these animals had been released with known pack members, a strategy aimed at enhancing reproductive potential from the start. Fifteen packs formed later on their own, only four from pairings of single wolves that had dispersed from their natal packs.

If the breeding unit of a typical pack consists of only two unrelated individuals, how can inbreeding among the rest, which are assumed to be siblings, be avoided? We know that the *effective population size*, defined as the number of breeders, is much smaller than the census population.[240] The long-term viability of wolf populations therefore depends on how effectively this exclusive mating system sustains genetic diversity.

Incest is more likely to happen in captivity[241] and in small isolated populations like that of Isle Royale where heterozygosity diminishes by 13% with each generation, or every 4.2 years (80% from founding in the late 1940s until 1997).[242] Social repression of subordinates by the dominant pair ordinarily prevents any mating by siblings. This structure crumbles if one of the breeding pair is somehow removed, and at such times incest is particularly striking in captive groups.[243]

8   Reproduction and parenting

Spontaneous maternal care is unusual in mammals. The behavior we think of as nurturing requires a flood of priming hormones during pregnancy, compounds produced or regulated by the *placenta*. "Hence, the onset, maintenance and termination of maternal behaviour are controlled by hormones which, in turn, are released in response to stimuli from the foetus."[1] Being helpless, altricial young (Chapter 5) require lots of attention. The hormones of pregnancy (see below) induce denning, develop the mammary glands, and ready the brain for maternal care, which to continue through weaning and beyond requires both a fetus and later a neonate. Intensity of maternal behavior becomes associated inversely with development of the young: the mother leaves her pups longer once they can thermoregulate consistently and become less dependent on her warmth; her milk production diminishes concomitantly with decreased nursing.

8.1   The reproductive cycle – part 2

The discussion in this section is limited to the dog unless otherwise stated. *Diestrus* comprises the stage in which corpora lutea are completely functional;[2] that is, the *luteal phase* of the female reproductive cycle.[3] It follows estrus and extends 55–75 days.[4] *Behavioral diestrus* is the period starting at the end of estrus when the female refuses to let the male mount.[5] Her restlessness subsides along with the vaginal discharge and swelling of the vulva.[6] External signs as diestrus progresses are those of pregnancy or pseudopregnancy (see below). About 20 days after initiation of diestrus the corpora lutea start breaking down (*luteolysis*), and the endometrial lining of the uterus begins to regress; later in pregnant females and some that are pseudopregnant, the mammary glands mature and milk-secreting tissues develop.[7]

The early luteal phase starts the first day of ovulation and continues about 5 days.[8] Most of the follicles (>90% in one study) will have ovulated by 96 h following the LH peak, the majority within 24–72 h.[9] *Endocrinological diestrus* is characterized by a rise in progesterone that begins 6–10 days after LH spikes,[10] persists through pregnancy and *pseudopregnancy* ("false") pregnancy, and is the distinguishing feature of diestrus.[11] Endocrinological diestrus is what I mean by diestrus. Signs of *clinical (overt) pseudopregnancy* include distended abdomen, aggression, licking, digging behavior, "nesting" behavior, anorexia, whimpering, maternal behavior directed

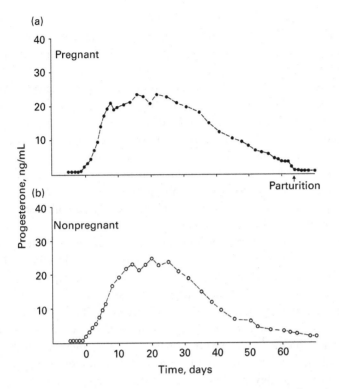

Figure 8.1 Mean plasma progesterone in nonpregnant and pregnant beagles. Values for the 14 days prepartum are aligned to a common day 64 parturition.
Source: Concannon, P. W., W. Hansel, and W. J. Visek. (1975). The ovarian cycle of the bitch: plasma estrogen, LH and progesterone. *Biology of Reproduction* **13**: 112–121. Copyright by Society for the Study of Reproduction, Inc.

toward objects or other animals including phantom or surrogate pups, weight gain, and swelling of the mammary glands sometimes with milk production.[12] Lactation is stimulated and sustained by self-nursing or adoption of unrelated neonates.[13]

Cellular changes in vaginal smears are reliable markers of when diestrus begins and ends.[14] The path traced by progesterone is also useful for defining its temporal limits.[15] Principal endocrinological differences between pseudopregnant and pregnant dogs during diestrus involve LH and FSH. The concentration of FSH, which had fallen to baseline values at the end of estrus, now increases and remains steady throughout diestrus and the beginning of anestrus during *covert* (*endocrinological*) *pseudopregnancy*.[16] In pregnant dogs, FSH increases steadily to about day 60, declining with parturition and remaining low through lactation.[17]

The gradual decline in progesterone over the 8 weeks of pregnancy ends abruptly 24–48 h prior to parturition[18] (Fig. 8.1a) and signals onset of anestrus.[19] Progesterone is required to sustain pregnancy,[20] and when the concentration falls to 1–2 ng/mL parturition occurs.[21] Progesterone differentiates and modulates the functions of the *endometrium* (lining of the uterus) and attachment of the placenta, and prevents premature uterine contractions.[22] Birth is induced by a sharp increase in the estrogen/progesterone ratio caused by the drop in progesterone to <2 ng/mL beginning 24–36 h prepartum (Fig. 8.1a).[23] Its rapid decline culminates in destruction of the corpora lutea.[24] Estrogen, which has remained slightly elevated through parturition, then declines.[25] The progression is similar in pseudopregnant females (Fig. 8.1b). Diestrus continues until progesterone production subsides during luteinization, peaking in early to mid-diestrus and declining gradually to baseline concentrations 51–82 days following the spike in LH.[26]

Progesterone is perhaps the only ovarian steroid needed to sustain pregnancy.[27] Elevated estrogen during diestrus has negative effects. Inserting estradiol implants into pregnant females to keep levels abnormally high induced abortion, resorption, or retention of dead fetuses *in utero* at days 36–48 prepartum.[28] Females that carried fetuses nearly to term died along with them unless saved by Caesarian section. Maintenance of progesterone during pseudopregnancy is thought to depend on LH.[29] However, LH can rise as progesterone is falling in both pregnant and pseudopregnant dogs, suggesting that cessation of diestrus might not result from insufficient LH.[30]

Uterine implantation of the dog embryo is delayed compared with many species, not occurring until 17–22 days after the female is first mounted,[31] at which point estrogen and progesterone secretion increase.[32] The fetus is protected because estrogen does not rise above proestrous levels, perhaps a result of the increased plasma volume.[33] The corpora lutea meanwhile regresses in three luteal phases each taking about a third the length of pregnancy or pseudopregnancy: 0–21, 22–43, and 44–63 days.[34] Remnants of former corpora lutea are still detectible after 2–3 reproductive cycles. About a month postpartum, or 90 days after onset of estrus, the endometrium is sloughed.[35] Sloughing is less extensive in pseudopregnant dogs and completed about 2 weeks sooner.

Prolactin, like LH and FSH a gonadotropin, is the principal pituitary hormone sustaining steroid production by the corpus luteum.[36] Prolactin is modulated by progesterone, and its hormonal function is to induce lactation.[37] *Relaxin*, produced by the placenta,[38] is the sole protein associated with pregnancy in the dog.[39] Its concentration increases in synchrony with prolactin (Fig. 8.2) and might aid in promoting progesterone by the luteal cells; alternatively, it could function indirectly through prolactin mediation. Relaxin's specific role is unclear.

Rhythms of prolactin secretion in mammals can generally be changed by altering photoperiod or *melatonin* concentration or by removing the *pineal gland*.[40] Lengthening daylight presumably reduces melatonin production thereby permitting a rise in secretion of *gonadotropic hormones (gonadotropins)*.[41] With the possible exception of the basenji, which cycles annually,[42] the domestic dog's reproductive cycle does not appear to be regulated by photoperiod.[43] The wolf might be similar. Removing the pineal gland of captive wolves failed to affect reproductive timing of either males or females.[44] The wolf's secretion of prolactin appears to be photoperiodic, peaking just before the summer solstice,[45] but photoperiod was not considered the causative agent behind reproductive cycling. That changes in day length have no effect on wolves seems strange, and this experiment should be repeated. If later results are the same then reproduction in

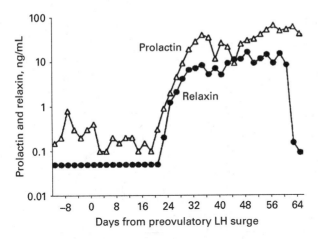

Figure 8.2 Mean concentrations of prolactin and relaxin during pregnancy in beagles. Ordinate is a log scale to clarify the extent of the concomitant rise of relaxin and the initial pregnancy-specific increased in prolactin.
Source: Concannon, P. W. (2009). Endocrinologic control of normal canine ovarian function. *Reproduction in Domestic Animals* **44** (Suppl. 2): 3–15. This material is reproduced with permission of John Wiley & Sons, Inc.

wolves and dogs appears to be regulated instead by neuroendocrine components modified by timing of the prior luteal phase, by hormonal spikes, and evidently unknown mechanisms.[46] Dogs and wolves are the same species,[47] making common endocrinological patterns likely.

Most rodents and many other mammals are long-day breeders, the onset of reproduction timed with the lengthening days of spring. Many ungulates (e.g. deer, moose) and others are short-day breeders, having cycles that commence with the shortening days of autumn. Wolves fall conveniently into neither category. They breed when daylength is shortest in mid- to late winter, a time when the rate of changing daylength is also slower.[48] Nonetheless, aspects of the wolf's life history seem adapted to photoperiodic effects. Like other wild canids they breed seasonally, with timing of mating and parturition becoming later with increasing latitude, and some extrinsic factor must be a physiological cue to end anestrus. However, the most complete test so far of the photoperiod hypothesis failed to affirm it.

Pinealectomy of captive pup wolves (age 5 months) and cervical-ganglionectomy of adolescents (age 16 months) of both sexes did not change attainment of puberty, which occurred on schedule along with sham-operated controls.[49] They matured, went through normal reproductive cycles, and displayed hormonal profiles no different from control animals. Dates of ovulation in treated versus untreated females were similar. Surgically induced anosmia performed on one male and one female with previous pinealectomies to test for a critical olfactory component somewhere in the reproductive cycle (Chapter 3) had no effect.

Prolactin levels in dogs start to increase 30 days after the first mating, rising abruptly in a transient surge a day or two before parturition (Fig. 8.3)[50] and is important in

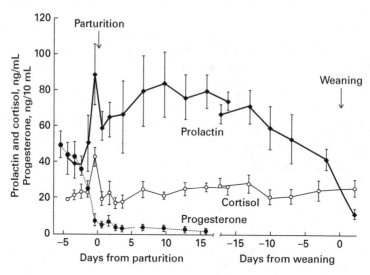

Figure 8.3 Mean (±SEM) serum concentrations of progesterone, cortisol, and prolactin during peripartum and lactation in beagles (*n* = 6–7).
Source: Concannon, P. W., J. P. McCann, and M. Temple. (1989). Biology and endocrinology of ovulation, pregnancy and parturition in the dog. *Journal of Reproduction and Fertility* (Suppl.) **38**: 3–25. © Society for Reproduction and Fertility (1993). Reproduced by permission.

developing and maintaining pseudopregnancy.[51] Pseudopregnant females experience a spike 2–3 times above ambient around day 57, or coinciding with the projected day of parturition.[52] Its rise might be a response to declining progesterone.[53] Thereafter the level varies with frequency and duration of nursing by the pups, dropping slowly as the nursing period proceeds before falling abruptly after weaning.[54] Besides initiating and maintaining lactation prolactin is involved in molting of the winter coat in wolves.[55] Because the seasonal spike occurs in all pack members – males, females, dominants, subordinates – prolactin might be important in sustaining parental care and inducing helping behavior (see below) by the rest (Figs. 8.4 and 8.5; note the higher prolactin concentrations in pregnant females and mated males). Even castrated and ovariectomized animals in captive groups show a seasonal peak in prolactin.

Cortisol (also called *hydrocortisone*), a corticosteroid, spikes the day before parturition, although its rise is not a prerequisite for parturition.[56] Part of its concentration in the mother's blood might represent fetal secretion.[57] Stress is not the causative agent, and the spike appears to be a normal physiological response.[58] Plasma LH remains steady through diestrus. However, estradiol rises again early in diestrus and stays high through the luteal phase (21–42 pg/mL),[59] probably originating from the ovary or corpora lutea.

Gestation in both wolves and domestic dogs is commonly said to be 60–65 days.[60] This refers to *true gestation length*, a definition based on endocrinological events, not external observation. *Apparent gestation length* (time from a fertile mating to parturition), which is based on observation, averages 64 days in

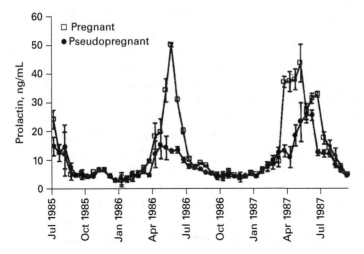

Figure 8.4 Mean (±SD?) prolactin concentrations of pregnant (*n* = 3) and nonpregnant (*n* = 3) wolves.
Source: Kreeger, T. J., U. S. Seal, Y. Cohen, E. D. Plotka, and C. S. Asa. (1991). Characterization of prolactin secretion in gray wolves (*Canis lupus*). *Canadian Journal of Zoology* **69**: 1366–1374. Copyright nrcresearch press. Reprinted with permission.

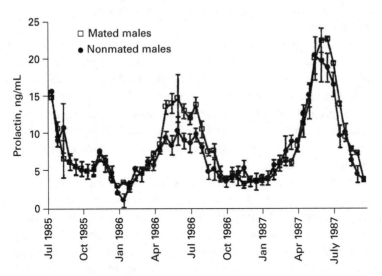

Figure 8.5 Mean (±SD?) prolactin concentrations of intact males paired with pregnant (*n* = 3) and pseudopregnant (*n* = 3) females.
Source: Kreeger, T. J., U. S. Seal, Y. Cohen, E. D. Plotka, and C. S. Asa. (1991). Characterization of prolactin secretion in gray wolves (*Canis lupus*). *Canadian Journal of Zoology* **69**: 1366–1374. Copyright nrcresearch press. Reprinted with permission.

the dog but ranges from 56 to 68 days, and parturition might not occur until 72 days from the first mating.[61] In captive dingoes, apparent gestation is 61–69 days, or longer than domestic dogs and dingo-dogs.[62] In eastern coyotes the average is 63 days.[63]

The extended range in dogs is attributable to variable time intervals between mating and peaking of LH, which influences all subsequent factors (e.g. ovulation, sperm penetration of the ovum, fertilization, passage of developing embryos into the uterus). Matings up to 8 days following the LH surge (i.e. 8 days before diestrus)[64] are often fertile, but a pregnancy after that is unusual, often resulting in an apparent gestation length of 55–57 days and the birth of only one or two pups.[65] Normal fertility results when breeding is 3–10 days prior to diestrus, or across an approximately 8-day span.[66] Conception within this interval can exceed 95% regardless of whether mating occurs on the first or the seventh day of estrus, and length of gestation is nearly identical in females bred early or late. In this same study the largest litter sizes were seen in females mated 4–10 days before the onset of diestrus.

The female's food intake fluctuates during estrus and early pregnancy. Her body mass increases over the gestation period (often by more than a third), with most of the gain in the second half.[67] One effect of this is a substantial increase in plasma volume that dilutes concentrations of circulating hormones.[68] In late pregnancy food intake is proportional to body mass. Also during the second half of pregnancy a dog's energy needs to rise by 30% to 45 grams of dry food per kilogram of body mass. Protein requirement increases by 50% to 15% of the diet. There is a need for carbohydrates, without which pups could be stillborn or die as early neonates,[69] although the danger can be circumvented by supplying a minimum of 50% protein in the diet.[70]

A female dog becomes restless 2–3 days prepartum. She might pant, scratch the ground repeatedly, and enter the den or birth location. Her appetite often diminishes. The signs are inconsistent and variable.[71] The birth of a litter is ordinarily completed in <6 h but can extend to 24 h; about 40% of pups are born in posterior presentation. The female eats the placenta and licks the pups clean. As the pups start to nurse, nervous impulses from the nipples trigger a reflexive ejection of milk "and set in train [the] series of endocrine events involved in the maintenance of lactation."[72]

No clinical signs mark the end of diestrus and beginning of anestrus, but the first day on which progesterone returns to baseline concentrations is sometimes used as an arbitrary break.[73] *Anestrus*, the fourth and last stage of the female reproductive cycle, is obligate,[74] lasts longer in monestrous than in polyestrous species[75] (2–10 months in the domestic dog), and ends at the start of proestrus and commencement of a new reproductive cycle.[76] Length varies considerably among individuals and by breed – about 36 weeks in collies but 20–22 weeks in the Alsatian.[77] Dogs that have become pregnant have a slightly shorter anestrus than pseudopregnant dogs.[78]

Throughout this part of the cycle the reproductive system moves toward stasis as the corpora lutea continue to regress, often called the time of "ovarian quiescence" because no visible signs of reproductive activity are evident.[79] An anestrous dog exhibits no interest in courtship and sex. She has no vaginal discharge, and the vulva shrinks to normal size. Her coat often becomes glossier; she gains weight and becomes more alert to her surroundings.[80] The tissues remain responsive to stimulation by LH and FSH,[81] which in the cycle just ended had pulsed in concert

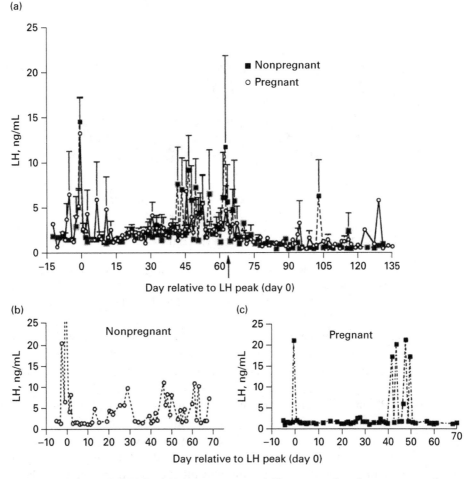

Figure 8.6 (a) Mean (±SEM) of 10 nonpregnant and 10 pregnant beagles over a complete reproductive cycle. Arrow corresponds to mean day of parturition in the pregnant group (day 65 after the LH peak). (b) Pattern of LH secretion for one nonpregnant dog. (c) Pattern of LH secretion for one pregnant dog.
Source: Onclin, K., B. Murphy, and J. P. Verstegen. (2002). Comparisons of estradiol, LH and FSH patterns in pregnant and nonpregnant beagle bitches. *Theriogenology* **57**: 1957–1972. Copyright by Society of Theriogenology. Reprinted with permission of Elsevier.

through proestrus and estrus.[82] Estrogen and other hormones remain at low levels while secretions of them continue, and the pituitary becomes increasingly sensitive to *gonadotropin-releasing hormone (GnRH)*[83] in preparation to release LH, FSH, and prolactin. Concentrations of FSH necessary to initiate the growth of new follicles double until diminishing early in proestrus.[84] A week or two before onset of proestrus the levels of LH and estrogen rise, initiating a new reproductive cycle.[85]

As shown (Fig. 8.6), LH returns to baseline levels following the surge associated with ovulation on day 0 (Chapter 7), but the concentration is lower in nonpregnant dogs through the normal time of parturition. Between days 40 and 65 (the

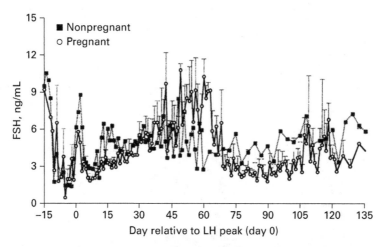

Figure 8.7 Mean (±SEM) daily plasma concentrations of FSH in 10 nonpregnant and 10 pregnant beagles.
Source: Onclin, K., B. Murphy, and J. P. Verstegen. (2002). Comparisons of estradiol, LH and FSH patterns in pregnant and nonpregnant beagle bitches. *Theriogenology* **57**: 1957–1972. Copyright by Society of Theriogenology. Reprinted with permission of Elsevier.

last third of pregnancy) the levels were baseline and pulsatile in both groups, the amplitude of pulses in the pregnant group more muted. From days 70 to 135, or well into anestrus, LH concentrations were <1 ng/mL in both groups with occasional low-amplitude spikes.[86]

Plasma FSH varied considerably among dogs, although a between-group pattern was evident (Fig. 8.7). In nonpregnant females concentrations rose from the end of estrus to 3–6 ng/mL and remained steady. In pregnant dogs FSH increased steadily to 10.3 ng/mL from days 40 to 65, declined rapidly as parturition approached, remained low during lactation, and then increased to values similar to the nonpregnant group.[87] The trend of baseline LH through diestrus was increasing concentrations (pregnant animals) and pulsatility (nonpregnant animals). The pulses are concordant in anestrus, and as this stage proceeds FSH increases but LH does not.[88] Thus FSH is necessary to initiate follicular development at commencement of the next reproductive cycle.[89] Nonetheless, LH alone can stimulate proestrus: injecting anestrous females with LH induced proestrus within 7 days, fertile ovulations about 16 days later, and six of the seven dogs treated delivered typical litters.[90] This indicates that in normally cycling dogs anestrus is caused by inadequate LH secretion, and follicular development might not require increases in FSH greater than levels normally present throughout most of anestrus.[91]

8.2   Wolf dens and rendezvous sites

The opportunity to breed is short for most wolves. Reproductive success is sometimes lower in both wild and captive younger wolves.[92] Average breeding tenure even for a competent pair is brief, 4 years in Denali.[93] Neonatal wolves are under threat of predation in many locations. A breeding female remains at the den almost continuously until her pups are about 25 days old, when she might leave for up to 12 h to hunt or feed at a carcass.[94] Minnesota females were sometimes absent for as long as 17 h.[95] The female's time away depends on such factors as whether other pack members are providing adequate food for her and the young, game is plentiful (or adequate game is nearby), and how many in the pack are available to hunt.[96] Two wolf packs in southcentral Alaska left pups between ages 2 and 7 weeks unattended about 5% and 15% of the time.[97] At least two reasons for this variation are pack size and the nearness and availability of prey. Breeding females in SNF regularly left their dens starting in early May.[98] Dens in Denali were attended most of the time,[99] maybe because of a constant threat of bears. The danger can be immediate: a breeding female in the Finlayson Lake region was killed by a bear,[100] and bears also kill and eat pups, sometimes excavating the den to extract them.[101] In the Nelchina Basin two wolves were observed harassing a female bear (sow) and her cubs until they left the den area.[102]

The urge to den is hormonal. Corpora lutea are functional early in diestrus, and the progesterone they manufacture is responsible for denning behavior in female dogs.[103] The same is no doubt true of wolves. Most of what we know about den-digging has come from watching captive canids. This description is based on observations of an adult male and female and two adolescent female wolves housed in a 0.1 hectare enclosure.[104] Excavation of the first den started a month before parturition, and the work took several days. Labor on the second and third dens began shortly after the first was completed and was not finished until the pups were born. The male did most of the digging. The adult female helped occasionally, but the adolescents contributed very little. Digging activity was highest during twilight. The animals worked intermittently, alone and together. Digging sessions lasted from a few seconds to 5 minutes.[105]

Dens vary in shape and size even when made by the same individuals. These had entrance tunnels 138–183 cm long × 36–41 cm wide × 31–38 cm high, sloping to a depth of 0.5 m. At the base of the entrance tunnels was a transverse channel about 5 cm deep and banked slightly along the far edge that collected rainwater and helped keep the end chambers dry. The end chambers where the pups stayed measured 45–127 cm long × 70–117 cm wide × 36 cm high with a domed ceiling and floor that was slightly dished.

Having dug these dens, the wolves slept in them before and after the pups were born. The two adolescents at first slept in den 1 until the adult female displaced them and gave birth there. The male had initially preferred den 3, but relinquished it to the adolescents following the birth of the pups. On day 10 postpartum the mother moved her pups to den 2 and thereafter moved them often among all the dens.

Dens ordinarily are located near the core areas of territories.[106] A pregnant wolf in the wild starts digging dens 3–5 weeks before parturition. Many – sometimes most – dens at certain locations are appropriated fox dens that have been enlarged and otherwise renovated.[107] Like those of captive wolves, these can take several forms depending on terrain. In a flat landscape they can be dug directly into the ground, but otherwise a burrow is excavated from the side of a bank or ridge or underneath a rocky outcrop. A den might be simply a rock cave, a hollow log, a hole in a dead stump or tree, or an enlarged and modified rabbit, marmot, badger, or fox burrow.[108] One Idaho wolf gave birth in the chamber of an abandoned beaver dam.[109] Wolves on Vancouver Island denned at the base of a wind-felled tree or excavated caves at the bases of large living trees.[110] On Russia's open steppe "the wolves arrange their dens at the bottom of gullies or crevices with numerous secluded spots, in pits or precipitous banks surrounded by bushes, grass and hop plants."[111] Finnish wolves often use protected sites under the drooping branches of large spruces.[112]

Denali wolves denned in holes dug into sandy hillsides, underneath the bottom branches of conifers, in modified tunnels made by beavers, in natural caves and crevices, and even in the open in shallow pits.[113] Some sites had been used to rear generations of wolves, and new packs often use the dens of those that had occupied the territory previously.[114]

Wolves seem to prefer open den sites atop bluffs and along rivers[115] or fronting meadows.[116] The use of more than one den is common,[117] which might be in the same vicinity or 8–16 km apart. The preferred substratum is sandy or loamy. The entrance is oval, about 35 cm high × 63.5 wide. Tunnels are generally similar in size to the opening, the spaces seldom large enough for an adult wolf to stand, although some are big enough that two adults can pass. Typically, the entrance tunnel is 1.8–4.3 m long. An occasional tunnel might extend 9 m. No bedding is used, and the pups are reared on the dirt floor of the end chamber. Whatever form a den takes, its location is usually near water.[118]

An abandoned den on Isle Royale had a tunnel 51 cm high and 36 cm wide and extended into the hillside for 3.6 m with no chamber at the end.[119] A den found in the Canadian Rockies had a descending tunnel 41 cm high × 46 cm wide extending 2.1 m and terminating in an enlarged chamber.[120] Another dug into the side of a ridge had a tunnel that penetrated for 1.5 m before turning parallel to the ridge line and extending another 2.1 m. Both dens had two entrances. The entrance of a den in Denali was 41 cm high × 53 cm wide, that of another 38 cm high × 51 cm wide.[121]

As noted, if undisturbed, the same dens might be used year after year.[122] In the high Arctic where permafrost prevents deep excavation, the dens are often caves or spaces among rocks. Suitable sites are sometimes scarce[123] and good ones might be used by generations of wolves. The age of a musk ox bone dug up near a wolf den on Ellesmere Island was radiocarbon dated to 233 (±70) years.[124]

Migratory wolves that follow the Alaskan and Canadian caribou herds (Chapter 6) are territorial only while rearing pups. They prefer dens on the tundra to forested sites, and those near the tree line to all others.[125] Caribou are absent from boreal forests in early autumn, making wooded dens and rendezvous sites inconvenient, and dens on the tundra typically lack structural support and are more likely to collapse. The tree line is ideal. Caribou arriving from the north gather there preparing to enter the forest for the winter, making them available to wolf packs needing to feed large, mobile pups.

Neonatal wolves require food and warmth (Chapter 9), of which food is more important. Not all pup wolves have the luxury of cover. Some are born and raised in shallow depressions on open tundra, exposed from the moment of birth to snow, freezing rain, and cold wind.[126] In such cases the female is often alone. She leaves the pups unsheltered for long periods to forage, returning wet and muddy herself and ill equipped to provide much heat. Nonetheless, many of these pups survive and grow normally.

During the pups' first 2 months the female might move them periodically to other dens.[127] Only the mother and rarely a post-reproductive female carry the pups when changing den sites,[128] although in a captive pair of eastern coyotes both parents did this.[129] Dens are abandoned during June and July when the pack moves to a first rendezvous site.[130] *Rendezvous sites* "are similar to above-ground dens" where pups stay while the other pack members are hunting[131] and often used into autumn. As the name implies they serve as a gathering place for the pack. While pups are still at the den, and later at the rendezvous site, pack members often sleep and rest nearby when not foraging.[132] Occupancy of specific sites ranges from 2 to 4 weeks,[133] and a female and other pack members intermittently occupy one or more of them,[134] quickly shifting the pups to another if disturbed, as by humans or bears.[135] Rendezvous sites are not large: three used by a pack in southern Ontario averaged about 0.4 hectares.[136] Typically they are near water.[137] A rendezvous site can be an open meadow bordered by forest, even an emergent gravel bar in a river.[138] At some locations wetlands (i.e. "wet meadows") are selected preferentially.[139]

Wolves in summer are more solitary,[140] and ranging is often restricted.[141] A lactating female in southern Ontario used a mere 18.3 km^2.[142] The summer separations are usually temporary, pack members meeting intermittently at the den or rendezvous site.[143] A pack without pups often remains together through the summer, its movements differing little from those in winter.[144] Minnesota wolves attended their rendezvous sites mostly at night.[145] The dominant male was the main provider for his mate and the pups, and his schedule was irregular, as was the female's once released from nursing. The adolescents seemed to have no schedules, coming and going irregularly. Tundra wolves, in contrast, attended mostly during the day.[146] However, cover is scarce in the high Arctic, and summer diurnal temperatures can discourage activity. Moreover, the extended daylength is sufficiently long to permit sight hunting at all hours.

Starting in autumn, Great Lakes wolf litters sometimes split up during excursions away from the rendezvous site.[147] By late August and into early October, the pups are ranging widely on their own, often far from other pack members, and any rendezvous sites not abandoned by that time are not occupied much longer. Final departure depends on the development of the pups.[148] Once a pack leaves the last rendezvous site in autumn it becomes cohesive and nomadic again in preparation for winter, the pups now traveling along.[149] Pups in southcentral

Alaska begin traveling regularly with the pack even earlier, from mid-August to mid-September.[150] Pack sizes are usually largest in winter because pups born that spring are included. Most are now indistinguishable from adults.[151] Traveling becomes extensive, and in early winter the packs investigate their territorial boundaries and scent-mark the peripheries once again,[152] repainting the social fence (Chapter 5).

8.3   Dens and rendezvous sites of free-ranging dogs

Free-ranging dogs can acquire wolfish habits, one being denning. According to Darwin, "the feral dogs of La Plata ... are of large size, hunt singly or in packs, and burrow holes for their young."[153] Wolfdogs living near Voronezh and Belgorod, Russia, dug dens adjacent to urban areas.[154] Female free-ranging dogs do not usually dig dens, preferring caves (Fig. 8.8), rocky clefts, spaces under exposed tree roots, underground burrows already dug by other animals, and waste timber dumps.[155] Bali street dogs are exceptional by digging dens into the earth.[156]

Female free-ranging dogs usually reproduce within the home range of the group[157] or leave the group to rear their pups.[158] Usually a female stays by herself, detached from the companions with which she associates. Some groups make use of selected locations analogous to wolf rendezvous sites while pups are being reared.[159] Groups of free-ranging dogs in rural Alabama sometimes shifted the core areas of their home ranges,[160] moves that appeared to be seasonal and based on ambient temperature.

Dingoes, like other free-ranging dogs, and like wolves, choose den sites opportunistically.[161] Dingoes in central Australia mostly occupy enlarged rabbit burrows, ordinarily with rabbits living in adjacent burrows throughout the warren. Others find sites in wombat burrows, in caves and under ledges, beneath

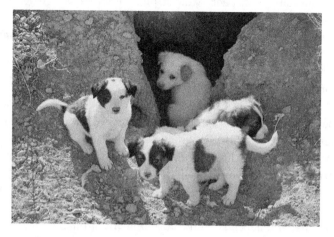

Figure 8.8 Free-ranging urban dog pups in a makeshift cave.
Source: Vladimir Melnik|Dreamstime.com.

debris and tussocks of spinifex (*Triodia* spp.), among exposed tree roots, and inside hollow logs. In northwestern Australia dingoes den in rock piles, underneath ledges and outcrops, inside hollow logs, and in one instance used the enlarged burrow of a sand monitor (*Varanus gouldii*).[162] High elevations near water were preferred. Many of the dug dens had multiple entrances, the dimensions of the entrances and chambers variable, although "most were large enough to allow a human to crawl into the [main] chamber."[163]

Before pup wolves are mobile, the activity of the pack is restricted to a core area in the vicinity of the dens and rendezvous sites, a pack not becoming nomadic until its pups are nearly adult size and able to keep up. Range restrictions during the dingo breeding season apply only to females with litters, and other group members continue to travel as usual.[164] While the pups observed were <3 weeks old, the only dingo found near the den consistently was the nursing female, making this situation no different from that of a free-ranging domestic dog.

8.4   Wolf litters

Wolves can breed to at least 9 years of age in captivity.[165] In the wild a few might reproduce through age 11,[166] but the normal reproductive life is short, probably no longer than 4 years or so, and most individuals in unexploited populations probably fail to even live 4 years (Chapter 7).[167] On rare occasions a wild wolf might survive to age 15.[168] Maximum longevity in nature of Minnesota wolves is about 13 years and 16 years for captive specimens.[169] A male of unstated origin at an Italian zoo died at age 17.[170] Of 86 wolves radio-collared in northwestern Alaska, 3 survived past age 9 and 1 past 14 years.[171] Survivorship is lowest in those younger than 3 years.[172] Not included in these estimates is prenatal mortality, which in dogs and wolves is estimated at 16–20%.[173] Therefore, none of the information commonly cited for "litter size" reflects mortality from conception to emergence from the den when pups are usually counted.

Females breeding for the first time generally have fewer pups than older females.[174] Litter size averaged 6.1 in an exploited population of wolves in south-central Alaska,[175] 5.7 in an expanding population in the Yukon,[176] and a typical litter is 4–7 everywhere.[177] Litters of wolves born to established packs in BISF averaged five pups,[178] those elsewhere in Minnesota about six or seven and mortality by mid-November was 50%.[179] A litter of Russian wolves reported in 1904 was said to number 13,[180] and another comprising 14 was taken in May 1939 from a den near Chatinika, Alaska.[181]

Litter size declines in saturated populations, especially in times of game shortages. During the early 1970s white-tailed deer in SNF became scarce. By 1974 the average litter was 1.5 pups compared with 6.4 pups per litter in the 1950s when the wolf population had been much smaller.[182] We might think of these 1950s wolves as having been more fit in the evolutionary sense, but in my opinion this would be inaccurate. The risk of mortality is greater after pups are weaned and start to wander on their own.[183] Furthermore, litter size alone is a measure of fecundity. *Fitness* is often defined as an individual's expected number of offspring,[184] and indeed it might be used as a synonym of fecundity in species that provide no parental care. However, in animals such as wolves in which parental care is complex and energy-intensive, fitness is better defined as the number of reproductive descendants an individual generates in its lifetime.[185] Litter size does not provide this information, nor can it predict eventual survivorship and reproduction if the fates of dispersing animals are unknown. Thus a wolf that produces two pups, one of which lives to reproduce, is more fit than a wolf with a litter of four all of which die before they can breed.

Ordinarily a den is occupied by the dominant female of the pack, the only pregnant animal. Packs in which more than one female reproduces are unusual. For example, this was never observed in the wolf population in the Finlayson Lake region.[186] On rare occasions two females share a den;[187] a male has two mates and maintains two dens (each with a lone female);[188] a pack has two den sites and raises two litters;[189] or a subordinate female mates with the dominant male, dens separately, and attempts to rear her pups alone.[190]

Multiple litters by a pack in the same year are atypical and might be more common in exploited populations.[191] The first published observation was Murie's from Denali,[192] then 40 years later came a report from the Nelchina Basin.[193] Multiple litters were seen or inferred in nine packs of Denali wolves between 1988 and 1994, one producing three litters.[194] A multiple litter was thought possible for a Yellowstone pack (the dominant male was seen to mate with two females),[195] and in later years several females of a Yellowstone pack gave birth in a common den.[196] There were, in addition, nine instances of subordinate females mating with a dominant male, and in all cases they were related to the dominant female as a sister, daughter, or niece. Multiple litters seem superficially to be more prevalent in North American wolves from high latitudes than in wolves comprising the Great Lakes and eastern populations, but this is speculation. Multiple litters also consistently recur in some groups of captive animals but not others.[197] It would be interesting to compare their origins, assuming genetic lines have not become too mixed.

Subordinate wolves in captivity mate readily when the existing dominance order breaks down,[198] and the same might occur in exploited populations of wild wolves,[199] although this would not account for multiple litters reported in areas such as Denali where wolves are protected. A pack on Isle Royale was said to have two or three breeding males subordinate to the dominant male, but the report included no confirmation.[200]

Natural mortality and restriction to a single annual reproductive cycle make breeding success and the rearing of pups without incident all the more urgent. An important factor in failure to breed is mate mortality.[201] However, if the female dies after her pups are weaned the male can sometimes rear them to adolescence.[202] Single wolves, both male and female, have been known to rear pups alone after losing a mate.[203] Wolves and dogs nurse their young for about

7 weeks[204] and thereafter wean them on vomited food.[205] However, observational evidence indicates weaning might be accomplished in half this time,[206] in which case even young pups could survive without a mother. Some female wolves reportedly start weaning their pups at about 4 weeks.[207] Supplemental feeding by regurgitation can start even earlier, at 22–24 days. Captive eastern coyotes raised by their parents were eating regurgitated food by 21 days.[208]

Pup wolves emerge from the den at about 3 weeks,[209] are moved to rendezvous sites at 4–6 weeks,[210] and soon become weaned on regurgitated food delivered mostly by the parents but sometimes other pack members (see below). In some wolf packs nearly all adult members and adolescents regurgitate for the pups at one time or another,[211] but mostly it is the breeding pair. The urge must be deeply ingrained. The Crislers already had two adolescent wolves when they acquired five pups. Upon seeing them for the first time the adolescent female vomited, and soon after being fed the male went to the shed where the pups were housed and regurgitated his stomach contents for them.[212] Other wolves the Crislers raised regurgitated spontaneously in front of uninterested pup dogs if they had no pups of their own. Within an hour of being placed with a strange adult female, six-month-old wolves raised in various states of isolation behaved submissively toward her and solicited regurgitations.[213] She initially bit and pinned them and then complied.

When pups are young and the female is attending them her mate does most of the provisioning.[214] A wolf returning from a hunt is met by the present year's pups, often adolescents from previous litters that have not yet dispersed, and the breeding female, all of which might solicit regurgitations.[215] The female is especially aggressive, rushing to meet her mate and snatching any uneaten food he carries if he fails to drop it for her.[216] If he is not carrying food in his mouth she eagerly solicits him to regurgitate. In doing so she becomes like a pup herself, crouching and licking-up.[217] Others wanting food also crowd around the returning hunter, wagging their tails, nose-pushing, whining, and licking-up.[218] The singular conclusion to be drawn is this: unlike many mammals *offspring are not required to elicit parental behavior in wolves.*[219]

The behavior of crowding around a returning hunter to solicit food has been termed *beggar harassment* in other contexts, and "when beggars harass, owners may benefit from sharing part of the food if their consumption rate is low relative to the rate of cost accrual."[220] *Food sharing*, if defined broadly as joint use of a food source that can otherwise be monopolized,[221] includes regurgitated food. Among chimpanzees the most aggressive beggars are most likely to be "paid" by the food's owner, ostensibly to go away.[222] To my knowledge no canid that regurgitates food for its pups or brings uneaten food to the den makes an effort to distribute it evenly. Mech described the free-for-all that occurs among pup wolves, and "he or she who hesitates is truly lost."[223] Littermate aggression over food has important survival implications and might account for the large size disparity sometimes seen among littermates (see above).[224]

A wolf returning from a hunt is mobbed by pups as it approaches the den.[225] Sometimes it rushes away a short distance wagging its tail and hindquarters, then returns with head lowered. The pups follow closely trying to lick-up. The wolf moves a few meters or sometimes up to 0.4 km before regurgitating meat, which is consumed quickly by the pups. Three-fourths of regurgitations occur on the spot when a donor wolf meets its solicitors. Most regurgitations are single events (61%), but some (24%) were seen to occur twice and in 12% of cases a wolf regurgitated three to five times. The average regurgitation contains 1.25 kg of undigested meat. Pups received 81% of regurgitations, the breeding female 14%, and helpers (see below) 6%. Donations by the breeding female and helpers went mostly to the pups, but the female might regurgitate to a helper left home to babysit or rarely into a cache. Helpers seldom regurgitated to the breeding female or other helpers. The male delivered 57% of his regurgitations to the pups, 32% to his mate, 5% to helpers, and 5% into caches. Sometimes the younger and most timid members of a pack stay near the den or at rendezvous sites to solicit food from returning hunters and trying to nurse from the dominant female, competing with the current year's pups.[226]

8.5   Free-ranging dog litters

Litters of owned dogs documented in the scientific literature have been as large as 20–22[227] and 23.[228] Litter size in free-ranging dogs varies widely but probably averages five or six,[229] and commonly more males are born than females.[230] The significance of this fact, if any, is unknown. Average litter size of dingoes is about five in Australia and Thailand.[231]

Dogs on the loose are more promiscuous than a stable wolf pack. An estrous group of free-ranging dogs is a disorganized scrum of impending paternity confusion. If pair bonds are rare, paternal care is rarer still. A male wolf attending his pups and supplying them with food has no consistent behavioral counterpart in dogs,[232] which have cut ancestral ties to fatherhood. Having deposited his sperm a dog has no notion of whether he has even fathered pups, never mind where they might be. Naturally, there are exceptions (see below).

Females have been known to nurse each other's pups.[233] Females in a group are known to give birth almost simultaneously and rear their pups communally.[234] Perhaps communal rearing in the absence of a reliable mate increases survivorship, but this is speculation. Females might nurse pups for the first 10–11 weeks and remain with their litters for 13 weeks.[235] Among street dogs in Bhabanibera, India, mothers spent the most time with the pups when they were young, tapering off until they became completely mobile at 10 weeks.[236] Females are usually more aggressive when their pups are young. Aggression is directed not just at other dogs but at other animals too (e.g. cattle, goats, humans). Females in Katwa, India, guarded pups aggressively mainly during the first 2 weeks.[237]

Data are thin on survivorship of pups born to free-ranging dogs, but the numbers are typically low, about a third living into early adulthood.[238] In Katwa, 63% were dead by 3 months.[239] In Italy, only 5% survived to age 1 year, with 70% dying during the first 70 days.[240] Another study found that just 12 of 76 dogs (16%) survived to early adolescence (20 weeks).[241] Causes were attributed to pups being left behind during den changes, becoming lost, predation by other canids, and inclement weather. Survivors were ordinarily recruited into their natal groups.[242] The idea that pups born free-ranging might be more susceptible to cold than young wolves and coyotes[243] is not necessarily true. Four of five young born into a group in interior Alaska in September 1979 survived to at least 1 year (the fifth was killed by a car), and mother and offspring were seen foraging in temperatures of −45°C when the wind speed was 6–8 km per hour.[244]

The survivorship of adults is also poor. A few owned dogs have lived for nearly 30 years,[245] but a free-ranging one of 5 years is a true Methuselah. Most adults are probably <3 years old.[246] Village dogs in rural areas of the world suffer comparable high mortality if veterinary care is unavailable or withheld. In the Isoso Indigenous Territory, Bolivia, annual mortality (presumably of adult dogs) was 34%, that of neonates 73%.[247]

Chances are slight that rural and wild areas are in danger of being overrun by unowned dogs. Sustainable populations must rely on outside recruitment because of low survivorship. At least four factors account for early high mortality:[248] (1) without a reliable mate the female must abandon her pups intermittently to find food and water; (2) at 6–8 weeks the pups begin to explore, which exposes them to predation and the risk of becoming lost if the mother is absent; (3) irregular breeding cycles can risk exposing at least one litter to unfavorable weather or distracted care; and (4) the mother's interest in her current litter wanes as she enters estrus again.

The mother might remain with her pups nearly full time for the first 6 weeks, then leave them intermittently to forage with the group.[249] Like wolves, free-ranging dogs feed their weaned offspring regurgitated food.[250] This was observed in Katwa when the pups were 6–10 weeks old.[251] Limited evidence implies that in dingoes other group members regurgitate for the current year's litter and might also help provision the breeding female while she is confined to the den,[252] although confirmation is lacking. Regurgitation for pups is not uncommon even in owned domestic dogs. More than 60% of Swedish dog breeders surveyed reported having witnessed it, ordinarily being carried out by the mother (78% of cases).[253] In just 3% of cases it was the father, and in the remaining instances (19%) the regurgitating dog was a relative (sister, maternal grandmother or great-grandmother, an uncle, sometimes more distant relatives) or unrelated dog. Regurgitation was more likely if the pups displayed food-solicitation behavior. Owned pups can be weaned artificially at 4 weeks without weight loss.[254] Weaning without human interference can be abrupt[255] or barely noticeable if solid food is made available continuously starting early.

It is sometimes stated that domestic dogs are the only canids in which males do not participate in rearing the pups.[256] However, certain male street dogs in Katwa stayed near their litters for the first 6–8 weeks, driving off other dogs,[257] and one even regurgitated for his pups.[258] These males were in monogamous relationships with the mothers, indicating that exclusive mating privileges might increase fitness of the offspring. At other locations males were reported remaining near the female and playing with the pups.[259] Sometimes the apparent father hangs around the vicinity, but whether he actually babysits is uncertain.[260] On two rare occasions a male that stayed after the pups were born played with them and slept near the mother, although he never regurgitated or delivered food to any of them.[261] Another male remained in the vicinity of a mother rearing pups for the first 3 weeks but seemed uninvolved in their care.[262]

The rearing of dingo pups to some extent parallels that of wolves. Pups first appear at the den's entrance when 20–22 days old, are perhaps moved to one or more secondary dens up to 1.4 km away before age 8 weeks, and transferred eventually to one or more rendezvous sites up to 5.9 km distant.[263] Older group members supposedly bring them pieces of prey, and at 9–14 weeks include them when feeding on nearby kills. At 9–24 weeks they start traveling with the group. Use of rendezvous sites lessens until at 16 weeks the last is abandoned.[264]

Lack of care-giving by male dogs and a general reluctance of the mothers to regurgitate food for their pups are considered a result of human interference substituting for these duties,[265] but such explanations fail to account for the impermanence of any such loss and its possible mechanism. Behaviors are just as phenotypic as morphological characters like floppy ears or short hair, and no situation alters phenotypes more relentlessly than prolonged captivity. Impoverished sensory stimulation and a restricted environment can prevent normal social behaviors from being released. The mere absence of a social phenotypic expression in captivity is not evidence of its extinction, which is why free-ranging dogs make such interesting subjects.

The pekin duck (the Chinese dish is Peking duck), a mallard (*Anas platyrhynchos*) domesticated in China, makes a good example. The pekin looks nothing like a mallard, yet it is one, just as a poodle looks nothing like a wolf. Placed in the wild, pekins mate with mallards and display all the aspects of species-specific social behavior seldom seen in a barnyard.[266] The pekin's natural behaviors have not been lost or rendered "degenerate", but simply repressed or restricted. They arise from different developmental processes during ontogeny at the individual level and are not necessarily the result of genetic contingencies. "Thus, identical genotypes in different contexts will have different developmental histories, just as different genotypes in the same environment will develop differently."[267]

When placed together in a wild setting, female mallards prefer to mate with male mallards,[268] just as wolves prefer other wolves over dogs, but pekin–mallard crosses are common.[269] Pekins released from the barnyard display all the intricate courtship behaviors of wild mallards. And just as dogs seem to have lost certain care-giving behaviors or display them in halting abbreviation (e.g. regurgitation for pups, male parental attentiveness), female pekins in captive settings are often indifferent mothers, failing on occasion even to incubate their eggs.

8.6   Helping and the altruism dilemma

As just described, a mother wolf with young pups ordinarily stays at the den while the rest of the pack hunts.[270] Parents rearing their own offspring are altruistic by imposing asymmetric fitness on the parties involved: pups receive free protection while the parents pay the costs of feeding them and increased physical danger by being present at the den. In terms of absolute fitness, protecting the pups probably costs the parents little more than it costs to protect themselves.[271] What I mean here by altruistic behavior is not specifically that of parents feeding or defending their young, which is actually *nepotism*;[272] rather, *altruism* is any act by which an individual relinquishes potential benefits of its own direct fitness to enhance the fitness of another individual indirectly. Such acts might be costly to self while benefiting others of the group.[273]

Sometimes another female relieves the mother of babysitting duties, freeing her to hunt with the pack or forage alone.[274] A *helper* (also called *alloparent* and *auxiliary*) is a nonbreeding member of a social group that does surrogate parenting of the breeding pair's current young.[275] *Helping behavior* in wolves includes feeding the younger ones (usually siblings) by bringing game, regurgitating food, or babysitting.[276] Sometimes it includes deferring to a mate, as when the male of a breeding pair of captive eastern coyotes allowed the female to feed first and helped clean the pups until they were weaned.[277]

Helping is thought to enhance the reproductive potential of the breeding pair and ultimately increase fitness of the lineage. Group living in wolves is both sustained and constrained by factors other than hunting (Chapter 6), and since the early 1960s altruism channeled through helping behavior has been a prominent hypothesis designed to answer the general question, why do some animals live in groups?

Kin selection is believed to drive sociality by promoting friendly interactions, thereby reducing intragroup strife. Its theoretical efficacy is based on the segregation of genotypes, widening variation among groups.[278] Kin selection derives from *Hamilton's rule*, which posits that natural selection favors individuals carrying out altruistic acts benefiting relatives, and its expression is the inequality $rb - c > 0$, where b is the benefit in fitness to the recipient, c represents cost in fitness to the altruist, and r is the *coefficient of relatedness* – the fraction of genes shared with relatives.[279] Before kin selection can function, an animal must be able to distinguish kin from other individuals (*kin discrimination*), and for us to test its validity we need evidence that individuals recognize relatives (*kin recognition*) and treat them differently from familiar but unrelated conspecifics. Whether wolves and most other animals can do this is doubtful.

Social mammals that practice helping have certain criteria in common. They typically live in closed groups of related individuals (often families) that are social, cooperative, and retain their young for a year or two after weaning;[280] that is, dispersal is delayed. At least 120 species of mammals spanning most major zoological orders practice helping in some form, and a lesser number has been shown to adopt.[281] Altruism in animal societies has always been enigmatic: why would an individual relinquish reproduction – and thus compromise its direct fitness – to help rear another's young? *Direct fitness* is gained when an individual reproduces and passes genes directly to its descendants. *Indirect fitness* derives from the effects of an individual's activities (e.g. helping) on relatives that are not its own direct descendants. Hamilton's rule provided a framework within which to examine altruism empirically. It showed that if helper and beneficiary are closely related the helper still passes along its genes, if indirectly: loss of direct fitness is compensated by the enhanced fitness of a relative's offspring brought about by helping.[282] An individual's *inclusive*, or *total*, *fitness* is the sum of its fitness, direct and indirect.[283]

The contribution of nonbreeding relatives to inclusive fitness varies with r. A female that delays her own reproduction to help rear a sister's offspring makes no impact unless the sister's litter is twice as large, or equal to their combined reproductive potential (assuming fecundity is a valid measure of fitness).[284] Furthermore, an apparent altruist's contribution must double for each halving of r as kin relatedness becomes more distant.

Kinship theory attempts to explain such altruism in nature, but the concept is understood best if partitioned. *True altruism* is the permanent loss of direct fitness by the altruist and a gain in fitness by the recipient; in cases of *apparent altruism* an individual (the helper) might temporarily lose direct fitness while gaining time to enhance its own survival or reproductive potential.[285] Only the true altruist loses something tangible; the apparent altruist loses nothing except a little time during which its own fitness can be enhanced.

Wolves that remain to help feed and protect another's pups are potentially apparent altruists. By staying with the pack, an adolescent wolf gains size, strength, prowess as a hunter, and general experience, all presumably advantageous when it eventually emigrates. Whether fitness is actually enhanced is questionable. For example, helping supposedly allows future parents to develop the skills necessary for rearing their own young.[286] However, first-time breeders raise their pups as successfully as those with parenting experience.[287] Ecological explanations for the timing of dispersal are sometimes just as plausible, and "it seems reasonable to infer that a period of reproductive flexibility in younger individuals is an adaptation to environmental unpredictability, and not a mere preparation for later activities."[288]

The importance of indirect fitness might have been overestimated.[289] At a fundamental level, many investigations have failed to show a direct association between helping and fecundity (assuming fecundity is the criterion of measure).[290] Helping is also not restricted to kin, and in some birds and mammals kinship appears to be unrelated to helping behavior,[291] posing the question of how helping actually influences fitness in animal societies. "That help is sometimes withheld from relatives or directed at nonrelatives, combined with the lack of a helper effect, suggests two challenging possibilities for many cooperative breeders: either that helping is selected against even when kin might benefit, or that kin selection is not the driving force for many helpers."[292]

The disconnect between altruism and relatedness is not unusual.[293] The meerkat (*Suricata suricatta*), a social mongoose, was long thought to represent a prime case of indirect fitness in action. However, helping in this species correlates with size, sex, and age of the helpers, not kinship ties.[294] Older full siblings were no more likely to babysit their younger brothers and sisters than other group members, including unrelated immigrants.[295] In fact, there was no consistent relationship between contributions of meerkat babysitters and their relatedness to young they helped rear.

Social familiarity based on individual recognition – not kinship – appears to be the glue holding animal societies together. Animals as diverse as desert isopods (*Hemilepistus reaumuri*),[296] Columbian ground squirrels (*Spermophilus columbianus*),[297] vampire bats (*Desmodus rotundus*),[298] and to a large extent humans base their societies on social familiarity. An urban street gang is territorial. It marks its neighborhood boundaries with paint, patrols and defends them, and acts aggressively toward gangs occupying adjacent territories. Trespassers are threatened or punished. Most members of a gang are genetically unrelated yet refer to themselves collectively as a "family."

Claims that mother dogs and pups separated when the pups are 8–12 weeks still recognize each other after 2 years[299] are doubtful. Most altricial mammals produce several young, failing to distinguish them as individuals or even appearing to notice if one is removed.[300] In tests of choice, female beagles are no more likely to retrieve one of their own pups removed from the litter than a strange pup of the same age.[301] Neonate wolves taken from natal dens and switched to unrelated nursing females grow up in their new "step-packs" not knowing the difference. Just as important, neither do their step-parents, step-siblings, or any step-aunts, step-uncles, step-cousins, or step-grandparents that might also be pack members. Dogs commonly nurse strange pups placed with them. Lawrence K. Corbett told the story of two dingo mothers with pups of approximately weaning age that arrived at the same location to hunt grasshoppers. The groups remained together for an unstated length of time, but apparently long enough to become familiar. "When the local supply of grasshoppers declined, the mothers departed in separate directions, but each with a mixture of both litters; this was deduced from their coat colours (one litter was black-and-tan, the other ginger)."[302] In another account, dingo females moved their pups to den sites 20 m apart, at which point the litters became intermingled to the evident unconcern of all.[303] Observations like these undermine the power of kinship theory as applied to canid societies and strengthen the idea that familiarity is the stronger bonding agent.

Subordinate male wolves experience spermatogenesis and the same endocrinological cycling as the dominant male, and females pass through all four stages of reproduction including pseudopregnancy in concordance with the dominant female's term of gestation. Pseudopregnant female wolves have even been reported to lactate at the end of diestrus,[304] although I came across no confirmation of it in the mainstream literature. "Hormonal priming" as the causative agent of helping behavior fails to illuminate why wolves will not only nurse strange pups but regurgitate food for them even when they have no offspring of their own or are reproductively out of phase.[305]

As I repeat later in a different context (Chapter 9), at 4–5.5 weeks pup dogs are supposedly able to recognize their mothers and littermates based on olfaction alone, and the mothers can recognize them in return.[306] After wallowing in the same birth site over days and weeks, pups and mother smell the same. Thus putative kin recognition is more likely to be olfactory imprinting brought about by mutual bonding and sharing the same location, or perhaps based on recognizing a component in the major histocompatibility complex (Chapter 7). The real question yet to be tested is whether the pups recognize this particular female *as their mother* and if she in turn recognizes them specifically *as her own offspring*.

Dogs might have limited capability to distinguish others of different breeds, but the basis of it is unknown. Aggressiveness was tested in male and female basenjis and cocker spaniels exposed to strangers of their own and the other breed. The groups (three males and three females of each breed) were littermates reared together from birth.[307] Aggressiveness to strangers decreased in this order: (1) same sex and breed, (2) same sex but different breed, (3) different sex but same breed, and (4) different sex and breed. To speculate, highly evolved breeds might recognize and interpret their own signals more clearly than those received from dogs not like them, especially if the strangers have docked tails or other physical features that make signaling abbreviated or misleading.[308]

Were helping entirely a matter of free choice it would be a poor one in many cases. For example, it imposes an energy deficit and the consequent impairment of self-maintenance. To wolves, regurgitated food represents lost energy. A study of meerkats showed that babysitters lost 1.3% of their body mass over 24 hours compared with members free to forage, which gained 1.9%.[309] The effect is cumulative: during the rearing period babysitters lost an average of 3.8% of body mass, and 20% of them lost 6–11%.

It seems probable that social organizations evolve to maximize the direct fitness of its individuals, and whatever indirect manifestations add to inclusive fitness comprises the remaining few genetic scraps. Infanticide (Chapter 5), reproductive suppression of competitors (Chapter 7), and expulsion of the competition by forced emigration would all seem to lower the benefits of indirect fitness, but not if outweighed by gains in direct fitness.[310] In such cases the loss to inclusive fitness would be nonexistent or negligible. Black-tailed prairie dogs (*Cynomys ludovicianus*) represent an extreme example of direct fitness before all else: more than half of litters are killed by other lactating females in the same colony, most often close kin.[311] Social canids are large and slow to mature compared with many other group-living mammals, and delayed dispersal is the foundation of their societies. In fact, delayed dispersal is ordinarily considered a prerequisite to the evolution of helping behavior.[312] Therefore, whether an individual immigrates, cooperates by helping, or competes by breeding depends ultimately on which best suits the opportunities to maximize its individual fitness directly.[313]

According to kinship theory, under certain conditions natural selection can increase the genetic frequency of altruism within a population. One of those conditions is that an animal assisted by an altruistic act must be the altruist's relative because the probability is high that relatives carry the same genetic component. Despite deferring its own reproduction to help raise a relative's offspring, copies of this "altruism gene" are still spread through the population. However, an accurate accounting must also consider the probability of successful reproduction versus reproductive failure if a potential helper emigrates instead of remaining to assist others rear their young.[314]

In practical terms, animals living in social groups could enhance their inclusive fitness by adding more close kin to the regional population.[315] Limited dispersal, however, might nullify kin selection for altruism[316] by raising the level of competition among relatives.[317] Territories of African lions are usually contiguous with those of close kin. When a pride splits the dispersing females nearly always take up occupancy adjacent to their natal territories.[318] Afterward, kin discrimination is not apparent during perceived intrusions (recordings played to them) into natal areas,[319] and dispersers are treated the same as other interlopers. In like manner the intrapack friendliness characteristic of wolf societies seldom applies when rules of territoriality are violated.[320] New territories in Yellowstone, Denali, and elsewhere are often established adjacent to a natal pack, but if relatedness perhaps dampens conflict at first such ties are ultimately irrelevant (Chapter 5).[321] Where kinship is involved all competition is local.[322]

The obvious prerequisite for kin selection is the capacity of individuals to discriminate kin from not-kin.[323] I found no evidence that wolves and dogs can do this. Any beneficial effect of limited dispersal also assumes later recognition of dispersed relatives and subsequent resumption of kin discrimination long after familiarity has waned. Neither capacity has yet been shown once an emigrant joins another pack or group or forms a new one. As just mentioned, kinship in wolves, as in African lions, seldom ameliorates territorial aggression. Having once dispersed, adolescent wolves are often no more acceptable to the natal pack than a stranger.[324] There are exceptions, of course. Four dispersing wolves in SNF traveled 183–494 km from the sites where they were radio-collared.[325] All returned to their natal territories or nearby, one after 179 days. Two subsequently dispersed again. A wolf dispersed in November from its natal pack in Algonquin Provincial Park and returned the following June.[326] A 2-year-old female dispersed in May and returned after 7 weeks, remained through the summer near her mother's den, and stayed with or near the natal pack or along its territorial peripheries until the following February when she was killed, presumably by humans.[327] This is evidence of recalled familiarity but not necessarily memory of kinship.

Pack budding (Chapter 5) is sometimes tolerated. A wolf pack in BISF allowed three offspring to colonize an area straddling its territory.[328] Still other territories in BISF overlapped temporarily without obvious aggression. These events probably would not have happened at population saturation (Chapter 5). The budding and splitting of packs and acceptance of unrelated wolves into established packs results in closer populational ties than would occur if the founders consisted of unrelated pairs from distant locations.[329] In Denali the genetic links are closest among neighboring packs.[330] If adolescents that leave home to form a budding pack had previously served as helpers then the help provided was not wholly altruistic.[331]

Wolves of a pack are typically related, sometimes all of them except the breeding pair (Chapter 5). They tolerate fellow pack members and express aggression toward packs occupying adjacent territories. The question is, do wolf packs perceive other wolves solely as competitors and potential interlopers or as not-kin? Saying both might be true fails to partition the hypothesis into testable components. Assume pack members recognize each other by phenotypic traits (e.g. unique aspects of appearance, odor, voice, posture, predictable responses) and myriad other phenomena acting alone or in combinations. Perhaps these merge into phenotypic patterns, or "templates," specific to each individual. There is still no reason to think such signs arrive bearing detectable genetic tags.

Any behavioral elements of kin recognition are confounded by social familiarity. Both require use of the senses, the capacity to interpret and categorize signs, and memory in which to store and retrieve pertinent data, but true kin recognition in wolves – if it occurs at all – operates simultaneously at a deeper and more fundamental level. I say this because evidence of it has remained hidden whereas obvious links exist between familiarity and sociality.

Alan Grafen argued convincingly that few animals have been shown to recognize kin based strictly on genetic relatedness,[332] and this includes us.[333] Try this streamlined thought experiment. Wolf Pack A is a family of parents and offspring. Pack B has the same familial composition, and none of its members is related closely to any wolves of Pack A. When coming together at a territorial boundary the wolves behave differently toward each other than toward their own family members. It could be inferred that each pack senses the genetic difference, thereby accounting for aggressive responses on both sides. This might lead to a mistaken assumption that kin recognition and kin discrimination are functional synonyms. However, because recognizing kin is a neural process its outward expression is not always released, "just as recognizing a fruit as an orange does not necessarily lead to us eating it."[334] Failure to verify kin recognition based on observations of putative kin discrimination is not necessarily evidence of its absence, but neither are apparent expressions of kin discrimination indication of anything other than familiarity until these concepts have been separated and tested.[335]

Two things are apparent from our imagined scene. First, wolves recognize other wolves as like themselves (species recognition). A species recognition system requires conspecifics to understand all signals and respond predictably. It functions in this context *because all participants are the same*; that is, members of a single species. Second, wolves recognize other wolves as individuals (individual recognition). A system in which individuals or finite social groups (e.g. wolf packs) recognize each other functions in this context *because all participants are different*; that is, single wolves are individuals, and identifiable packs of individuals are themselves individuals.[336]

Together, these factors could account entirely for the friendliness among pack members and aggression toward strangers. Neither suggests recognition based on kin versus not-kin. Grafen's statement, "to show kin recognition it is necessary to show that the ability is used to assess kinship,"[337] is both logical and reasonable. Demonstrating it unequivocally in *diploid* populations is exceedingly difficult, not least because the coefficient of relatedness represents a continuum along which genetic distance starting with first-generation offspring diffuses rapidly. This is described by 0.5^n, where $n =$ the number of generational links: $r = 0.5$ (parents to offspring, sibling to sibling), 0.25 (to nieces and nephews or to grand-offspring), 0.125 (to first cousins or to great-grand-offspring), 0.03 (to second cousins), 0.008 (to third cousins), and so forth.

According to kinship theory, animals should recognize their closest kin most readily because of shared genes, but even if kin recognition occurs, at what genetic distance would it quit working? Is a diploid animal that passes along 50% of its genes twice as likely to recognize its own offspring than a niece or nephew with which it shares 25%? In Japanese macaques (*Macaca fuscata*) the distance of recognition does not appear to extend past $r = 0.125$,[338] assuming the factors assessed were true measures of kin discrimination. Savannah baboons (*Papio cynocephalus*) form tight female–female bonds with close kin, but in the absence of relatives a female will bond readily with an unrelated female,[339] indication of a social need extending beyond kinship. Aggression among captive red deer hinds extends to third-degree relationships and beyond, but the experiment did not account for familiarity as a confounding variable.[340]

Other hypotheses have been proposed to explain altruism, although like kin selection, none seems a comfortable fit for group-living canids. One alternative is *group augmentation*, in which survivorship of individuals is increased in large groups and it becomes advantageous to recruit new members either through reproduction or immigration.[341] In the group augmentation model large group size enhances survivorship and reproductive capacity, and even unrelated individuals benefit from helping to rear new recruits.

Three conditions are explicit. First is *delayed reciprocity*, in which the new recruits being helped will in turn aid others in the group at some later time. The term can be misleading by implying a closed loop between recruits and the specific individuals helping them. If the helpers emigrate they receive no reciprocal benefits from those they helped. The ultimate beneficiary of reciprocity in this case is the group.[342] The second condition is waiting in a queue for a future breeding position. The third is a general absence of cheating, such as being a distracted or inconsistent helper while inheriting helpers raised by others upon obtaining a breeding position. Being a *cheater* in this context means refusing to help as a nonbreeding member of a group and accepting help later upon achieving breeder status.[343]

Although scrounging (Chapter 6) is not formally a part of the group augmentation model, it represents a form of cheating. Adolescent wolves sometimes try to scrounge regurgitations meant for the current year's pups or wait at the den or rendezvous site anticipating a returning parent with a full stomach. Observations of two packs in SNF monitored over a summer indicated that subordinate wolves did not help feed the pups and often left them unattended while the parents foraged.[344] Their rendezvous site visits suggested they might have been soliciting regurgitations themselves. "For example, [adolescents] that spent considerable time at [homesites] and may occasionally chase off a bear ... can hardly be called 'altruists' if the primary reason they are there is to intercept food intended for the pups."[345] The nonbreeding contingent can be largely unaffected by the presence of pups, often traveling throughout the territory and rarely visiting them.[346] A study on Ellesmere Island produced opposite results: nonbreeders were a positive force in food transfer to the current year's pups,[347] sometimes caching food for later delivery.[348]

Group augmentation theory applies best to large animal societies that are stable over time, those in which security in numbers makes helping a viable alternative to breeding. Wolves are a poor fit. At least three problems arise in applying group augmentation to social canids. First, canid groups are small and unstable compared with meerkats, bats, and many rodents,[349] and long-term benefits of indirect fitness seem more remote. Adolescent members, both male and female, are therefore less inclined to stay with their natal packs and more likely to disperse and try to reproduce. Their annual loss and a general absence of queuing (see below) undermine group augmentation theory unless the definition of "pack" is expanded to include all wolves in the region. In other words, the prospects of delayed reciprocity to future members of the original pack (the unborn and immigrants) vanish when pack members emigrate, and any later contribution would have to appear somewhere else in the population.

Second, because group augmentation is modeled on large group size, stability, and immigration, it incorporates a social queue, a presumption that helpers accede to breeding status by waiting their turns. In such instances delayed reciprocity might apply to the same individuals and not simply the group; that is, a helper accedes to breeding status, and the young it helped rear now assist in feeding its own young.[350] As discussed, mating among wolf pack members other than the breeding pair is unusual.[351] Social dominance delays functional maturity (Chapter 7), and inbreeding avoidance (Chapter 7) renders queuing for eventual reproduction unlikely. The inheritance of territories by full siblings is infrequent. Vacancies are filled instead by unrelated wolves seeking breeding opportunities. Rising to reproductive status within a pack is uncommon unless one of the dominant pair is replaced by a step-offspring or unrelated immigrant. Third, per capita food intake correlates inversely with pack size (Chapter 6), which selects against packs becoming large and stable and works in favor of small packs and pairs.

Wolves in nature ordinarily mature late, and staying with the natal pack to help rear younger siblings could make more sense than venturing forth with raw survival skills.[352] In an unusual situation a wolf might remain at home for 4 years without breeding.[353] Altruism seems inconsistent with the fact that social repression – not the lack of physiological preparedness – keeps subordinate wolves from mating and having pups of their own (Chapter 7). Instead, an adolescent's regurgitating for younger siblings and babysitting them seem more "pay to stay" so long as the dominant pair's fecundity is sustained.[354] "Pay to stay" is about the only situation that might incur a cost to the helper.[355] Its importance is unknown, but "it seems reasonable to infer that a period of reproductive flexibility in younger individuals is an adaptation to environmental unpredictability, and not a mere preparation for later activities."[356] For an old animal the situation might be different. Maybe a "pay to stay" arrangement was in force in an Ellesmere Island pack when the breeding female "retired" and became a helper in her post-reproductive years, replaced by her daughter as the dominant male's mate.[357]

A dispersing wolf assumes risks by leaving home, two being early mortality and reproductive failure, but these are also risks if it stays. Dispersal is often associated with decreased survival, especially if emigrants must compete for space to establish territories.[358] This is the situation in saturated populations (Chapter 5), and such extrinsic factors are thought to predispose species to altruism.[359] Competition is subsequently heightened by a jamming of the outbound conveyor as parents live on and their offspring delay dispersal. While perhaps valid, the argument is hampered by circular reasoning: vacancies outside the natal territory are restricted only because the other spaces are occupied.[360]

Assuming the dominant pair in a wolf pack is monogamous, an adolescent is related as closely to its younger siblings as to its own potential offspring. If reproductive opportunities are fewer elsewhere its fitness might be enhanced indirectly by helping its parents. What a dispersing wolf potentially gains is fitness, both direct and indirect, the first by reproducing, the second by improving the fitness of relatives left behind (i.e. one fewer mouth to feed, reduced social competition).[361] The qualifier "potentially" is the key, notably in the case of improved group fitness. Indirect fitness of the natal pack could be compromised by loss of a helper and defender of its territory. The emigrant can lose direct fitness too if the choice is exchanging a slight future chance to breed in the natal pack for maybe none at all somewhere else. Adolescents (females in particular) might still reproduce by staying behind after maturity. In any case, the possible benefits to a wolf of delaying emigration instead of attempting to maximize its direct fitness are questionable. Immediate enhanced survivorship and later reproductive success, the two main arguments favoring indirect fitness,[362] have not been demonstrated in wolves.

For some species of social birds and mammals the normal condition is to delay dispersal without helping, evidence that the link between staying and helping is not always tight.[363] Helping in wolves is facultative too, some adolescents declining to regurgitate for the current year's pups or babysit them (see above), and yet the dominant pair tolerates their presence. It seems likely that helping is generally more effective in cooperative breeders living in large societies. Pairs of stripe-backed wrens (*Campylorhynchus nuchalis*) with two helpers were more fecund than pairs with no helpers or just one.[364] In this species helpers assist in feeding the young and also defend the nest against brood parasites (see below) and predators. Small groups lack the reproductive success of large ones, and males demonstrate higher fitness by waiting in queue to reproduce. Delayed dispersal provides helping opportunities, adding to the benefits of philopatry and making larger stable groups possible,[365] in addition to decreasing competition for breeding vacancies.[366]

Kinship theory requires that helpers boost the dominant pair's reproductive success. Consequently, helpers should enhance the survival of pup wolves and younger adolescents. If so, then survivorship ought to increase with pack size as occasionally claimed.[367] Field data have yielded mixed results,[368] some of it showing that neither size of the pack nor litter size consistently affects pup survival.[369] At a time in SNF when ungulates were scarce and the wolf population was declining, litter size and pack size showed an inverse correlation: more pups were produced by pairs than by larger packs containing potential helpers, although mean pup weights were similar.[370] With ungulates comparatively abundant in BISF and wolves increasing, litter size and pack size correlated directly. Investigators posited that helpers with full stomachs might be more inclined to share food with younger siblings, noting that experiments to assess costs and benefits provided by helpers had not been done.

Assuming they help at all, adolescent wolves are not always accomplished hunters (Chapter 6), and remaining with the pack offers assurance of regular meals. A dominant male on Ellesmere Island caught young Arctic hares (leverets) and gave them to the adolescents that had chased them unsuccessfully.[371] Pursuing hares is useful: adults can reach 5.3 kg.[372] During the same hunt the breeding female captured two, but attempted to eat them herself. When no pups are present the dominant male is a major provider for adolescents. Sometimes this takes a ritualized twist and one of the parents regurgitates for them.[373]

In wolves, evidence that altruism extends benefits to either the helper or recipient has not been demonstrated, and whether helpers exert a positive effect on fitness is unknown. Studies in which "helper" has been defined simply as adolescent and nonbreeding adult pack members failed to find a survival effect on pups.[374] In no way do the sparse data now available confirm that "wolves have evolved their social structure with some selective pressure for traits of value to the group, and not just the individual."[375] As put forth previously, we have little evidence that animal societies are constructed for the good of the species and much evidence showing they serve just its individual members. As Michael T. Ghiselin wrote, "the evolution of society fits the Darwinian paradigm in its most individualistic form."[376] The bias is clearer if viewed through teleology's lens: "Many who have written on 'reproductive strategies' have been concerned, not with the actions of individuals, but with the good of the species, for no more basic reason than the tendency to view the struggle for existence as a contest between 'teams' rather than 'athletes.'"[377]

Why believe that helping behavior evolved as a result of natural selection and serves an adaptive function with the payoff being direct or indirect fitness? The body of work is unconvincing, as argued persuasively by the ornithologists Ian G. Jamieson and John L. Craig.[378] From their viewpoint, tests of kinship theory place undue emphasis on ecological facets of helping that seem malleable to theory and not enough on the behavior itself. A community member need not be in "hormonal breeding condition" or even sexually mature to help, as shown in wolves and many other mammals and birds. The courtship and mating stages of the reproductive cycle are distinct both physiologically and behaviorally from those occurring later such as incubation of eggs, lactation, and rearing young. Nor is it necessary that helpers and those receiving help be related. Pup dogs have been nursed and reared successfully by female wolves[379] and even lactating domestic cats.[380] Such cross-fostering experiments pose an unexplained problem for kinship theory.

Nature's own cross-fostering experiments are hardest to explain. Among birds *brood parasites* lay their eggs in the nests of other species, leaving these "hosts" to incubate them and rear the young.[381] The eggs of brood parasites often differ noticeably in shape, size, and color from the hosts' eggs. Despite obvious differences in body size, morphology, vocalization, and aggressiveness of these unwanted guests the hosts nonetheless foster them along with their nestlings, often at a cost in direct fitness when the guests steal food from their own nestlings or push them out of the nest. Neither kin recognition nor kin discrimination plays a part in this arrangement. Brood parasitism occurs in about 1% of bird species including all honey guides (Indicatoridae), almost half the 130 species of cuckoos (Cuculidae), two genera of finches (Ploceidae), five species of cowbirds (Icteridae), and a duck.[382] Offspring of the brown-headed cowbird (*Molothrus ater*), the only widespread avian brood parasite in North America, have been reared successfully by at least 139 of the 216 species it has been reported to parasitize.[383] So how can helping behavior be explained? According to Jamieson and Craig, "it is proposed that the feeding of nestlings in communal breeders is maintained by the same stimulus–response mechanism that results in parents feeding their own young or host species feeding parasitic young, a situation where there is no reasonable adaptive explanation."[384]

My description of wolf societies so far has demonstrated that dispersal can be inhibited where habitats are saturated, and adolescents might be inclined to stay with the natal pack longer or make only temporary forays outside the territorial boundaries. These stay-at-home wolves could be inclined to help, but if they disperse the parents can easily raise any offspring alone. Helping in this case is facultative, its fitness advantages problematic. We should consider this uncertain context as unusual, not the helping behavior itself, which under different circumstances would not be elicited.

Obligate helping is more likely to contain a fitness component, although species depending on it like Australia's white-winged chough (*Corcorax melanorhamphos*) are rare.[385] Taking into account its broad diversity of form and inconsistent pattern, helping might be a stereotypical response and not a genetic trait selected for and sustained by inclusive fitness. Stated differently, the current perception of helping as atypical behavior expressed only in social animals could have a more parsimonious explanation. This would take shape as signal ↔ response triggered by behavior of the young and sustained through mutual reinforcement (double arrow) by helper and beneficiary. The initial stimulus might be food solicitation or something else. As mentioned before, wolves sometimes regurgitate at the mere sight of unrelated pups. In a similar manner, a helper bird is stimulated to drop insects into a nestling's gaping mouth.[386] Thus "if provisioning behavior occurs regardless of genetic relationships, then the feeding of closely related kin may be more simply explained as a consequence of the type of social system, that is, one in which juveniles do not disperse from their natal territories."[387]

Care-giving behavior comes naturally to canids. One of the Crisler's male wolves "kidnapped" a pup dog, apparently just to take care of it.[388] A similar incident was witnessed in a captive group of Great Lakes wolves: when a female left her pups momentarily to chase away other members of her group they were carried off and tended by an adolescent female.[389]

Direct correlation between reproductive success and the presence of helpers is just that – a correlation. A large pack could simply reflect the high reproductive success of the dominant pair. In many species of birds only the breeding female incubates the eggs, rendering helpers useless for this function.[390] As mentioned, some early mortality in wolves and dogs occurs in utero when helping is irrelevant. Breeding female wolves and dogs are typically the only lactating members of the pack or group and usually exclude others from the den or birth location. Occasionally, two female wolves or dogs give birth together and rear their litters communally, but both are lactating and still provide complete early care including feeding and cleaning the pups. Auxiliary help in dogs is rarely extended to breeding females. Among wolves the dominant male and sometimes other pack members regurgitate for the breeding female, bring game, or cache meat nearby where she can get it without traveling far from the den.[391]

How does it happen that dispersing individuals from animal societies are offspring and not the parents? To reply that such a system functions in inbreeding avoidance simply begs the question. Specifically, why does the dominant pair in a wolf pack stay behind instead of emigrating and bequeathing the territory to its offspring? A pair of adults is certainly better equipped to establish and defend new spaces than naïve adolescents dispersing alone.

From models based on game theory came the concept of the *evolutionarily stable strategy* (*ESS*).[392] Simplified, if individuals from population A disperse at rate D then A's "strategy" is an ESS if it proves superior to that of another population, B, the members of which disperse at rate D'.[393] If v represents the proportion of dispersing offspring and p the fraction surviving, the ESS dispersal rate is $v^* = 1/(2-p)$, with v^* decreasing as the survival interests of parents and offspring come into conflict.[394] This occurs when the young approach sexual maturity and delay dispersing if doing so compromises their future fitness through early death or reproductive failure. To increase their own fitness, the parents must then force at least half their offspring to emigrate despite the (presumed) reduced probability of them surviving. Although more fit at this point than their young, the breeding pair jeopardizes its own continued fitness by relinquishing an established territory.

9 Socialization

Humans name everything, living and dead. We name our pets and the wild animals we come to recognize while conducting field research. In doing so we bestow on them a human-centered individuality, an epibolic trap from which they can never escape. Animals, of course, are individuals without us.[1] In the following pages I hope to shed light on the factors necessary for *socialization*, the behavioral and ontogenetic progression through which young wolves and dogs become integrated into societies of their own kind – or alternatively, to human societies. Its rudiments appear early and are reinforced throughout life.

Wolves and African wild dogs are the most social of the canids by living in true societies. I define a *canid society* as a group of mostly related conspecifics that occupies a common territory, communicates in complex ways, and shares responsibilities, as in a pack. Domestic dogs interact more loosely, and their groupings do not constitute true societies as just defined. The objective here is to describe the socialization of wolves and of free-ranging dogs. The wolf section includes observations from both captive and wild animals, and the findings do not always apply mutually.

Nearly all domestic animals are social species that form bonds with conspecifics, a quality that makes them more manageable, or tame. Tameness has been interpreted as "an ontogenetic phenomenon facilitated through artificial selection."[2] This might explain how it came to be, but not what it is. Tameness, defined earlier as the absence of conflict behavior (Chapter 2), can also be thought of as the absence of fear, and a tame dog or wolf is one that does not fear humans. Feralization is then equated with the absence or loss of tameness and its replacement by fear.[3]

9.1 The socialization sequence

As mentioned, almost all domestic mammals and birds are social, and so are their wild progenitors.[4] They have in common a brief period early in life when social relationships can be formed easily with their own kind or others, including us. Conceptually, socialization in wolf and pup dogs is a sequence of four ontogenetic stages – neonatal, transitional, critical, and adolescent – each arising and tapering off at predictable intervals.[5] These bracket and often overlap an optimal time for the acquisition or execution of specific skills or functions and depend on the state of maturation of the brain and other organs. It bears emphasis that although all stages are cresive, some begin and end more abruptly or over shorter intervals than others. This flexibility is inherent because "the important aspect of each developmental period [each stage] is not time sequence but the fact that each represents a major developmental process."[6]

The *neonatal stage* commences at birth and lasts about 2 weeks.[7] A newborn canid is altricial (Chapter 5), emerging blind, deaf, nearly immobile, and completely dependent on maternal care. Motor functions consist of twitching, sleeping, sucking, and elimination of wastes in reflexive response to licking of the anus, genitals, and lower abdomen by the mother[8] or stroking of these locations by a human caregiver.[9] Licking by wolf mothers to ingest the urine and feces of pups can continue for 5–6 weeks.[10]

Touch is the first sense to develop and the earliest means of acquiring information from the external environment,[11] and haptic learning in dogs might take place before the second week concludes.[12] The neonate's limited repertoire of behaviors comprises searching for a teat, vocalizing if stimulated by discomfort or pain, and crawling slowly toward the mother or littermates to seek warmth (*thermotaxis*) or comfort by touching the mother or conspecifics (*thigmotaxis*).[13] Both are important. Neonate dogs are unable to maintain normal body temperature in environments colder than 6°C until 28 days of age, or above 40°C until age 21 days.[14] Even at room temperature (21–25°C) they often have rectal temperatures several degrees lower than the mother's and little resistance to cold stress. The rate at which deep-body temperature changes during cold exposure parallels that of a beaker of stirred saline water placed in the same room and containing a mass of liquid equal to that of the pup.

A neonate's principal needs are food, warmth, and elimination of wastes.[15] Pup dogs whine continuously until starting to nurse or if cold or injured. Amelioration in all three situations is thought to be haptic,[16] but this supposition falls short: pups separated from their mothers at 3 weeks, hand-fed, and pampered vocalized more than controls fed by a mechanical device and reared without any contact.[17] A likely explanation is mutual reinforcement with caregivers. Nonetheless, human handling during the first 3 weeks postpartum has a calming effect thought to enhance later emotional stability.[18] Also at this time the pups vocalize if left alone, which has been interpreted as an indication they notice the absence of companionship; when placed in strange surroundings as evidence of attachment to familiar places.[19]

Early socialization is believed to be a two-step process: (1) pups become distressed when left alone, and (2) their cries bring the adults to relieve their discomfort. What a pup's vocalizations actually signify to the mother is uncertain. That pups of either dogs or wolves vocalize to attract the attention of their mothers[20] is a false statement by implication of intentionality (Chapter 3). More likely the cause is entirely affective, and any presumed intentionality is misplaced if interpreted by the mothers' behavior. A mother dog ignores whining pups and seems unable to locate them even a meter or so away from the rearing site, especially if a pup is placed behind a screen and can be heard but not seen.[21] A whining pup placed 3 m away brought the mother to the rearing box and her other pups instead of to the whiner.[22] In fact, a mother dog was much more likely to respond to a silent moving pup than a pup that was loud and stationary.

Movement during the neonatal stage is restricted to weak crawling. Movement toward the mother and subsequent success in finding a teat requires her preliminary arousal. The senses of smell and taste are likely active in neonates, although of unknown importance.[23] There is no startle reaction, no response to noise or visual stimuli, and no fear of falling; no fear of anything. A neonate is able to lift its head weakly; it can right itself if turned onto its back. Affective state in response to cold, pain, or hunger is expressed by whining and even yelping.

The neonatal experiences of canids do not necessarily serve as either the foundation of later behaviors or even bridges leading to them.[24] For example, no canid barks as a neonate, but the frequency of other vocalizations is not a predictor of future breed differences in domestic dogs. This is demonstrated by basenjis, which are among the most vocal of all breeds as neonates but largely silent at maturity.[25] In practical terms the maternal care provided by a mother wolf or dog can be adequately replicated by human caregivers without undue concern that normal behavioral development will be somehow altered or disrupted.[26] Even wolves taken from their mothers at 3–5 days and reared by hand can be successfully integrated into a group of captive wolves as older pups.[27]

A *transitional* stage follows, lasting from 10 to 14 days and ending at age 3–4 weeks.[28] Young wolves in nature meet the pack on emerging from their dens at 10–24 days postpartum.[29] This is a crucial time of socialization when bonds other than maternal are starting to form. Some adult behaviors now appear, their execution crude, abbreviated, not necessarily the tenuous foundations on which later behaviors will be erected. Modifications at the transitional stage might not influence how adults behave.[30] Substitution of the mother's teat by a rubber nipple, for example, and subsequent rearing by an alien species (us) will have little effect on future behavior.

Onset of the transitional stage is marked by the opening of the eyes at about 13 days (range 11–19 days), at which time vision is immediately functional. The neonate's haptic world during this time is increasingly supplemented by other senses. Hearing commences at 3 weeks (range 2–4 weeks) with the opening of the *external auditory meatus*. Startle reactions to sound are apparent including withdrawal, flattening the body against the ground, and erecting the ears. By close of the transitional stage all senses are functional with thermotaxis and thigmotaxis having attenuated sharply. Wolves appear to develop fear responses earlier than dogs.[31]

Pup dogs separated from their mothers readily take to bottle-feeding while in the transitional stage. They can lap milk awkwardly from a dish, but become undernourished if simply left with a dish of milk and not subjected to external stimulation and handling by a human caregiver.[32] Forced weaning during the transitional stage results in temporary *sucking-frustration*, behavior in which a pup is likely to suck the caregiver's finger or a littermate's appendage in the absence of a nipple. These effects are gone by 5 weeks, indicating that sucking-frustration is not the cause of later aberrant behavior known as *body-sucking*.[33]

Many adult forms of behavior appear. Maternal care slackens, and the female intermittently leaves the pups to themselves, probably strengthening bonds among littermates. Crawling ceases, and more time is spent awake. At about 3 weeks most pup dogs are standing and walking unsteadily (both events can start as early as 12 days) and beginning to notice human observers. Eastern coyotes walked by day 21 and ran by day 23.[34]

During the transitional stage the pups start to urinate and defecate without their mother's prompting, ordinarily away from the den (wolves) or birth location (dogs), although some captive-born pup wolves were not seen defecating outside the den until 49 days.[35] They investigate the environment using all their senses and can orient toward distant objects. Elements of play can appear in dogs at 14 days,[36] and near the end of the transitional stage both dogs and wolves begin to play-fight, pawing and biting the mother and littermates and sometimes growling. Pup wolves ambush littermates and tussle clumsily.[37] Play in wolves can be delayed until the next stage, or 21 days. Its beginning, as described from observation of captive pups, consisted of face-paw and lick-up of conspecifics, sometimes chewing on an ear or the neck, and they licked and nibbled the observer's hand.[38]

The *critical stage* (also called *sensitive stage*) is third and most important in the socialization sequence because it envelopes a critical window of time during which emotional bonds are formed to individuals and places.[39] In social canids these are necessary for normal socialization. The critical stage in dogs commences at an average age of 19.5 days (range 16–22 days) and ordinarily extends 5–6 weeks, ending at 7–10 weeks.[40]

For wild canids the opening might be narrower. Pup eastern coyotes hand-reared through the critical stage socialized to humans, but pups reared by their parents were unapproachable, becoming more wary with age.[41] The critical stage started slightly earlier than in dogs and lasted only half as long. Fear in captive pup eastern coyotes was seen at 21 days, about the time they also responded to sound. They stiffened when picked up, crouched with wide open mouths and tails tucked between the legs, and refused to eat if humans were nearby unless the parents were there too. Pups removed during the third week could be socialized to humans successfully. They became friendly but responded negatively to even gentle discipline, sometimes with aggression. Past 21 days was too late. Two 5-week-old pups taken from their parents had to be returned at feeding time because they refused to eat. Although handled many times daily they never became tame and were eventually placed back with the litter where they behaved like the others – wary, wild, and stiffening when handled. On seeing a stranger their immediate response was to escape and hide.[42]

As mentioned, by this time pups can perform awkward equivalents of some adult behaviors: locomotion, feeding, defecating and urinating on their own, play-fighting, tussling, and barking. Play near the end of the critical stage includes maladroit attempts to mount other littermates. In wolves, adolescents sometimes join pups in play.[43] Pups removed from familiar individuals or locations express their discomfort by vocalizing. Barking begins at 18–24 days in dogs[44] and as early as day 1 in wolves.[45] Through the first 4 weeks or so the pups continue to be nursed. The end of the critical stage therefore coincides with weaning. Also about this time (21 days) the canine and incisor teeth appear in dogs,[46] and pups start to chew on littermates and to eat supplementary dry food if provided as a mash.

At 24 days captive pup wolves display a startle response and try to avoid unfamiliar stimuli by running away and hiding.[47] They show active submission by approaching a conspecific or human caregiver with tail-low and wagging rapidly, ears-folded, tongue-flicking, and wearing a submissive-grin.[48] The *exaggerated look-away* becomes apparent at 30 days during play-solicitation. In this behavior the play solicitor turns its head and neck to the side while watching its potential playmate from the corner of its eye. The soliciting pup approaches another with ears-flat and lips retracted in a submissive-grin then jerks its head suddenly to one side and slightly backward. Sometimes this move is accompanied by pawing and licking-up.

At 43 days pup wolves are observed *jaw-snapping* (an aggressive behavior sometimes seen in adults) along with ears-flat, yelping, and growling. At about the same time pups chewing on each other during play perform vigorous *head-shakes* as if killing small prey. Jaw-wrestling has become well developed and used during play and fighting, often in conjunction with growling, whining, and ears-flat. At 8 weeks pup wolves begin to nose-push, directing this behavior at conspecifics and caregivers during greeting and play solicitation. In the latter application "the push may take the form of a more intense stab."[49]

What has been thought of as play "is performed during social interactions in which there is a decrease in social distance between the interactants, and no evidence of social investigation or of agonistic … or passive-submissive behaviors … although these actions may occur as derived acts during play."[50] This definition fails by stating what play is *not*, and by excluding other instances of social distance diminishing and not normally associated with play. Examples are when animals rest or sleep next to each other, feed peacefully shoulder to shoulder, and one grooms another.

Many definitions of animal play have been suggested, and all are deficient.[51] For purposes here *play* can be considered "all locomotor activity performed postnatally that appears to an observer to have no obvious immediate benefits for the player, in which motor patterns resembling those used in serious functional contexts may be used in modified form."[52] Until this point most of the play discussed has been *social play*, which involves direct interaction between or among conspecifics or other animals, including us. Authorities also consider two other categories. *Locomotor play* is usually performed by young animals when alone and involves such activities as tail-chasing, jumping, and so forth, none having any immediate benefit. During *object play* (Fig. 9.1) an animal paws, bites, chews, chases, or pulls an object (e.g. a ball or stick).

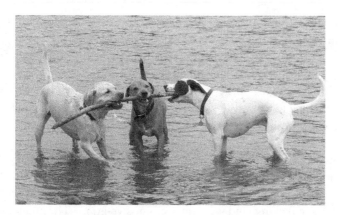

Figure 9.1 Object play: three dogs with a stick.
Source: Ljung|Dreamstime.com.

The incidence of barking in pup dogs during social interaction with littermates starts to rise at 5 weeks, peaks at 11 weeks when maximum breed differences are also apparent, and begins to decline at 15 weeks.[53] Pups left with the mother through weaning but handled regularly from age 5 weeks emerge from the critical stage with the same low timidity as pups fed exclusively by human caregivers.[54] Therefore, the feeding process is an important factor in socialization, but not the only one.

By 6 weeks of age, or 3 weeks into the critical stage, pup dogs are attempting to follow scent trails.[55] They can run, although coordination is not yet fully developed. *Allelomimetic behavior* (coordinated group activities) appears; for example, the pups run to greet a human caregiver or the mother if she has been absent, or one pup is attacked by its littermates during play-fighting.

Toward the end of the critical stage pup wolves start to feed on opened carcasses.[56] Pup dogs start taking solid food of increasingly coarse consistency, defecate in specific locations, and sleep apart from the mother and littermates. Agonistic behavior intensifies. Whining when approaching a human or another dog is accompanied by tail-wagging, pawing, and attempting to lick-up. This behavior, thought to be infantile and representing food solicitation, persists into adulthood and often throughout life. Wolves socialized to humans also behave this way toward human companions.[57]

From 3 to 8 weeks is the window of time for establishing bonds with a pup dog or pup wolf. Weaning is complete by 8 weeks, at which time all basic adult behaviors are in place and social relations have become established. In dogs this important event peaks between 6 and 8 weeks, the ideal time to remove a pup from the litter and make it a pet.[58] Pup wolves raised starting at 3 weeks bond easily with humans and domestic dogs.[59]

During weaning a mother dog growls at her pups if they seek her nipples.[60] She might shake them or shove them away, teeth-bared, and by week 10 most pups have abandoned any further attempts to nurse. They now display aggression toward littermates during feeding.

Socialization in the wolf might peak a week or so earlier than in the dog, and unless efforts are made to overcome signs of the fear apparent at week 6 or 7 a positive response becomes progressively more difficult, requiring considerable effort by the end of week 8. If the critical stage passes, by week 12 "the fear responses are developed to the point where strange objects, loud noises, or strange people usually elicit urination, defecation, salivation, crouching, piloerection, pupillary dilation, tail-ducking, trembling, and a laying back of the ears."[61] The socialization process takes increasingly longer at 6 months and older.

Wolves reared in captivity – and domestic dogs in particular – are not necessarily damaged when something goes awry during the critical stage. Both show considerable ontogenetic flexibility. Single pup dogs reared with domestic kittens and nursed by the mother cat from age 25 days through 16 weeks seldom vocalized and rarely wagged their tails.[62] After 2 weeks of living with dog-raised pups the same age they behaved no differently than their peers and were socialized completely.

The effects are similar on wolves raised with varying degrees of interaction with humans, wolves, and dogs, as demonstrated in isolation experiments using a litter of six pups reared with minimal human contact.[63] One pup was isolated from age 27 days to 6 months and during this time had daily contact with people but not wolves. Two others were isolated from days 27 to 43 without human contact except when removed from their cages for caretaking; after day 43 they received no contact at all from humans or wolves. Two more were caged together from day 27 to age 6 months with humans but not wolves visible to them. A final pup was raised in a home with an owned dog. The isolated pups displayed several self-directed behaviors (e.g. grooming the legs, chasing the tail, biting a hind leg, pawing water in the water dish, playing with a bone). When placed together after the treatment periods all wolves except one male showed initial fear manifested as tail-low, running back and forth and jumping at the walls, and drooling. This soon stopped, a dominance hierarchy emerged, and normal behaviors expected in a wolf sociogram appeared (Chapter 3).[64] These observations parallel others demonstrating that pup wolves reared in captivity without adult "tutors" assume appropriate roles and behave as members of an integrated social group.[65] As a consequence the social development of wolves and dogs is strongly buffered across a broad range of extrinsic conditions even during the critical stage, as shown by the restricted range of emergent phenotypic behaviors. Isolation and limited contact with other wolves did not produce creatures "unable or unwilling to interact appropriately with conspecifics, animals that are extraordinarily violent, socially incompetent, or ostracized from the group."[66]

A popular hypothesis proposes that the first wolves tamed by humans were those lurking around the campfire hoping to scavenge scraps. With the passing of time and through generations of wolves and humans a few animals eventually lost their fear and became tame. Such a progression is doubtful. Adult wolves are difficult to socialize (see below). The first wolves to interact fully with humans must have been taken from the den early and socialized while still young. Even a hand-raised wolf is an unreliable and often aggressive companion on reaching sexual maturity.[67]

The fourth stage of development, the *adolescent stage*, extends from weaning to sexual maturity, which occurs between 5 and 12 months in dogs, but usually 22–24 months in wolves (Chapter 8). Maximum physical development is attained at about age 2 years in dogs (males and females) and female wolves. Male wolves in northwestern Alaska reach full adult body mass at 11 months, females at 23 months.[68] Motor skills improve during adolescence, and males can balance on three legs and raised-leg urinate at 5–12 months.[69] Both sexes begin to ground-scratch and urinate on scent-posts. Food-solicitation and allelomimetic behaviors are still prominent. Play-fighting diminishes. Agonism takes the form of dominant ↔ subordinate displays, especially in dogs and captive wolves. Sexual maturity defines the arbitrary end of adolescence.

Among wolves, older pups and younger adolescents can be identified by their social behavior:[70] (1) higher frequency of play, (2) play at inappropriate times (e.g. while hunting), (3) limited participation in killing large game, (4) limited hunting skills,[71] (5) enhanced "freedom of behavior"[72] reflecting permissiveness of the dominant pair,[73] (6) fluid social rank among themselves,[74] (7) no expression of sexual behavior, (8) friendliness among themselves and submission only to older pack members,[75] (9) tendency to travel at the rear of the pack, and (10) often sleeping in contact with each other.[76]

Dogs taken from shelters bonded rapidly with their handlers, and their anxiety diminished.[77] However, a captive wolf that has not been socialized to humans is often sensitive to even minor external changes. One investigator wrote that moving such an animal to a novel environment disturbed it less than minimally altering its present surroundings by placing new objects in the yard.[78]

9.2   Play and bonding

My use of the term play has so far been descriptive and without comment about its possible function in animal societies. The subject is an epistemological minefield camouflaged cleverly through "the transfer of concepts derived from human experience."[79] For example, we could delude ourselves into thinking of play as practice for the adult activities it resembles, a teleological presumption that ontogenetic stages "exist for the sake of adult life."[80] The claim that play assists development is another teleological fallacy. Even if ontogenetic progression and play were to show strong correlation, this would not be evidence that animals play to develop socially.[81] Thus at a societal level the statement, "there has been a unanimous conclusion that the development of social behavior is intimately related to the ontogeny of social play"[82] appears to be unanimously misinformed.

Play might not actually be playful, but rather the antithesis of having a good time.[83] In other words, play is serious activity. Crisler believed that the dog's dependence on humans gives its life triviality. "There is no triviality about a wolf, even in play."[84] As Ghiselin noted, "animals at play behave very much as if they were at work."[85] He suggested that play functions to prevent agonism, and this might hold true in canid societies.[86] Perhaps more accurately it serves to nullify the aggressive components of agonism. Certainly some behaviors slide into different contexts when agonism and play overlap. Growling, barking, face-pawing, and submissive-grinning are seen during both activities. The growls emitted during aggression and play are similar, and other dogs and wolves are likely to recognize the differences by facial and body displays of the growler.[87] Two statements can be made with reasonable assurance.[88] First, play is not a "primary activity" because it seems to occur more frequently after an animal's physiological needs and drives have been satisfied. Animals that are hungry, sick, or cold tend to play less, although at least some play distracts even the disadvantaged: abandoned buildings occupied by urban street dogs often contain play objects, such as chewed balls and sticks.[89] Second, like other social behaviors play progresses ontogenetically, its normal development depending partly on social experience and conditioning. In domestic dogs it also depends on breeding. Golden retrievers displayed more wolf-like visual signals than Siberian huskies, but used them in play that seldom escalated into aggression.[90] In this instance agonistic signaling has been altered by behavioral paedomorphism to mimic continuous infantile behavior.

Play also depends on species. Behavioral development starting at about 21 days differs noticeably among dogs, coyotes, eastern coyotes, and wolves.[91] Early on, coyotes are the most aggressive. Social relationships are established by day 30 and involve severe fights after which aggression diminishes and social play becomes prominent. Dominant coyotes are least successful at initiating play. Dogs (beagles in this case) were the least agonistic and most playful, engaging in play bouts three times more often than wolves and seven times more than coyotes. Wolves were slightly more agonistic than dogs, but the aggression took the form of threats, never fights. Agonistic behavior declined and social play rose between days 43 and 50. In general, its early social development was similar to the dog's.

Play is an integral part of wolf societies. Following a successful hunt there can be much gamboling, chasing each other singly and in groups, ambushing, and wrestling.[92] After sighting or scenting a moose the large Isle Royale pack was seen to "assemble closely, sniff noses, and wag tails before starting toward the prey."[93] Wolves also assemble just before setting out to hunt, a ritual that includes enthusiastic sniffing of noses, tail-wagging, romping, and occasional chorus-howling.[94] Even those left behind to babysit might participate by following the others a short distance before turning back. Murie reported a thrilling scene as the pack he was monitoring gathered before an evening hunt.[95] The pack stopped to play after having gone about 0.4 km. The female doing babysitting duty ran to them and joined the pushing and clasping. After a few minutes the hunting pack of four set off again. The female followed a short distance, lay down briefly, and returned to the den.

Wolves attack bears and other potential predators that wander near their dens, but when humans remove their pups they howl and leap about at a distance, signs not of aggression but of anguish.[96] The notion that wolves past a certain age

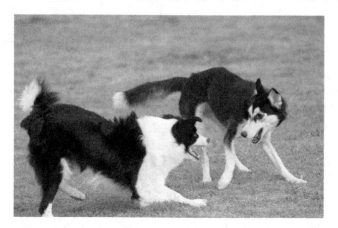

Figure 9.2 Play-bow used during play-solicitation.
Source: Raywoo|Dreamstime.com.

(about 3 months) are resistant to socialization[97] might hold true for their interaction with humans, but as noted previously is refuted each time an individual disperses and immigrates into an alien pack. Here, play appears crucial to successful integration. A loner observed by Murie attempted to play with members of the resident pack in Denali before being driven off.[98] Acceptance of a new breeding male into a Yellowstone pack was preceded not just by displays of dominance and submission by the various individuals, but extended displays of play-solicitation initiated by the stranger.[99]

Wolves also play before facing a formidable foe. Two adult and two adolescent wolves in the Nelchina Basin surrounded an adult brown bear feeding on a moose carcass: "Three of the wolves huddled together touching noses and wagging tails, then separated and charged the bear, displacing it from the kill."[100]

Wolves give each other – and tame wolves give to humans – what Crisler called the "full wolf greeting." She never defined this term, but it seems to indicate play-solicitation. Evidently a wolf lays its chin on the ground followed by the rest of its body, the front legs splayed out at 45 degrees. The Crislers returned the greeting by mimicking this body posture.[101] Similar behavior termed the *play-bow* is commonly seen in dogs and wolves and considered play-solicitation. The dog soliciting play crouches, forelegs flat on the ground and rump elevated,[102] sometimes with the tail-wagging (Fig. 9.2). *Play-solicitation* includes behaviors like play-bow, prancing in front of the prospective playmate, licking-up, face-pawing,[103] exaggerated approach and withdrawal as if encouraging chase, exaggerated look-away, and rushing at a playmate and then running off. A play signal in dogs is often accompanied or followed by a bark.[104] Strange dogs might respond with conflicted behavior (Fig. 9.3). The spotted animal in the middle has solicited play from the dog on the right and is behaving submissively. However, the dog being solicited is conflicted about the other's intentions. Its ears and tail are erect in a dominant's posture, but its foreleg has also been extended in a tentative face-paw.

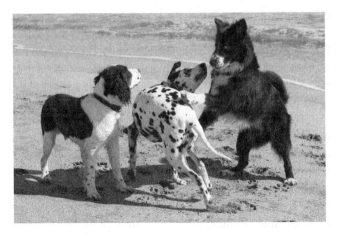

Figure 9.3 Conflicted behavior during play solicitation.
Source: Galena Barskaya|Dreamstime.com.

Tail-wagging is a general expression of excitement, not just part of a social greeting. Wolves wag their tails when closing in on prey after a stalk.[105] Wolves also tail-wag when alone and hunting mice: "When looking for a mouse – one for which it had pounced and not captured – it wagged its tail, the rate of tail wagging increasing with the rise of its excitement, which in turn was dependent upon the nearness of the mouse."[106] Twice while this wolf pursued mice it stopped to howl. In dogs play-bows and other play-soliciting behaviors are often accompanied by barking.

Wolves generally make comparatively poor candidates for socialization with humans, but there are exceptions.[107] A wolf named Lady Silver, taken as a pup from a Montana den in the 1920s, later performed in Hollywood movies.[108] Other wolves have been trained to pull sleds (no doubt poorly) and one, having been raised with a water spaniel, even performed as a field dog. This Great Lakes wolf × Canadian gray wolf cross named Big Jim, reared from a day old in a Detroit home, learned to retrieve ducks. When a TV station arrived to film Big Jim in action, "he retrieved everything, including the photographer's tripod – everything but a duck."[109] In 1952, at age 15 months, Big Jim was released onto Isle Royale. At 40 kg he had become too large to keep as an urban pet.

With diligence even adult wolves unfamiliar with humans and showing extreme fear can be socialized to some extent.[110] When the investigator initially enters the cage with a nonsocialized adult wolf and sits quietly in a corner the animal makes every effort to escape. It leaps into the air, digs at the floor, paws the doors, and retreats as far as possible. These responses continue for a month or so each time the investigator enters. Gradually the wolf's emotional intensity abates, replaced by a calmer avoidance. Escape attempts become less frequent, and instead of crouching and trembling in a corner it now sits with ears erect. Movement by the investigator, however, can instantly initiate the fear response with its attendant behaviors.

Several more months pass. The investigator and the wolf can slowly approach each other, provided the investigator looks askance. Activity stops on eye contact. The wolf sniffs the investigator, retreating if receiving a direct look. Later it chews and pulls his clothes and rubs against the place where he sat. Sometimes the wolf scent-marks this location with urine. Still later it might rub against the investigator, urinate directly on him, and often allow itself to be petted. These curious behaviors might represent efforts to make the intruder a familiar part of the habitat.

Wolves urine-mark territorial boundaries, but ordinarily only dominant wolves do this, and they preferentially mark prominent objects in the landscape. Much of this wolf's behavior was conflicted. To a wolf not yet socialized to humans the investigator's presence was confusing by being unfamiliar. Consequently, the wolf urine-marked him as it would a fence post or any landmark, but perhaps also because of his strange and frightening odor. Urinating on each other is not what wolves do, even to strange wolves, and this one doubtfully considered the investigator a conspecific. In fact, he might not have represented anything except an unnerving presence. Wolves have no way of responding to environmental stimuli except as wolves. They make the unfamiliar seem comfortable by urine-marking it, as this wolf over-marked the location recently occupied by the human intruder.

With confidence the wolf's fear and uncertainty morph into aggression. It bites and tugs the investigator's clothes. If he moves to stop this behavior the bites become harder, the tugs more vigorous. Attempts at domination can trigger an attack or else a reversion to an earlier stage in the sequence, making the recovery of lost progress difficult and extending the socialization process. During this important period the wolf, still unsure of itself, gives conflicted signals: a lip-curl, a growl, ears-flat. Another person should be present outside the cage and move forward if the animal becomes too aggressive, which causes it to stop and retreat.

More time passes, and aggressive behavior tapers off, replaced by timid friendliness. The wolf has now lost its fear and approaches the investigator when he enters the cage, allowing itself to be petted. It tail-wags on seeing him, licks his hands, licks-up at his face. It clasps the investigator, muzzle-grabs his chin or nose in greeting.[111] Complete socialization in this case took about 7 months of hourly sessions repeated every third day. Wild-caught adult wolves at Moscow Zoopark supposedly became socialized to humans. I found no description of how this was accomplished and how long it took, just the statement, "even adult wolves which entered captivity in a surly spirit and had appeared savage and ferocious may become tame."[112] A collaborating author in these studies later provided information indicating that wild-caught adults are trainable.[113]

Socialization of pup wolves requires continuous reinforcement or else tameness fades and is extinguished after 6 months of no human contact.[114] Despite the many months needed to socialize an adult, tameness is subsequently retained even after the animal is left in the company of nonsocialized conspecifics and been without human handling for 22 months.[115] Also in contrast with dogs, wolves apparently do not bond strongly with specific humans,[116] but all humans who "act appropriately towards them."[117] In wild wolves this behavior obviously does not extend unilaterally to wolves from alien packs (Chapter 5), nor in captive wolves to known conspecifics as described later.

Social bonds evidently are not dependent on food as innately rewarding but develop separately, suggesting that how food is delivered is irrelevant to their formation. To test this idea, dogs were separated from their mothers at 3 weeks and placed in two groups with the same amount of human contact through the critical stage.[118] One group was fed by mechanical devices, the other by hand. Both groups became equally attached to people. Food is a motivator in one respect: underfed pups bonded with their human caregivers more rapidly than overfed pups. Thus socialization proceeds whether or not food is used as a reward, although hunger can accelerate the process.[119] In fact, food seems less important than companionship during the socialization process. Pup wolves 6 weeks old and starved for 18 hours chose the company of a familiar adult malamute over a food reward.[120]

Not even punishment necessarily retards socialization. Fox terrier pups were separated into three groups, reared in isolation, and fed mechanically to eliminate food as a variable. All were taken from their isolation containers for regular human contact and treated as follows:[121] group 1 (always treated kindly), group 2 (treated kindly or punished at random), group 3 (punished for any movement toward the human caregiver). Group 2 pups were the most attracted toward the caregiver and showed the greatest dependency, probably the result of intermittent positive reinforcement. Group 3 pups showed the least. At the end of the critical stage these differences disappeared rapidly, and all pups approached the caregiver. Thus intermittent punishment does not impede socialization and might even accelerate it. Separating pup dogs from their mothers and littermates in a strange place for 20 hours each day hastened socialization to humans.[122] Experiments such as these are evidence that induction of strong emotion in young pups, "whether hunger, fear, pain, or loneliness, will speed up the process of socialization"[123] and might explain why the critical stage is delayed until pertinent emotional reactions are possible.

Early socialization depends on mutual reinforcement, strengthening the bond between adults and pups and especially between pups and their mothers. The bond is strong, as revealed by anecdotes of how parent wolves behave when their pups are taken away. When Parmelee and a colleague ran down and captured two pups on the tundra of Ellesmere Island, the mother came bounding toward them. Expecting to be attacked, Parmelee wrote, "what happened next was hardly predictable. The big wolf skidded to a full stop and whined pitifully. Ambling around the pup and me, she whimpered and emitted strange ululations. There were no fierce snarls – not even one good growl."[124] They released one pup and started back with the other. Along the way they shot some ptarmigans for museum specimens and tied them off to their rifle barrels They slung the rifles over their shoulders and trudged on, Parmelee still carrying the other pup with its mother following closely behind.[125] She stayed outside their tent that night, and the men subsequently gave her back the pup.

On 15 May 1940 Murie took a week-old pup from a den in Denali, leaving five others behind. The parents showed no distress other than to bark and howl from a distance until he left. Murie raised the pup and chained it outside his cabin. By June, members of the pack had found it and began visiting.[126] The Crislers took all five pups from a den in the Brooks Range while the parents "bounded around crying."[127] At no time did they become aggressive.

Bonding with littermates begins almost from birth. These relationships become more established during play, and even older pup wolves occasionally require mutual contact when sleeping. Other pack members, subordinate females especially, might babysit the pups while the mother hunts with the pack (Chapter 8).[128] Adult pack members returning from a hunt regurgitate recently ingested meat onto the ground, which weaned pups gobble up (Chapter 8). Thus adults and to a lesser extent adolescents from previous years are major influences in socializing the pups and facilitating mutually affectionate ties with pack members. "Very briefly, the wolf's bonds to other members of its pack seem to be about the same as a dog's bond to its master."[129]

According to Mech, "by the time the pups are traveling with the pack (about seven months of age), their ability to form new psychological ties, without the forced training of experimental conditions, is almost nil."[130] This might be the case with wolf–human interactions,[131] but were it true generally no wolf could ever disperse, pair with an unrelated stranger, or integrate into an alien pack. Wolves often pair long before the mating season, but this doubtfully constitutes extended courtship as claimed.[132] More likely it represents the formation of a long-term bond based on friendship. It has yet to be shown that any "expectation" of impending sexual contact, which is explicit in courtship, factors into friendships formed between wolves as pups or early adolescents. On the other hand, it could be argued that no such "expectation" is required if the courtship–mating–reproduction sequence is seamless, although believing this hardly constitutes a test of the prolonged courtship hypothesis. Until refuted the null – and simplest – hypothesis is friendship and mutual affection between wolves of opposite sex.

Pair bonds can form between adult wolves and dogs. I found one case especially interesting.[133] It occurred at Mishmar Ha Emeq, a kibbutz 20 km southeast of Haifa, Israel. A farmer living there identified only as Mr. Shamgar owned a male Alsatian mixed-breed that went with him into the fields. One day in February 1963 Mr. Shamgar saw what he thought was a jackal and signaled his dog to chase it away, but the animal was a female wolf, among the last survivors of a nearby pack. Dog and wolf sniffed each other and started to play, spending most of the day together. The next morning the wolf was waiting for them in the field.

There followed many days of play, mutual mountings, and copulations. The wolf began approaching the farmer within 20 m, but then disappeared to have her pups. During this time the dog also disappeared intermittently, sometimes for a few days. The pups were found dead when about 6 weeks old in an orchard that had been sprayed with insecticide. The wolf then returned and once again spent time with the farmer and his dog in the fields. She also began accompanying them back to the living area, often trailing only a meter behind Mr. Shamgar, although the distance lengthened if he looked directly at her. Some mornings she was waiting on his doorstep. During estrus in 1964 both the dog and the wolf disappeared, returned for a time, then disappeared for good. A home film showed the wolf to initiate most interactions with the dog, but the dog's activities were influenced mainly by Mr. Shamgar.

A pack of Ellesmere Island wolves consisting of an adult pair and three adolescents from the previous year produced no pups in 1993.[134] However, the parents treated the adolescents as if they were pups, hunting hares and regurgitating food for them and leaving them occasionally at a familiar rendezvous site. Once when the adults tried to depart the younger wolves refused to follow and started to howl. The parents gave in and returned. This pack was more nomadic without a den site to attend. Had there been pups, the adolescents might have matured faster, becoming better hunters and helping supply their younger siblings with food. They might even have dispersed.

Murie, among the first to unobtrusively and with limited bias observe a wild wolf pack, wrote: "The strongest impression remaining with me after watching wolves ... was their friendliness. The adults were friendly toward each other and amiable towards the pups ... This innate good feeling has been strongly marked in the three captive wolves which I have known."[135]

Play in pup wolves is precocial. By 4 weeks they display socially reciprocal behaviors: wrestling, mutual licking, tug-of-war, and rudimentary expressions of dominance $\leftrightarrow$ submission.[136] These activities diminish over the next 4 weeks but rise in pup dogs, increasing steadily through 16 weeks. With age the wolves became more aloof, the dogs more social. It should be mentioned that agonistic behaviors witnessed when pups interact are not necessarily evidence of actual dominance $\leftrightarrow$ submission, "only that these postures are correlated with dominant and subordinate status among adults."[137]

Wild wolves are not inherently aggressive toward humans and other pack members, but in socialized wolves this trait also extends to dogs. A wolf raised from a pup avoided aggressive dogs and refused to fight with them, "often turning his head and pressing his hips against the other animal."[138] Murie briefly described the growth and behavior of a female wolf he raised from a pup. He wrote, "she often cowered in a friendly way when I approached her, just as a wild wolf often cowers when approaching another wolf."[139] She liked dogs and enjoyed playing with them, always gently. She could easily have injured them but never did, even on occasions when the dogs became aggressive toward her. This seems typical of captive-raised wolves. Fentress' pet wolf Lupey was also friendly with dogs, greeting them with squeaks and pawing,[140] and the Crislers' wolves solicited dogs to play with them, what Crisler referred to as "courting."[141]

Wolves are reluctant to attack humans even when placed at a distinct disadvantage where escape is impossible. Biologists can often handle a wolf caught in a trap by simply pinning its neck to the ground using a forked stick or holding it firmly by the scruff of the neck. Mech and his colleagues used both methods on a trapped wolf to attach an ear tag and radio collar and examine the teeth. The animal remained "as docile as if anesthetized."[142]

So far I have discussed the bonds dogs and wolves form with each other and with humans but without mentioning their affective nature. *Infantile attachment* is a particular subcategory of bonding directed by an infant toward its mother.[143] A corollary requires that the mother serve as a *secure base* to which the infant returns for comfort and security, as seen in chimpanzee and human infants.[144]

By these definitions a bond does not qualify as infantile attachment unless it can be shown that an infant considers its mother a secure base. Several criteria determine this, one being recognition: the infant must be able to distinguish its mother from other conspecifics. At 4–5.5 weeks pup dogs purportedly recognize their mothers and littermates based on olfaction alone, and the mothers supposedly recognize them.[145] Whether either party recognizes the other specifically as close kin and not simply familiar conspecifics has not been shown (Chapter 8). An infant might demonstrate a clear preference for its mother over other adult females by staying in close proximity in her presence, displaying *separation anxiety* (e.g. increased vocalization when she leaves, increased activity) in her absence, and recognition when she returns.[146] Nonetheless, these behaviors are not evidence of kin recognition, as claimed. Cross-fostered pups behave identically.

Attachment to humans by dogs is evident starting at 16 weeks.[147] Bonds with humans come easier to pup dogs than to wolves the same age and appear to require less interaction. Pup dogs subjected to intense handling by human caregivers became attached no more strongly than pups simply reared by their mothers in a household,[148] suggesting that even casual contact is sufficient. Socialization of pup wolves to humans is generally a more rigorous process than it is with dogs,[149] and pup wolves show the same response to humans whether familiar or strangers.[150] Limited behavioral expressions were compared in dog and pup wolves at age 3, 4, and 5 weeks, all animals having been intensively hand-reared by individual caregivers.[151] Activity levels were similar. Dogs tail-wagged more and avoided humans less. Pup dogs were never aggressive toward humans, but in 26% of trials wolves growled at familiar humans and even tried to bite them, and aggression was more pronounced than in dogs over the whole period. Although at 5 weeks the wolves preferred their caregivers to other humans, the attachment was looser than it was with dogs, and the wolves were more easily distracted.

Wolves make the transition to solid food more slowly. During the first 10 weeks they develop more quickly, are more active, and overall motor performance exceeds that of dogs the same age. During bottle feeding they are more discerning about the size and texture of the nipple, and changing the formula can disrupt feeding and digestion. In the end socialization can be problematical: "From about 6 weeks of age to about 8 weeks of age, their orientation toward humans shifted from passive acceptance to indifference to tolerance to wariness, and even during [the critical] period they showed an unequivocal preference for canine social partners."[152] The group-ceremony observed in a pack of wild wolves for a returning member was not transferred to human caregivers, behavior the opposite allelomimetic displays by pup dogs.

9.3   Confinement and social order in wolves

To believe that a mirror held up to a zoo cage reflects back an image of nature is naïve. I say this confidently after spending much of a working life observing animals in the wild while also capturing and taking care of them at zoological institutions. As I argued elsewhere, the zoo is a simulacrum, its animals artifacts.[153] The philosopher Keekok Lee defined an *artifact* as "any entity or object which does not exist in nature (without human intervention), but is created by humans, according to human designs to fulfill human purposes."[154]

All domesticated flora and fauna are artifactual, and so are zoo animals. Those "rescued" wolves in captive breeding programs hardly qualify as *natural kinds*, entities capable of evolving or even existing as independent agents. Certainly their reproductive choices are not their own. Lee wrote, "any organism which has been deprived of its reproductive powers and success may be said to be ontologically different from other naturally-occurring organisms and, therefore, lack independence and autonomy in a radical sense."[155]

Behaviors have social relevance only when measured in context, and the interactions among captive canids give a fractured representation of freely roaming packs, groups, or individuals. Mech understood the situation clearly: "Such an approach is analogous to trying to draw inferences about human family dynamics by studying humans in refugee camps."[156] Prisons, where control is absolute and dispersal not an option, might be more appropriate. A refugee camp is similar to a landscape of saturated territories: everyone is free to leave, but few have anyplace to go.

The following observations hold more or less true for captive wolves. Dominant males generally tolerate subordinates except during the breeding season; dominant females are less tolerant of lower-ranking females at all times and across more contexts.[157] One dominant female, for example, was intolerant of her subordinates when they were eating and when they howled.[158] In other instances, captive females have killed rivals.[159]

A dominant female wolf can prevent the others from breeding, intimidating them into separating from the group and assaulting any subordinate in estrus attempting to solicit the attention of a male.[160] Specific mate preferences develop, and a dominant male might intimidate or briefly attack a subordinate attempting to mate with his favorite female, which might not be the dominant one.[161] Sometimes the dominant female joins him in these attacks despite having been rejected. Alliances can form. In one case a subordinate male always protected the dominant male while he was being attacked *in flagrante delicto* by another subordinate.[162]

Dominants ordinarily hold sway over members of their own sex, but if the dominant male is removed his female counterpart not only mates with one or more lesser males, but also intimidates them. Removal of one or both dominants from a captive group during the breeding season throws the social order into disarray, which can result in more subordinates mating.[163] Nonetheless, wolf–wolf relationships, once established, can remain stable through periods of separation of at least a year.[164]

Underlying most – perhaps all – of these exaggerated behaviors is the inability of young captive wolves to emigrate. Wolves start to disperse from the pack as young as 9 months, most are gone after 2 years, and few remain after 3 years (Chapter 5). Confinement promotes the continuous reinforcement of dominance ↔ submission. Agonistic behavior escalates, leaving no room for the natural attenuation of its aggressive components. What in the wild would be friendly displays and egalitarianism devolve into bickering, fights, and formation of alliances. Introduction of wolves from outside the familiar group is another factor likely to promote aggression. Incomplete habituation to humans undoubtedly makes captive wolves uneasy, and in situations of constant stress minor infractions within the social structure tend to become magnified. The emphasis on sustaining social hierarchies by captive animals of many species seems more pathological than natural.[165] Whatever its cause, the intense agonistic behavior reported in colonies of captive wolves is an aberration worth discussing for this reason.[166]

Erik Zimen published two studies of a group of anomic zoo wolves that read like lupine inflections of *In the Belly of the Beast*, Jack Henry Abbott's letters from prison.[167] Zimen's bland prose scarcely camouflaged the angst and violence brought on by confinement and a mix of animals with limited or no history of familiarity. Originally, 19 Eurasian gray wolves were squeezed into an enclosure of 500 m² (0.05 ha).[168] Four three-year-olds eventually got transferred to an enclosure of 65,000 m² (6.5 ha) where the pack was later "enlarged by 5," whether familiar wolves or strangers is not stated.[169] That same month four pups were born. The group now numbered 13. My narrative from this point is based on Zimen's 1975 report, which thoroughly and with considerable insight details the interactions among individuals.

Some pups (these and presumably others before them) were separated from their mothers at age 6 days to 3 weeks and hand-reared so they could later be leashed and taken for walks outside the compound. These animals seemed more active, their behavior less stereotyped than those left with their mothers, which in contrast "give one a rather apathetic impression."[170] The group thus comprised both tamed and untamed animals. When Zimen's observations commenced during October 1968 there were four males and three females.

Consistent with some other reports of captive wolves this group aligned itself into bilinear hierarchies of males and females.[171] Aggression within the male ranks ordinarily was subdued, no lower-ranking animal seeming to dominate any other consistently. The female hierarchy displayed a true rank order with the dominant holding sway over female number 2, and she in turn over female number 3.

The females were also more aggressive among themselves, especially in winter during the breeding season. The hierarchies were not completely independent. The dominant male out-ranked the dominant female, and she out-ranked the subordinate males, which out-ranked the subordinate females. Pups ranked lowest. Between-sex aggression was rarely observed. Ensuing altercations, presumably about rank, will now be described starting with the females. What follows is an abbreviated account of events paraphrased from Zimen's descriptions. As we shall see, motivation was noncompetitive unless possession of a mate is counted as object-directed.[172] In addition, aggression was highest during times when the hierarchy was unstable.

In a pack of wild wolves the rules of dominance "bear no resemblance to those of the pecking order, that of a group of similar individuals competing for rank."[173] In contrast, social competition can be an ongoing activity among those held captive. When observations of this group begin, Anfa, the oldest female, is slightly dominant over Andra, the next oldest, with Mädchen ranking lowest. Relations are friendly, and the three often play together. Starting in November 1968, during play Andra becomes increasingly aggressive toward Anfa. This apparently stimulates Anfa to direct her own aggression toward Mädchen. Play tapers off. By February 1969 Anfa and Andra are equals, and in March all three come into estrus. Without a fight Andra becomes dominant and suppresses any socializing with the males by Anfa and Mädchen. If a male approaches either of them Andra inserts herself between the pair and drives away her rival.[174] All play among them ceases; none mates.

Social suppression subsides after the breeding season, and in April play again commences. Andra still tries occasionally to dominate Anfa, but Anfa now resists. The situation remains uneasy into June, when Anfa begins to show signs of dominance. However, she approaches Andra in the guise of a subordinate with tail-low and head-low and then attacks her hesitantly. Remaining superior, Andra does not retaliate.

At the end of June a fight takes place. For an entire day Anfa attacks Andra, but Andra still does not respond. Then the real fight starts. The animals attack each other ferociously. The action is silent and brutal. Mädchen, showing allegiance to Anfa, joins her to fight the dominant Andra. Overwhelmed, Andra loses as the males stand around and watch. She retreats to a shallow depression in the ground.

Attacks continue the following day, Anfa once again the dominant female. She displays this new status by walking stiff-legged with tail-high and urinating with a raised leg. Andra skulks around the enclosure, occasionally attacked by the males, although the most intense attacks come from Anfa, and, to a lesser extent, Mädchen. Time passes (how much time is not stated) and Mädchen challenges Anfa, her former ally, for dominance. A fierce fight erupts in mid-July. The combatants stop after 15 minutes, seemingly by mutual consent. Neither is clearly the victor; both are hurt badly.

They resume the battle the next day, and Anfa's nose is injured. Although Mädchen appears to be winning, Anfa does not retreat. Mädchen now struts the postures of a dominant. Anfa, despite behaving as the subordinate, attacks Mädchen. Andra, suddenly in allegiance with Anfa, joins in, and the two drive

Mädchen into retreat after an attack lasting 10 minutes. Over the next few days Anfa continues to attack Mädchen, while Andra, having moved up a rank, becomes playful and submits to Anfa.[175] In mid-August Mädchen, for the first time, demonstrates submissive behavior toward Anfa. Play among the females resumes, and ranks have returned to the same order as the previous October: Anfa > Andra > Mädchen.

The four males were all the same age (1.5 years). Zimen's description of their interaction begins a year later, in October 1969. Grosskopf is dominant; Alexander, Näschen, and Wölfchen appear to have similar status as subordinates. Grosskopf plays with them all. Mutual interactions are cordial and any aggression is mild and rare.

Grosskopf is removed from the group at the end of October, at which point agonistic behavior among the remaining three commences almost immediately. Näschen, the most aggressive, is soon dominant, although his status is shaky. By January 1970 Näschen shows aggression only toward Wölfchen, directing at Alexander nonthreatening displays of dominance. Alexander, meanwhile, becomes increasingly aggressive toward Näschen. The anticipated fight takes place near the end of January, during which Wölfchen joins Alexander, and Näschen quickly surrenders.

Matters are still not settled. Wölfchen starts becoming aggressive toward Näschen, and he backs away. Wölfchen nonetheless presses the issue, and the two fight near the end of March with Näschen winning. Alexander is confined in a kennel at the time and unable to participate. Näschen now seems to rank higher than Wölfchen. When Alexander returns to the group he retains his dominant position. The males play together that summer, but Alexander now turns aggressive toward Zimen as well.[176] The other males are friendly with each other, as usual.

At summer's end Wölfchen, having leap-frogged over Näschen in rank, starts to challenge Alexander. In September, Alexander and Näschen form an alliance against Wölfchen, and he returns their aggression. Alexander and Näschen enjoy a cordial relationship with Alexander dominant. Wölfchen and Näschen still play together while Alexander, carrying the burden of authority, watches for Wölfchen over his shoulder.

At the end of September Wölfchen attacks Alexander. The fight is silent, vicious, and lasts 15 minutes. Alexander and Näschen continue their allegiance, but Alexander nonetheless receives serious injuries. Alexander then retreats to a kennel from which he defends himself for a month, well into October. Wölfchen assumes a dominant's pose – standing-taut, walking stiff-legged, tail-high – almost as soon as Alexander retreats to his bunker. On a leash he mimics Alexander's previous behavior, including aggression toward Zimen inside the enclosure. Alexander, having lost his status, becomes friendly once again, even greeting a hated keeper submissively.

Näschen stays close to Alexander after his deposing, sleeping near him, licking his wounds, and defending him in those rare moments when Wölfchen threatens. Despite these occasional aggressive encounters, Wölfchen, even during the winter breeding season, is far more tolerant of his male subordinates than the dominant female is of hers, and this appears to be true of captive wolves generally.

What seems strange is the impermanence of these dominant ↔ subordinate relationships, almost as if learning and memory were connected only tenuously. The pain inflicted on each other was intense, the attacks continuing for hours, days, weeks. In wild packs dispersal would have kept this from happening. Lacking any capacity to emigrate the recipients held out as best they could, sometimes forming alliances with previous rivals. Captivity appears to file down the normally sharp edges of signal and response until pain is no longer a useful memory.

Any dominant ↔ subordinate relationship has to involve agonistic behavior, and its perpetuation depends on learning: for example, one animal learns to dominate a familiar conspecific, which in turn learns (and remembers) to behave submissively. This particular relationship is one of mutual training (Chapter 3) based on intermittent reinforcement of such agonistic displays as cower ↔ threaten, run ↔ chase, and so forth. The subordinate has been conditioned to expect pain if given certain signals by the dominant. The dominant has learned that the subordinate responds to these signals.[177]

Rudiments of agonistic behavior appear soon after pups become mobile. Bites during rough play occasionally inflict pain, causing the bitten to yelp and roll over or try to run away. Learning associated with such experiences develop quickly: being bitten hurts, aggressiveness induces submission. The subsequent evolution of dominant ↔ subordinate rituals to prevent bloodshed probably derive from this mutual reinforcement. A subordinate wolf that rolls onto its back in passive submission seeks avoidance of pain by blunting aggression. Running away would excite the aggressor, encouraging it to give chase and perhaps cause greater pain.

Whether such incidents are actual evidence of future status even in captive conditions remains to be demonstrated convincingly. Wild and captive wolf societies are very different. The idea of parallel hierarchies – one male, one female – topped by a pair of dominant wolves was proposed by Schenkel based on observing zoo animals.[178] Later it was suggested that "alpha" status is a kind of essence, not stochastic but deterministic, and that potentially dominant animals might be identifiable in young litters of canids based mostly on precocial mobility and assertiveness.[179] Maybe wolves really are this transparent. On the other hand, they might be more opaque than previously thought, in which case such judgments are simplistic, analogous to observing a kindergarten class and predicting which children will become CEOs of corporations and which are destined to pick up litter along highways. Hugh Drummond cautioned that inferences drawn from behavior of young animals have limited predictive value. He wrote, "we may have to drop our rather Freudian assumption that such learning in infancy necessarily conditions competitiveness during adulthood, with dominants going on to be champions and subordinates facing a lifetime of surrender and defeat."[180]

Rank among wild wolves is subtle. Of a pack in the high Arctic Mech wrote, "other than the pack leader's position, which itself was not all that obvious, the other wolves' ranks on the social ladder took much watching for me to discern."[181] He noted that dominance ↔ submissive behavior was rare compared with observations of zoo wolves. Wild wolves rarely fight with pack members; rather, the norm is friendliness and good fellowship.[182] Crisler, who lived among wolves, had this to say: "The wolf is gentlehearted. Not noble, not cowardly, just nonfighting."[183]

Under natural conditions pack members rarely show aggression, in large measure because of the parent–offspring relationship. Parents and offspring live by a mutual code of passive inhibition based on parental dominance. Passive inhibition also allows littermates, or unrelated animals of the same age reared together, to remain peaceful, although dominant ↔ subordinate relationships can still develop with age. Mech, after years of watching wild wolves, proposed instead that pups enter the world more or less equal in social status and remain this way until they breed, at which time they automatically become dominants.[184] This is probably true in traditional packs composed of an unrelated breeding pair with offspring, but in others the dominant male also mates with one or more subordinate females, an event perhaps more likely if the dominant and subordinate females are related.[185] Despite being breeders their subordinate status remains unchanged.

Like all societies wolf packs are stable conceptual entities but labile and dynamic in their workings. Although a pack might occupy the same territory for years, its composition is always in flux as members are born, die, immigrate, change social status, and disperse. From the work of Mech and his colleagues has emerged the most focused and complete picture yet. Packs of wolves ordinarily are family units, not random assemblages of individuals, although their compositions are fluid. Multiple families might hunt[186] or den together,[187] or den nearby;[188] offspring eventually disperse and change a pack's composition;[189] an adolescent disperses temporarily and returns (Chapter 5);[190] two dispersing wolves meet and form a pack;[191] the dominant male might mate with more than one female[192] or more than one male breeds;[193] a single breeding female or male of a pack might not be dominant;[194] an unrelated loner joins an already stable pack after a member of the breeding pair dies;[195] some pairings are unsuccessful, and individuals separate;[196] a relative of one of a breeding pair might be taken in;[197] a young wolf immigrates into a pack as a subordinate;[198] a daughter replaces her mother and mates with her step-father;[199] or the offspring of a step-parent replaces its parent in the breeding pair.[200] Brother–sister pairings occur in the wild[201] but are rare. Regardless of how a pack is assembled it contains at its core the breeding pair and its offspring and functions as a unit the year around.[202]

Subordinate females sometimes mate with males outside the pack,[203] an indication that their reproductive lives are not controlled completely by the dominant female. Mech claimed that because nearly all wolves eventually disperse from their natal packs, all of them probably breed if they survive long enough.[204] He emphasized that dominance status even in captive packs is dynamic, not preordained, and that wolves in subordinate positions are not inherently non-breeders. In fact, subordinate animals in captivity breed readily if separated and paired apart from the main group.[205]

Mech considered that only a few body postures consistently reflect dominance ↔ submission.[206] The single posture of dominance is when a wolf stands-taut. Subordinate wolves lower themselves and cringe. Both dominance and submission are important in the maintenance of friendly social relations. Schenkel considered active submission and some aspects of passive submission derived from food solicitation behavior.[207] Certainly they seem similar. When a parent or other pack member returns from a hunt the pups surround it, eagerly licking-up, a signal for the adult to regurgitate its stomach contents (Chapter 8). Mech saw no difference between these forms of submission and soliciting food, although I can think of no reason why there should be. For a behavior to be derived only its application needs to be different. Whatever its origin, a submissive wolf often approaches the dominant with ears-folded, tail-low, and licking-up.[208]

Obvious expressions of dominance hierarchies in wolf packs are largely artifacts of captivity. Mech did not see even one dominance contest throughout 13 summers of watching his habituated pack on Ellesmere Island.[209] In wild packs the terms "alpha" wolf and "breeding" wolf appear to be synonyms. Dominance simply connotes parenting, the same as in a human family of two unrelated parents and their children.[210] Aggression, when it occurs at all, takes the form of interpack strife along territorial boundaries, and such encounters can be fatal (Chapter 5).

Except for these long-term observations by Mech and colleagues at Ellesmere Island we know almost nothing about the daily lives of wild wolves. Radio-collaring allows individuals to be located but does not reveal specific activity. Only by habituating a pack, as Mech did, and watching it year after year can natural behavioral patterns truly be identified and assessed.

9.4   Dominance in free-ranging dogs

Because dominance hierarchies are not unusual in captive wolves some have assumed *a priori* that a similar social structure exists among domestic dogs.[211] Does it? Apparently not as a matter of course in free-ranging dogs occupying urban and suburban areas. Dogs released into a large fenced field in a semi-stray state and monitored showed little evidence of social organization or leadership and scarcely any dominance behavior.[212] Truly free-ranging dogs might present a different situation,[213] but we have little evidence either way.

Free-ranging dogs are unlikely to meet all criteria of a pack,[214] defined earlier as a stable social unit with bonds of attachment, usually comprising related members that hunt, rear young, and defend a common territory together. The key word is *together*. Some picture a group of wandering dogs as no different from the standard wolf pack of a monogamous breeding pair with pups and related offspring of various ages,[215] but whether this model could withstand close scrutiny is doubtful.

Even if a monogamous pair were to form the core, free-ranging dogs traveling together are commonly unrelated[216] and maybe not even known to each other until joining forces. Pup mortality is high, and group membership is sustained by recruitment of outsiders.[217] Parental care is asymmetric with only the mother providing it. As with wolves, a breeder that dies is replaced by an outsider and accepted into the group.[218] Dominant ↔ subordinate relationships – and social bonds generally – often seem nonexistent.[219] The lack of a defined social structure, which assures maintenance of territories and group assistance in pup rearing, make self-regulation of free-ranging dog populations inefficient (Chapter 5). Group members seldom help a female guard her pups and even more rarely assist with rearing them.

Urban street dogs are barely social (Chapter 5), which is not surprising. Group living offers little selective advantage in urban settings.[220] Scattered resources, as noted before, favor individual exploitation.[221] Cooperative foraging is unnecessary if the major food source is garbage or small prey. Communal hunts make sense only if the prey is larger than the hunter and able to feed the group (Chapter 6). Wolves hunt in concert if pursuing caribou but act alone when searching for mice or foraging at a dump. Also, most evidence indicates that urban strays occupy home ranges but do not defend territories (Chapter 5). Home ranges can be patrolled safely and effectively alone; territorial defense ordinarily is a group activity. The situation might be a little different for rural dogs, which have an increased tendency to establish less fluid groups and consequently become more social than those on city streets.[222] Group living has some advantages for dogs not fed by humans, such as guaranteed access to concentrated food sources (e.g. garbage dumps) and maybe even protection of litters,[223] although this last is problematical (Chapter 8).

Urban dogs are characterized by six factors:[224] (1) most live solitarily except when in estrous groups or gathered at a communal food source, (2) adult ratios are generally skewed toward males, (3) activity is most frequent during crepuscular periods, (4) all are indirectly dependent on humans for food (handouts, garbage), (5) most depend on human-made structures for shelter (e.g. abandoned buildings, junked cars), and (6) their populations are probably not sustainable without recruitment from the pool of free-ranging owned dogs.[225]

Rural free-ranging dogs are less inclined than urban street dogs to be solitary.[226] Females typically leave the group to give birth and rear their pups alone,[227] and the pups are not incorporated into the group until about 4 months of age.[228] Group composition is more facile than in wolves, sources of recruitment being unrelated (and perhaps initially unfamiliar) free-ranging dogs or pups born to females of the group.[229] Continuing recruitment of outsiders is probably necessary to maintain populations in the face of high pup mortality (Chapter 8).[230] Transient recruitment occurs too: owned dogs perhaps join a group for several hours and then return home;[231] other transients might stay a day or a week.[232]

9.5   Leadership

When you open the front door do your dogs greet you as a fellow "pack member?" Probably not. Pack behavior is a misty genetic memory. Furthermore, owned dogs live in perpetual puppyhood. More likely they perceive you as their dog-parent.[233] Announcing yourself by saying, "Mom's home" is more accurate than telling them, "Hi gang, I'm back in the pack," although I suppose this is open to interpretation. The Crislers clearly believed their pet wolves accepted them socially as "part of their pack,"[234] and in the sense that they served a parental function the assessment might even be true. But did this make them the leaders? As discussed below, the breeding male and female of a wolf pack serve more as parental guides than either leaders or dictators.

Lick-up, muzzle-grab, and face-paw are subordinate behaviors, part of the repertoire young wolves and dogs use when greeting their parents. Adult wolves socialized to humans greet them in like manner: licking-up, face-pawing, using human chins or noses as substitute protuberances for muzzle-grabs, and, in wolves, clasping.[235] Licking-up to human caregivers appears early (21 days) in the behavior of hand-reared wolves.[236] The association of paedomorphic behavior with infantile attachment in adults is evidence that humans still serve as substitute parents.[237]

Leadership at its most elementary might be defined simply as departing to find food, as when a few experienced fish "lead" naïve conspecifics to a feeding station.[238] Right away a problem arises: are the followers truly being led, or is the experienced fish simply swimming off to eat? Conceptually, leadership comes very close to implying intentionality. However, we have no evidence that any animal recruits followers purposely, or recruits them at all.[239] Perhaps an animal departing from the group to feed is hungry with no motive (and certainly no intention) of recruiting followers. So is leadership among social animals nothing more than selfish behavior, an individual acting alone to fulfill its individual needs? If true, then followers are incidental. Leaders by definition require followers; conversely, there can be no followers in the absence of a leader. We often think of a leader as physically leading: first in line at the head of the group, but a problem arises here too. Order in a pack of wolves moving single-file through snow is unrelated to dominance; that is, the dominant wolf – the obvious candidate to lead – is not necessarily the one in front, making leadership so defined *mis*-leading.[240]

A dominance hierarchy is not necessarily a chain of leadership. A wolf pack displays little evidence that certain animals actually "lead" activities, even those involving parenting.[241] That wolf packs are "led" by the breeding male, or by the male and his mate, seems generally accepted.[242] One early assessment presented them as providers: "Pack leaders are those individuals which have demonstrated repeatedly their ability to provide their followers with game."[243] But what if leadership among wolves is merely dominance cleverly disguised?[244] Then the idea becomes a tautology unless the two concepts are based on different premises. Dominance implies control over others, often against their will. Leadership seems imbued with a quality, or trait, that induces others to follow. Leadership among wolves has been defined as "the behavior of one wolf that obviously controls, governs, or directs the behavior of several others."[245] This actually describes dominance behavior.

According to a more egalitarian definition used by primate behaviorists, leadership is "deciding where to move next, initiating travel, and leading a group between food, water sources, and rest sites."[246] Note that initiating group movement followed by leading the group away from its present location have been combined. Another definition, applied to bar-headed geese (*Anser indicus*), states that leading is "causing the departure *or* [emphasis added] determining the direction of movement of the whole group." Here, initiation of movement and movement itself have been separated, and either supposedly defines leadership.

Any accurate definition depends on group organization, mechanism of communication, and process of decision making. An aggregation of migrating wildebeests contains thousands of individuals, none in communication with all the others. Herds of some ungulates, flocks of birds, and schools of fish are *self-organizing groups*, a pattern requiring individualism to be subsumed in the collective response.[247] Members are mostly unrelated and free to join or leave.[248] Affective ties are minimal or nonexistent. Transfer of information is by *local communication*; that is, by monitoring and then reacting to the behavior of the nearest neighbors based mainly on spacing.[249] If a few fish on the periphery of a school turn suddenly all the rest turn with them (*combined decision*). If the change of direction is 180 degrees, those previously in front now bring up the rear. No individual leads, nor is any a follower in the sense of being led. Think of yourself in a huge crowd at a concert when you notice a disturbance some distance away. You ask the person beside you what happened, but instead of answering she begins to push toward the exit. Suddenly everyone is pushing for the exit. No one is either leading or following. Self-organization prevails, all communication is local, and the crowd has made a combined decision to stampede for the doors.

Alternatively, groups can be organized and coordinated by the leadership of one or a few. A *leadership group* is small compared with those that are self-organized, its members familiar to one another. Communication is *global*, not local, because each individual is available to interact socially with any of its comrades, and decisions are made either by the leader or by consensus (see below).[250] Pack-forming social canids like wolves are leadership groups. Most members are related or at least mutually familiar, and each individual from pup to breeding male is in contact with the others. This leaves only the type of leadership that best describes how wolves make decisions.

Leadership can be partitioned and defined in various ways, but two accepted categories are personal and distributed.[251] *Personal leadership* is unshared and involves a single dominant individual imposing its choice, in which case leadership and dominance are not different.[252] Early observers thought they saw personal leadership in wolf packs and presumed the dominant male to exert his will on the rest.[253] Gorillas evidently live in personal leadership societies,[254] but not wolves. Personal leadership in social mammals is actually rare.[255]

Distributed leadership is far more common. Here leadership is shared and some or all members of the group "negotiate" a decision, which is then accepted.[256] White-faced capuchin monkeys (*Cebus capucinus*) make use of this mechanism,[257] as do domestic sheep[258] and some primates like the chacma baboon and hamadryas baboon (*P. hamadryas*).[259] An important component involves decision making. Social animals organized around distributed leadership rely on *consensus decisions*, a process by which members of the group select from two or more mutually exclusive actions before accepting one of them.[260]

Where wolves are concerned, our concepts of dominance and leadership have traveled parallel tracks with little effort made to distinguish them. The autocratic behavior described in captive groups did little to clarify things, serving instead to solidify the idea of wolf societies as aggressive and rigid. Observations of wild wolves by Allen, Crisler, Mech, and Murie softened this image, depicting wolf packs as friendly family groups.[261] Mech pointed out that his own observations of wolves on Ellesmere Island had been made in summer when reproductive hormones are still at low ebb.[262] Nonetheless, in his opinion dominance actually holds little sway, and leadership is embodied in the protection required of parenting.[263] Leadership in packs of wolves and groups of dogs appears largely unaffected by dominance, just as it is in many other social mammals including sheep.[264]

In trying to identify leadership criteria in Yellowstone wolf packs, Rolf O. Peterson and colleagues monitored scent-marking (Chapter 4), *frontal leadership* (frequency and time leading the pack while traveling and hunting), initiation of group activity, and *nonfrontal leadership* (exerting leadership while not in front of the pack during its movements). Scent-marking constitutes dominance behavior, and nonfrontal leadership was eventually dismissed as rare or too difficult to observe, leaving frontal leadership and initiation of group activities as the remaining. Breeding pairs initiated activities of their packs most often (75% of cases),[265] but this option seemed open to other members. Frontal leadership was divided almost equally between the dominant male and female (78% of the time combined), although subordinates led occasionally too. Any of several individuals might lead when a pack is traveling along a well-used trail, and frontal leadership has been dismissed in these situations.[266] Leadership *seems* evident during attacks on large prey. The most aggressive wolf is often first to attack and sometimes continues to harass a prey animal that stands its ground after the others have given up.[267] What passes superficially for leadership as wolves close in for a kill might be little more than experience.[268]

As pointed out by Mech, wolf societies are neither autocratic nor democratic but a sort of hybrid.[269] Pack members do not follow blindly, nor are they coerced to follow. In some situations (e.g. crossing a frozen lake) they might even decline to accompany the breeding pair.[270] Nonetheless, the best predictor of leadership is dominance status.[271] Wolf packs in nature appear to be organized around a system of distributed leadership with the breeding pair at its center.

Some elements of what have been termed leadership and division of labor with overlap are evident in wolf packs.[272] The breeding pair dominates offspring of all ages in addition to any unrelated subordinates. The male is dominant over the female. He is principal provider for the female and pups while the female is nursing, and he sometimes feeds adolescents still with the pack. He typically is first to leave on hunts, appears to determine the direction of travel, and usually is most aggressive in defense of the den and rendezvous sites. The female also defends the den and rendezvous sites, protects the pups, and assists in hunting when the pups are old enough to be left alone at the rendezvous sites or in the care of other pack members. The expression of dominance is subdued, however, not explicit as often seen in captive wolves.

Going hand in hand with leadership is the notion of *teaching*, defined as directed instruction of one individual by another and usually incorporating the assumption of intentionality (i.e. the attribution of mental states).[273] Accordingly, the notion that canids – or any other animals – actively "teach" their offspring to hunt or do anything else is doubtful[274] despite the concept's widespread (and undemonstrated) repetition in the literature.[275] That animals can learn from associating with conspecifics (e.g. *observational learning*) is undisputed, but learning and teaching are not linked ineluctably. No evidence exists that even chimpanzees instruct others in the use of tools.[276]

Observations of one animal "teaching" another have more parsimonious explanations even assuming, as some have argued,[277] that teaching can exist apart from intentionality or attribution of mental state. The idea that certain carnivorans, notably the cats, actively "teach" their young to hunt is more easily explained by instinct, ontogenetic timing, or mimicry.

Some have wondered how young wolves learn to hunt if they leave the natal pack before acquiring sufficient skills.[278] Having been born with the innate motivation, highly evolved physical features needed to chase down and subdue large prey, and a brain and sensory systems hardwired for predation, "learning" to hunt might simply be another level of practice. Just 2 of the 41 gray wolves introduced into Yellowstone in the 1990s had ever seen a bison. Neither of these animals was present when 21 days after release into the park eight naïve 1-year-olds killed an emaciated calf bison; 2 years later Yellowstone packs were attacking and killing adults.[279]

Leadership defined similarly to that of wolves appears to characterize groups of free-ranging dogs, and dominance might not be a factor. A trio of adult street dogs in St. Louis that lived and foraged together most of the time comprised two large males named X and Y and a smaller female designated F.[280] Both males urine-marked often, the female rarely, yet she appeared to initiate most of the group's activities. Eye contact was frequent. Two animals would look back if the third was lagging, then walk on and look back again.[281] Another time F awoke at 3:55 a.m. on a porch where the trio had been sleeping and stood up. Y immediately sat up. F moved to the sidewalk where she turned and looked back at Y and the sleeping X. She started down the road. Y stood while F looked back at him. Y looked at X (still asleep) and followed F. Five minutes later both return to the porch where Y tail-wagged at X, which finally sat up. Y moved down the steps while F waited beside X. Y returned and tail-wagged at F. She descended to the sidewalk and looked back at X. Y crossed the road and looked back at F now standing in the middle of the road; she in turn looked at X. X joined her. She gave him a tail-wag and led him across the road to Y. With F going first, X and Y followed her off to forage.[282]

However, F's "leadership" was sometimes rejected by the males. On one occasion she crossed a main highway while X and Y stayed behind on the sidewalk. F then returned to them, and they went off in another direction. Another time Y crossed the highway and headed toward a park, but F and X stayed on the sidewalk. Y looked back and then rejoined them. No displays of dominance or submission were ever observed, although Y was aggressive toward strange dogs. All direct interactions were friendly (e.g. tail-wag, play-bow, nose-push).

These sequences show distributed leadership predicated on a form of decision making while attempting to maintain group cohesion. There was no evidence of the leader at a given moment actually trying to lead while expecting others to come along. Roberto Bonanni and co-authors reported that leadership measured as first to move off during group departures is fluid and only vaguely predictable, and made the points that "leadership is not an inherent property of individuals," and "individual variation in leadership ... at the time of group departure was significantly affected by dominance relationships."[283] This tells me that development of leadership in dogs (and wolves too) is certainly less refined than dominance, tied in with dominance ↔ subordinance, and perhaps not a distinguishable quality at all. In wolves especially the potential for dominance is inherent in every animal but expressed only with attainment of social stature. A formerly submissive wolf that achieves dominance begins instantly to act the part (Chapter 3). If it then shows signs of leadership using current criteria, how can these attributes be separated?[284]

Every adult and juvenile dog in this group studied by Bonanni and co-authors could initiate collective movement,[285] just as in wolves.[286] In some groups of dogs certain ones behave as leaders more often than others,[287] which behave as followers more often, although distributed leadership is not in doubt.[288] Being a leader appears to offer no special advantage, nor does being a follower diminish social status as would be expected were leadership personal.

Animal studies have involved measuring easily observed behaviors putatively associated with leadership while failing to isolate those traits that distinguish leaders. Any leader, as mentioned, requires followers, but when does follow-the-leader in wolves and dogs advance conceptually beyond what happens in a school of fish? The observation of a dog awaking from a nap and trotting off with one or two others behind could be evidence of many things besides leadership, including having been first to detect a signal and move toward it.[289] More likely this dog was simply hungry and set off in search of food. Free-ranging dogs in a loose group often forage alone, as noted. More important, does any dog demonstrating putative leadership behavior have an *expectation* of followers at any cognitive level, or is leaving the group temporarily merely leaving and followers are irrelevant?[290] The difference is important. If a dog gravitates toward a known food source followed by others of less experience – and what we observe is all there is – then an experienced fish swimming toward an established feeding station followed by naïve conspecifics demonstrates an equal degree of leadership. Later, after all group members have become conditioned (dogs or fish), how do we know that the first individual in line is not just the most aggressive or the hungriest?

Wild wolves have given observers a general impression of friendship and even a certain egalitarianism. When approached by a subordinate wagging its tail, the dominant wolf might respond simply by standing-taut and wagging his own tail.[291] Similar behavior occurs in groups of free-ranging dogs. Males and females in the group studied by Bonanni and co-authors were equally likely to behave as leaders.[292] Older dogs that received many acts of paying homage were more likely to behave as leaders; younger dogs that received submissions based on aggression were not. Dogs that were consistent followers appeared to stay closer to those that were leaders more often. Like wolves, whether these dogs were leaders or dominants is often unclear from observational evidence.

We might expect a leader to be the most aggressive dog when interacting with a rival group, but even this is unclear. Aggressive behavior between groups of free-ranging dogs plays out as follows.[293] One approaches the other aggressively (or they approach each other) until separated by about 20 m. Individuals posing with tail-high lunge toward their opponents while barking, snarling, and growling. Actual fighting is unusual, and most activity takes the form of threats. *Cooperators* participate in these demonstrations; *cheaters* stay behind, avoiding the fray and showing neither aggression nor submission. Perhaps not surprisingly the proportion of cooperating members diminishes with group size. Of the cooperators an actual leader is difficult to identify because most lunge and retreat an equal distance from the opposition.

Leadership in this case, if it exists at all, is a combined display. Some dogs cooperated most often both when their group was outnumbered or they outnumbered their rivals. These were usually dogs to which the others paid homage the most. Curiously, they and high-ranking younger dogs did not usually stay at the front of the group in the heat of the action. In other words, individuals that consistently displayed the presumed qualities of leadership did not lead, unless part of being a leader is just showing up. Still other dogs cooperated when outnumbered but avoided the front lines entirely, and some were habitual cheaters.[294]

9.6   Dingoes

The dingo has never been truly domesticated either in New Guinea or Australia by aboriginal peoples.[295] It took up life on its own after being brought by island-hopping mariners from southern Asia and the Indonesian archipelago[296] and remained that way despite a 5000-year association with humans.[297] Any traits selected during that interminable opportunity to make dingoes better "camp dogs" are minor.[298] Dingoes in Thailand and elsewhere had long since been domesticated (Chapter 2).

Socializing dingoes to humans is more difficult than it is with other dogs,[299] and the relevant question here is why they were never incorporated into human society. Although a domestic dog by ancestry, dingoes even today retain a reputation of being aloof and intractable. The fact that foxes can be domesticated within 40 or so generations (Chapter 4) makes the dingo's situation especially curious.[300] How could so much time go by without dingoes becoming socialized to humans?[301] No other animal in Australia offered as much potential to early aboriginals. In a land where foraging is difficult, it seems incredible that tame dingoes were not on hand to greet the first Europeans.

The reason, of course, is because dingoes were never really tamed, or even bred consistently in the camps with a purpose in mind, but simply replaced annually. At the end of winter men would find the birth sites used by female dingoes and take a few pups to rear.[302] One anthropologist concluded that as a conservation measure the aborigines declined to kill or capture the mothers, thus assuring an endless supply of young.[303] The aborigines have never been considered conservationists, and this is a doubtful assessment of motive unless payment is involved. When bounties were being offered for dingo scalps the reward applied to pups and adults alike, and pups were far easier to capture. The aborigines knew that "as the labour of tracking up and spearing a single adult dog is as great as, or greater than, that involved in locating a litter, they do not molest the breeding [females], but when the time is ripe, descend upon the family and secure a haul of six or eight instead of one."[304]

Why bring a pup dingo back to camp when chances are it would eventually escape into the bush? The dingo's function in early aboriginal societies has never been settled. The more modern the observation or opinion the least helpful it is likely to be: aboriginal people today have been living in camps for many years, have adopted western ways, and the dogs they keep are seldom pure dingoes. It appears that dingoes originally served any or all of six possible functions: (1) detectors and executioners of evil spirits, (2) watchdogs, (3) food, (4) pets, (5) warmth during cold nights, and (6) hunting aids.

The first two are not in question.[305] History shows that dingoes, like dogs everywhere, raise the alarm at any unusual disturbance whether caused by tribal enemies or advancing demons. In Walbiri culture the *djanba* (Fig. 9.4) are "malicious, indeed malevolent beings, who on occasion seem to be wholly immaterial and to possess miraculous powers, yet have many human qualities and frailties."[306] *Djanba* were invisible to all except dogs, medicine men, and totemic heroes. Medicine men made them visible by the use of magical quartz crystals. Originally dingoes, and later dingo-dogs and dogs of European breeds, could see *djanba* too.[307]

In Wolmadjeri culture neither dingo nor any other dog was a completely reliable demon detector, and in some animals this ability waxed and waned.[308] Demons disguised as dogs might sneak close to their victims unless the real dogs and dingoes could see them and attack, making it necessary to keep lots of semi-tame canids around to assure even modest security. Native Australians had mixed

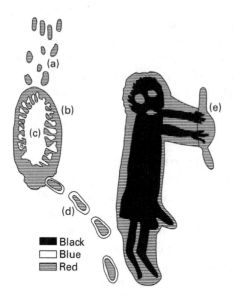

Figure 9.4 *Djanba* searching for victims at night. (a) *Djanba* feces. (b) Trees. (c) *Djanba* camp among the trees. (d) *Djanba* "boot" tracks. (e) Jara bag.
Source: Meggitt, M. (1955). Djanba among the Walbiri, Central Australia. *Anthropos*
50: 375–403. Reproduced with permission of the publisher.

feelings about the dingo, which in mythology is tied to the supernatural more than any other animal.[309]

According to some sources dingoes were rarely eaten by native Australians either before or after Europeans arrived except during times of scarcity.[310] Here the information conflicts, perhaps because customs differ throughout the country. Scott Nind, a medical officer assigned to a post near King George's Sound in 1827, wrote, "in the wild state [dingoes] are sometimes killed by the natives, who eat their flesh, but of the skin no use is made."[311] Domestic cats introduced by Europeans soon turned feral and were considered edible.[312]

Dogs were once common food throughout the Americas.[313] They are still eaten in southeast Asia, and dingoes have no doubt always been a menu item there if not in Australia. It seems odd that a ready source of protein would be ignored, and aborigines in New Guinea and Australia had probably always eaten dingoes until modern times.[314] Gerard Krefft, writing in 1866, stated, "the natives, who hate the Dingo most cordially for his living on the fat of the land, kill him on every opportunity and eat his flesh, which is by no means of ill flavour, though I have partaken of it under stress of hunger, and I will not vouch that I should sit down to roast Dingo with the same gusto now as ten years ago in the Murray scrub."[315]

The idea that dingoes have historically been worthless hunting companions also seems inconceivable, particularly in hunter-gatherer societies, but maybe it was true. A man using stone-age weapons accompanied by a dog with any training and sense of loyalty at all is surely more efficient than a man hunting alone. Macintosh claimed his investigations into the aborigine–dingo relationship were "divisible into half alleging Aboriginal use of the dingo as an aid in hunting, and half alleging the uselessness of the dingo for any purpose at all."[316] I suspect much of that confusion arose after dingoes started mating with European breeds, some of which had a long history of training as hunting dogs. Perhaps the conceptual image of the dog – if not the dingo – changed, and they were seen to have utilitarian uses other than nocturnal bed warmers[317] and food when the hunters could not find game. Australian aborigines supposedly kept dingoes around for warmth, huddling with them on cold nights, but the dingo-as-blanket function is controversial. Old reports described Aborigines huddled at night under their kangaroo-skin mantles, and "the dogs also are admitted to a share of their bed."[318]

We have anecdotal evidence of dingoes participating in hunts, but never with the perseverance and skill of trained European hounds and spaniels. Whether they were ever used consistently as hunting aids is undecided. Early accounts of aborigines training and using dingoes to hunt are brief (ordinarily a sentence or two), vague, and doubtfully reliable. In different parts of Australia trained dingoes putatively tracked game or ran it down, even dropping the catch on command. The more valuable animals were fed, given names, and permitted to sleep with their owners. "Thus, there is little we can construe as real evidence of the effectiveness or otherwise of such training, of the efficiency of dingoes as hunting aids, or of the amount game they brought in to the camps."[319] Most who wrote about them were explorers and settlers having limited interest in nature and native cultures.

One conclusion: "I suspect that some observers tended to confuse exoticism with utility."[320] It seems reasonable. Dingoes reared in the camps as wild-caught pups ordinarily returned to the bush, especially in the breeding season, and most did not come back. One early nineteenth century writer claimed a greater degree of loyalty: "At some periods [the food provided] is so scanty as to compel the dog to leave his master and provide for himself; but after a few days he generally returns."[321] Dingoes were at best semi-tame, as proved by the maiming of pups to keep them from deserting. Casual neglect, starvation, intentional crippling, and selecting animals randomly from the wild are unreliable techniques for molding good hunting dogs. Captive breeding was obviously rare or nonexistent; otherwise, the dingo supply would not have required regular replenishment. Without inbreeding over generations there could be no selection for useful traits like tameness or hunting prowess.

Accounts of dingoes kept as pets make clear that socialization was not part of the process. In southwestern Queensland women broke the forelegs of dingo pups to prevent them from later escaping into the bush.[322] As mentioned, semi-tame dingoes often ran away, usually for an opportunity to eat regularly because their owners seldom fed them. The result of staying was fierce competition for the few scraps available. Foraging and probably life in general was better away from the camps. Early explorers remarked on the thin and unthrifty appearance of camp dingoes compared with wild ones. What we read about the modern aborigine's love for his dog refers to European breeds and mongrels, not dingoes.

Historical hunting methods have been described, for some of which an untrained dog would be a liability. For example, aboriginal men sometimes hid behind blinds at waterholes waiting for kangaroos to come close enough to spear.[323] They also stalked kangaroos patiently, spearing or killing them with clubs or surrounding them (again using silence and patience) until getting within spearing range.[324] Pitfalls were also constructed, and here too dogs would be superfluous. Eggs of birds, nestlings, and opossums were collected by climbing trees.

Dingoes were supposedly used when driving game with or without burning the grasslands, and for chasing down bandicoots, small kangaroos, and opossums but supposedly proved too slow to capture emus and large kangaroos.[325] Today we know that dingoes can indeed capture and kill large kangaroos (Chapter 6). Brian Hayden, a Canadian anthropologist, disputed Meggitt's claim that dingoes were generally useless as hunting dogs, citing reports to the contrary.[326] However, these too are anecdotal and thin on details. He presented brief comments that dingoes were good at finding small game like snakes, rats, and lizards but not good at killing kangaroos. One second-hand report claimed that dingoes were actually good at running down and killing kangaroos, although the writer did not witness this personally. Dingoes were sometimes valued because they seldom barked and foraged for themselves.

Because camp dogs will attack a night-stalking *djanba*, "for this, among other reasons, dogs are highly prized by the Walbiri; a man would be very hungry indeed before he ate his hunting dogs."[327] These "other reasons" have never been explained adequately. Whether the dogs were dingoes or European mongrels (probably both), and how the Walbiri used dogs in hunting, remain mysteries. Art left by early aborigines offers no answers. Australian rock engravings and paintings commonly depict two – rarely three – dingoes hunting kangaroos, but none of which I am aware show dingoes and humans participating in a hunt together.[328] Dingoes are missing from the earliest art. They figure prominently in myths and legends but are rarely mentioned in a pragmatic role.[329] Finally, dingoes themselves were often the prey of humans, hunted not for food but for their tails, which were used as ornaments by aboriginal men.[330]

Notes

Preface

1 Knell (2009).
2 Wang *et al.* (2004).
3 Wayne (1993), Wayne and Jenks (1991), Wayne *et al.* (1992).
4 Wayne (1993: 220).
5 Genetically a dog is indeed a wolf. The dog genotype differs from the gray wolf's only by one or two restrictions, or by approximately 0.2% sequence divergence (Wayne *et al.* (1992)).
6 Aggarwal *et al.* (2007).
7 Wang *et al.* (2004).

Chapter 1: What makes a wolf

1 Wang and Tedford (2008: 7).
2 Dragoo and Honeycutt (1997). More specifically, the lineages probably began to diverge 12–15 million years BP and split into the red fox-like canids, the wolf-like canids, the South American foxes with a few others (e.g. the raccoon dog, *Nyctereutes procyonoides*) continuing along original trajectories (Wayne and Ostrander 1999).
3 Wayne and Ostrander (1999).
4 Vilà *et al.* (1999a and reference). Scott (1968) stated that dogs, wolves, coyotes, and jackals can interbreed but did not cite a source.
5 The older literature contains anecdotal evidence of jackal × domestic dog crosses (Iljin 1941: 361). Lorenz (1953: 11–12) believed jackals were ancestral to the domestic dog but later recanted (Lorenz 1995). See Matthew (1930) and Reed (1959) for traditional views of the dog's ancestry. Vilà *et al.* (1999a) cited Coppinger and Schneider (1995) as suggesting the golden jackal as an ancestor of the domestic dog, but they were wrong. The legend below figure 3.9 of Coppinger and Schneider (1995: 34) was clear that the dendrogram depicts cranial similarities, not evolutionary relationships. Variation in skull formation among domestic dogs exceeds that of any species of wild canid.
6 Allen (1920), Arnason *et al.* (2007), Leonard *et al.* (2005), Li *et al.* (2008), Miller (1920), Vilà *et al.* (1997, 1999a), Wayne (1993), Wayne and Ostrander (1999), Wayne *et al.* (1992, 2006), Wood Jones (1921). Some genetic sequences between gray wolves and domestic dogs are identical, but their sequence divergences are also nearly the same, meaning that genetic diversity among dogs is as great as it is among wolves.
7 Koler-Matznick (2002), Wayne *et al.* (2006), Wayne and Ostrander (1999).
8 Degerbøl (1961).
9 *Canis simensis* has a wolf lineage and is not descended from the lineage that gave rise to the jackals (Wayne 1993).
10 Wang and Tedford (2008: 58).
11 Wang and Tedford (2008: 52).
12 Savolainen *et al.* (2002: 1612 and references).
13 Wayne *et al.* (1992, 1995). Also see Vilà *et al.* (1999a). Any such time-scale analyses based on mutation rates should be viewed skeptically. Ho *et al.* (2005: 1566) wrote: "Taking rate variation

into account is particularly important for analyses of sequences on timescales [*sic*] of less than about 1–2 [million years BP], such as studies of populations, domestication, and conservation genetics, which often incorrectly apply phylogenetic substitution rates to population-level analyses." Wang and Tedford (2008: 52) claimed twice that length of time in North America alone: "Finally, the gray wolf (*C. lupus*) reached midcontinent North America in the last glacial cycle (100,000 years ago) after a much longer residence in North America above the Arctic Circle (since 500,000 years ago at least)."

14 Vilà *et al.* (1997), Wayne (1993).
15 The red fox (*Vulpes vulpes*) has taken over this distinction in recent times (Careau *et al.* 2007 and reference).
16 Hatt (1959), Mech (1974), Nowak (1983: 10, figure 1), Wronski and Macasero (2008). In recent times the only mammal with a natural range that has exceeded the wolf's was the lion (*Panthera leo*), also a large, mobile, adaptable carnivoran (Nowak 1983).
17 Hedrick and Fredrickson (2008), Nowak (1983: 12, figure 3).
18 For a brief early history of federal wolf control, see Young (1944: 369–385).
19 Aspi *et al.* (2006), Blanco *et al.* (1992), Randi *et al.* (2000).
20 Gier (1975).
21 Gier (1975).
22 Gier (1975).
23 Fener *et al.* (2005), Gier (1975).
24 Gehrt *et al.* (2009).
25 Bekoff and Wells (1986), Bowen (1981).
26 Gehrt *et al.* (2009), Gompper (2002), Koblmüller *et al.* (2009), MacCracken (1982), Morey *et al.* (2007).
27 Bowen (1981), Fuller and Keith (1981), Paquet (1992).
28 Bekoff and Wells (1986), Bond (1939), Bowen (1981), Gerads *et al.* (2001).
29 Vaughan (1983).
30 Boisjoly *et al.* (2010).
31 Brown and Lanning (1954), Boisjoly *et al.* (2010), Kays *et al.* (2008), Severinghaus (1974).
32 Lehman and Wayne (1991), Wayne *et al.* (1992).
33 Lehman and Wayne (1991), Vilà *et al.* (1999b).
34 Lehman and Wayne (1991), Roy *et al.* (1994).
35 Wayne (1993).
36 vonHoldt *et al.* (2011).
37 For lists of subspecies considered valid at one time or another, see Goldman (1944), Mech (1970: 349–353; 1974), Miller (1912), and Pocock (1935).
38 Fritts (1983), Kuyt (1962), Mech (1987), Merrill and Mech (2000), Van Camp and Gluckie (1979).
39 Wayne *et al.* (1992).
40 Ciucci *et al.* (2009), Kojola *et al.* (2006), Wabakken *et al.* (2007).
41 vonHoldt *et al.* (2011).
42 Boitani (1992), Ciucci *et al.* (2009), Ellegren (1999), Flagstad *et al.* (2003), Jhala (1993), Lehman *et al.* (1991), Randi (1993), Randi *et al.* (2000), Theuerkauf *et al.* (2003), Vilà *et al.* (1997, 1999b, 2003a), Wayne *et al.* (1992, 1995), Wronski and Macasero (2008).
43 Wayne *et al.* (1995).
44 Aggarwal *et al.* (2007).
45 Fox and Chundawat (1995).
46 Aggarwal *et al.* (2007), Sharma *et al.* (2004).
47 Aggarwal *et al.* (2007).
48 Aggarwal *et al.* (2007: 168).
49 Sharma *et al.* (2004).
50 The authors spelled the proposed specific name two ways: first as *himalyaensis* then *himalayensis* (Aggarwal *et al.* 2007: 170).
51 Kolenosky and Standfield (1975).
52 Koblmüller *et al.* (2009).
53 Kolenosky and Standfield (1975).
54 Goldman (1944), Mech (1974), Wilson *et al.* (2009 and references).

55 Wilson *et al.* (2009).

56 von Schreber (1775); with skepticism by Pocock (1935).

57 Goldman (1944: 437–441) summarized the early taxonomy of *C. lycaon.*

58 Grewal *et al.* (2004), Rutledge *et al.* (2010a, 2010b), Wilson *et al.* (2000, 2003).

59 Kyle *et al.* (2006), Wilson *et al.* (2000).

60 Rutledge *et al.* (2010c) analyzed skull samples recovered from an Iroquois village midden dated to 1530, or about 481 years BP. Genetic analysis yielded two ancient domestic dog and coyote haplotypes, but nothing indicating gray wolf ancestry. The teeth were too large to be dog or coyote. Rutledge and co-authors concluded that the animals must have been indigenous wolves.

61 Fain *et al.* (2010), Hedrick *et al.* (2002), Kyle *et al.* (2006), Rutledge *et al.* (2010c), Wilson *et al.* (2000, 2003, 2009).

62 Fain *et al.* (2010), Kyle *et al.* (2006).

63 I use the term admixing instead of hybridization and reserve hybrid for the tangible product of admixing (i.e. the admixture of genetic components from diploid animals of genetically distinct populations). See Glossary entries for admixing, admixture, hybrid.

64 Mech and Federoff (2002), Wheeldon *et al.* (2010). Fain *et al.* (2010; 1760) pointed out that admixing might not be recent but either generations removed or occurred over multiple generations. Moreover, some of these genetic components are dynamic, "raising questions as to how the loss of rare mtDNA haplotypes over 100 years of extirpation and recovery should be interpreted with regard to the comparability of the ancestral pedigrees of historical and recolonized [western Great Lakes] wolves." Others have argued that the Great Lakes wolf has not been restored because this animal was originally *C. lycaon*; that is, gray wolf mtDNA occurs in the current population but was absent from historical samples (Leonard and Wayne 2008), indicating that gray wolves moved into empty habitats after *C. lycaon* had been eliminated.

65 Goldman (1944: 393–395, 437–441). Also see Kolenosky and Standfield (1975). The Great Lakes wolf has long been regarded as among the smallest of North American wolves (e.g. Goldman 1944: 437–441).

66 Goldman (1944: 439).

67 Kolenosky and Standfield (1975), Leonard and Wayne (2008), Wheeldon and White (2009: 103, figure 2), Wilson *et al.* (2009).

68 Koblmüller *et al.* (2009), Kyle *et al.* (2006), Mech (2010), Mech and Paul (2008), Rutledge *et al.* (2010b), vonHoldt *et al.* (2011).

69 vonHoldt *et al.* (2011).

70 Lehman *et al.* (1991), Pilgrim *et al.* (1998), Roy *et al.* (1994).

71 Miller (1912), von Schreber (1775).

72 Goldman (1944), Kolenosky and Standfield (1975), Nowak (1983, 1995, 2002). Koblmüller *et al.* (2009: 2323) recognized the Great Lakes wolf as a coyote × gray wolf (particularly eastern coyote) hybrid, but nonetheless consider it a "discrete wolf taxon," presumably an entity something like a subspecies, *Canis lupus lycaon.*

73 Nowak (2002).

74 Roy *et al.* (1994), Wayne *et al.* (1992).

75 Sears *et al.* (2003).

76 Kyle *et al.* (2006), Leonard and Wayne (2008).

77 Koblmüller *et al.* (2009), Schmitz and Kolenosky (1985), Schmitz and Lavigne (1987). Koblmüller *et al.* (2009) found no genetic evidence that the Great Lakes wolf arose from a unique episode of admixing, nor did their findings indicate uniqueness. To them it is a gray wolf ecotype.

78 Kyle *et al.* (2006), Wilson *et al.* (2000, 2003).

79 Pocock (1935).

80 vonHoldt *et al.* (2011).

81 Kays *et al.* (2010), Wilson *et al.* (2009).

82 vonHoldt *et al.* (2011).

83 Voigt and Berg (1987 and references).

84 Leonard and Wayne (2008), Koblmüller *et al.* (2009).

85 Rutledge *et al.* (2010c).

86 Voigt and Berg (1985 and references) mentioned that no coyotes existed in the northeast by about 1830.

87 Lehman and Wayne (1991), Lehman *et al.* (1991), Pilgrim *et al.* (1998), Roy *et al.* (1994), Thurber and Peterson (1991), Vilà *et al.* (1999b), vonHoldt *et al.* (2008).
88 Adams *et al.* (2003a).
89 Wilson *et al.* (2009: S87). Kolenosky (1971) described two hybrid litters from the captive mating of a female Great Lakes wolf and male coyote.
90 Carrera *et al.* (2008), Parsons (1998).
91 García-Moreno *et al.* (1996), Hedrick *et al.* (1997), Lehman *et al.* (1991), Roy *et al.* (1996).
92 Goldman (1944: 437–441).
93 Koblmüller *et al.* (2009 and references).
94 Mendelssohn (1982).
95 Mendelssohn (1982 and references).
96 Kays *et al.* (2010), Koblmüller *et al.* (2009), Lehman *et al.* (1991), Leonard and Wayne (2008).
97 Wilson *et al.* (2009).
98 Grewal *et al.* (2004), Rutledge *et al.* (2010b), Wilson *et al.* (2000, 2003, 2009).
99 Analysis of lineages using mtDNA alone can skew evolutionary perspective by focusing exclusively on the maternal side. The use of Y chromosome markers and those inherited from both parental sides provide a more complete picture of inheritance (Leonard *et al.* 2005).
100 Wilson *et al.* (2003, 2009).
101 Koblmüller *et al.* (2009), Rutledge *et al.* (2010b).
102 Lehman *et al.* (1991).
103 Lehman *et al.* (1991), Wayne (1993).
104 Roy *et al.* (1994).
105 Lepais *et al.* (2009).
106 Differences in gene composition are certainly not evidence of different "species," the designation of which is arbitrary. Whether the determination to separate one "species" into two is decided by eye or based on rigorous rules makes the decision no more nor less a matter of opinion. Life is a continuum with no convenient breaks and fault lines, and what look to us like similarities and differences might be irrelevant to the animals involved. Certainly the historical notion of different "species" being unable to interbreed and produce viable offspring has been disproved many times, canids being just one example.
107 Reich *et al.* (1999), vonHoldt *et al.* (2011).
108 Roy *et al.* (1994).
109 vonHoldt *et al.* (2011).
110 Riley and McBride (1975).
111 Wayne and Jenks (1991).
112 Wayne and Jenks (1991).
113 Roy *et al.* (1996: 1422).
114 Fredrickson and Hedrick (2006), Phillips *et al.* (2003).
115 Adams *et al.* (2003b), Fredrickson and Hedrick (2006), Phillips *et al.* (2003), Wilson *et al.* (2009).
116 Nowak and Federoff (1998).
117 McCarley (1978).
118 Riley and McBride (1975).
119 Young (1944: 210–211).
120 Bond (1939).
121 Atkins and Dillon (1971), Paradiso (1968), Paradiso and Nowak (1971), Phillips and Henry (1992). Young (1944: 478–481) recognized the red wolf as *Canis niger* and three subspecies: *C. n. niger*, *C. n. gregori*, and *C. n. rufus*.
122 Brownlow (1996), Reich *et al.* (1999), Roy *et al.* (1994, 1996), Wayne (1992, 1993), Wayne and Jenks (1991), Wayne *et al.* (1995, 1998).
123 Bertorelle and Excoffier (1998), Hedrick *et al.* (2002), Wayne (1992), Wayne and Jenks (1991), Wilson *et al.* (2000). Goldman (1944: 488) believed some red wolf subspecies might be coyote admixtures.
124 Fredrickson and Hedrick (2006), Gipson *et al.* (1974), McCarley (1962), Nowak (1992, 2002), Nowak and Federoff (1998), Paradiso (1968).
125 Lawrence and Bossert (1967, 1975).
126 Bertorelle and Excoffier (1998) based on their reworking of data in Roy *et al.* (1994); Hedrick *et al.* (2002), Roy *et al.* (1994).

127 Lawrence and Bossert (1967).
128 Nowak (1979).
129 Kyle *et al.* (2006), Wilson *et al.* (2000, 2003).
130 Roy *et al.* (1996).
131 Wilson *et al.* (2000).
132 Wilson *et al.* (2000).
133 Way *et al.* (2010).
134 Nowak and Federoff (1998: 723, figure 1 showed historical northeastern extension of red wolves into Pennsylvania); also see Brewster and Fritts (1995) and Wayne *et al.* (1995 and references).
135 vonHoldt *et al.* (2011).
136 Hedrick *et al.* (2002), Roy *et al.* (1994), Wayne (1993), Wayne and Jenks (1991), Wayne *et al.* (1998).
137 Roy *et al.* (1994).
138 Wayne and Jenks (1991).
139 Reich *et al.* (1999).
140 Wayne (1992), Wilson *et al.* (2000). See Wayne (1992 and references) for genetic requisites of subspecies.
141 Red wolves, had they composed a distinct species, would have evolved in areas abutting or overlapping historical ranges of coyotes and gray wolves. Widths of *admixed zones* can be 50 times the distance individuals disperse in a generation (Barton and Hewitt 1989). Considering that gray wolves and coyotes often disperse hundreds of kilometers and easily traverse geographic barriers, the chances of early red wolves staying physically isolated were slim.
142 Wayne (1993).
143 Gipson *et al.* (1974).
144 Roy *et al.* (1996), Wayne (1992). As Wayne (1992) pointed out, that red wolf skulls can be distinguished from those of gray wolves and coyotes is predicated on phenetic similarity (i.e. similarity in appearance based on measurements of physical features). *Phenetics*, or *numerical taxonomy*, does not take into account evolutionary relationships, nor data indicating divergent or shared character states.
145 Wayne and Jenks (1991).
146 Wayne and Jenks (1991). The value of mongrel canids has been reassessed in recent years, some advocating that genetic "purity" be set aside in favor of ecological function. A similar case has been made for Australian dingoes and dingo-dogs (Daniels and Corbett 2003), which serve similar functions as top-down predators.
147 Lehman *et al.* (1991).
148 Roy *et al.* (1994).
149 Thompson (1952) reported that coyotes also occupied the home range of a pack of four Great Lakes wolves.
150 Hailer and Leonard (2008), Lehman *et al.* (1991), Pilgrim *et al.* (1998), Roy *et al.* (1994).
151 Wilson *et al.* (2000).
152 Murie (1940: 11, 17–18).
153 Connolly and Longhurst (1975).
154 The Allee effect is named after the ecologist Warder Clyde Allee, who first put forth its principles in 1931. Restated in the words of Courchamp *et al.* (1999: 405), "populations at low numbers are affected by a positive relationship between population growth rate and density, which increases their likelihood of extinction." Also see Wells *et al.* (1998).
155 Lehman *et al.* (1991).
156 Boisjoly *et al.* (2010), Kays *et al.* (2010).
157 Hailer and Leonard (2008), Lehman and Wayne (1991), Lehman *et al.* (1991), Vilà *et al.* (1999b).
158 Lehman *et al.* (1991), Wayne (1993).
159 Lehman *et al.* (1991).
160 Wayne (1993: 223). Silver and Silver (1969: 26) wrote, "There is some popular belief that size differential would prove a barrier to breeding between coyotes and wolves or some large dogs."
161 Rutledge *et al.* (2010b: 525).
162 Silver and Silver (1969: 26).
163 Berger and Gese (2007), Carbyn (1982), Cowan (1947), Fuller and Keith (1981). For anecdotes about coyotes killed by wolves see Mech (1970: 160).

164 Fuller and Keith (1981).
165 Berger and Gese (2007).
166 Lehman *et al.* (1991), Wayne (1993).
167 Hailer and Leonard (2008).
168 Hedrick *et al.* (1997), Vilà *et al.* (1999b).
169 Hailer and Leonard (2008).
170 Wilson *et al.* (2009).
171 Schmitz and Lavigne (1987).
172 Silver and Silver (1969: 39).
173 Moore and Millar (1986), Way *et al.* (2010).
174 Moore and Millar (1986), Way *et al.* (2010).
175 Silver and Silver (1969), Thurber and Peterson (1991).
176 Jackson (1922).
177 Parker (1995).
178 Wilson *et al.* (2003).
179 Parker (1995).
180 Compare the map in Leonard and Wayne (2008: 96, figure 1a) with that of Wilson *et al.* (2009: S81, figure 1A).
181 Parker (1995).
182 Kays *et al.* (2010), Lawrence and Bossert (1969).
183 Kays *et al.* (2010).
184 Slater *et al.* (2009).
185 Larivière and Crête (1993), Schmitz and Lavigne (1987).
186 Lawrence and Bossert (1969).
187 Sands *et al.* (1977).
188 Anonymous (2010a).
189 Estes and Goddard (1967), Gittleman (1985), Vézina (1985).
190 Lawrence and Bossert (1969), Thurber and Peterson (1991).
191 Gier (1975), Moore and Millar (1986), Parker (1995), Way *et al.* (2010). Gier (1975) reported some Alaskan coyotes weighing 18 kg.
192 Harrison (1992), Lavigne (1992), Moore and Millar (1986), Parker (1995), Pekins (1992), Larivière and Crête (1993 and references).
193 Lavigne (1992).
194 Larivière and Crête (1993), Wayne and Lehman (1992). Mengel (1971) proposed that the eastern coyote is a coyote × wolf hybrid and that the western coyote and what is now called the Great Lakes wolf were its progenitors. Such an animal, he noted: (1) would not have the liability of an offset breeding cycle, (2) would not lack for paternal care, (3) and seemed probable considering the recent and known migrations of western coyotes into regions occupied by Great Lakes wolves. He thus refuted Lawrence and Bossert (1969), who had suspected the eastern coyote of having arisen from coyote × domestic dog hybrids.
195 Kays *et al.* (2010), Larivière and Crête (1993), Parker (1995), Thurber and Peterson (1991).
196 Silver and Silver (1969: 28).
197 Silver and Silver (1969: 39).
198 Gittleman and Van Valkenburgh (1997).
199 Kays *et al.* (2010), Parker (1995).
200 Kays *et al.* (2008), Parker (1995).
201 Silver and Silver (1969: 40).
202 Lawrence and Bossert (1969).
203 Harrison (1992).
204 Silver and Silver (1969: 40).
205 Chambers (1992).
206 vonHoldt *et al.* (2011, figure S5A) based on previous microsatellite analyses of Carmichael *et al.* (2007), Koblmüller *et al.* (2009), Muñoz-Fuentes *et al.* (2009), Musiani *et al.* (2007). Support for boreal forest and Rocky Mountain forest clusters is weakest.
207 Rutledge *et al.* (2010a, 2010b), Wilson *et al.* (2009).
208 vonHoldt *et al.* (2011).

209 Goldman (1937; 1944: 393, 437).
210 Pocock (1935: 684).
211 Kolenosky and Standfield (1975), Mech (2010), Mech and Paul (2008).
212 Pocock (1935: 684).
213 Iljin (1941: 370).
214 Tome (1854: 112).
215 Silver and Silver (1969).
216 Peterson *et al.* (1984).
217 Boitani (1982). Randi *et al.* (2000: 465) briefly described these pups.
218 Silver and Silver (1969).
219 Melanism has long been a property of dogs. Australian dingoes are many-colored but even black specimens have a white tail tip (Macintosh 1975). Dingo pups are born nearly black with a white tail tip, white feet, and sometimes a white nape patch (see the photo of a female and her litter in Macintosh 1975: 95, figure 7–4).
220 Black (1936) referred to them as timber wolves and called them *Canis nubilis*. He noted that no museum specimens had been preserved.
221 Schmutz *et al.* (2007).
222 According to Riley and McBride (1975), melanistic red wolves had been reported but were rare. None had been seen in recent years.
223 Anderson *et al.* (2009). Also see Kerns *et al.* (2003), Schmutz *et al.* (2007).
224 Anderson *et al.* (2009). Of three melanistic Italian wild wolves, two were genetically intermediate between wolves and dogs; the third tested as completely wolf (Randi and Lucchini 2002).
225 Mech and Paul (2008).
226 Parsons (1998).
227 MacFarlane (1905: 692).
228 Ognev (1931: 126).
229 Allen (1979: 11).
230 Mech (1970: 16 and references).
231 Cowan (1947).
232 Murie (1944).
233 Mech *et al.* (1998: 40).
234 Ballard *et al.* (1987).
235 Lentfer and Sanders (1973 and references).
236 Peterson *et al.* (1984).
237 Jolicoeur (1959), Musiani *et al.* (2007).
238 Anderson *et al.* (2009).
239 Lentfer and Sanders (1973).
240 Mech *et al.* (1998: 40).
241 Critchell-Bullock (1930: 208).
242 Gipson and Ballard (1998).

Chapter 2: What makes a dog

1 See Goodwin *et al.* (1997) for a discussion of how paedomorphism and neoteny differ.
2 Taylor *et al.* (2009).
3 Scott (1950: 1019). Not until the sixteenth century did the dog (among other animals) shed its purely utilitarian function and become "an object of emotional investment" (Boehrer 1999: 153); that is, a pet. The substantive "pet," connected with animals, first appeared in the *Oxford English Dictionary* in 1539, its derivation Scottish (Boehrer 1999).
4 Leonard *et al.* (2005).
5 Parker *et al.* (2004). Also see Irion *et al.* (2003).
6 Parker *et al.* (2004). The Kennel Club of England was founded in 1873, the American Kennel Club in 1884 (Scott 1968).
7 At least one (the Kintamani dog from Bali, Indonesia) has evolved haphazardly from free-ranging dogs; in other words, without human interference and the crossing of existing breeds (Puja *et al.* 2005).

8 Wildt *et al.* (1982).
9 Savolainen *et al.* (2002).
10 Price (1984: 3).
11 Daniels and Bekoff (1989c).
12 Savolainen *et al.* (2002, 2004), Verginelli *et al.* (2005), Vilà *et al.* (1997).
13 Savolainen *et al.* (2004).
14 Parker *et al.* (2004).
15 Boyko *et al.* (2010: 8).
16 Wayne (1993: 222).
17 Leonard *et al.* (2005), Vilà *et al.* (1997), Wayne *et al.* (2006 and references).
18 Germonpré *et al.* (2009).
19 For example, domestic dogs were living in both Europe and Asia about 15 000 years BP (Wayne *et al.* 2006 and references). By 10 000 years BP there were dogs in western Europe, north Africa, and North America (Verginelli *et al.* 2005 and references).
20 Vilà *et al.* (1997); also see Schwartz (1997).
21 Savolainen *et al.* (2002).
22 Okumura *et al.* (1996).
23 Puja *et al.* (2005).
24 Wayne and Ostrander (1999).
25 Parker *et al.* (2004). Also see Koskinen (2003), Ostrander (2007).
26 Leonard *et al.* (2005), Parker *et al.* (2004).
27 Neff *et al.* (2004). Dogs carrying this mutation (*mdr1–1Δ*) are sensitive to the parasiticide invermec-tin and often succumb to a fatal paralysis when administered the drug.
28 Lindblad-Toh *et al.* (2005: 811) wrote that the boxer's genome is constructed of large blocks of haplotypes, and "the long stretches of *homozygosity* indicate regions in which the sequenced boxer genome carries the same haplotype on both chromosomes." (Italics added to indicate a Glossary entry.)
29 Lindblad-Toh *et al.* (2005 and references).
30 Leonard *et al.* (2002). Koler-Matznick (2002) argued that domestic dogs did not evolve from wolves but from a dog-like canid ancestor. In her opinion, this "generalist canid" would have resembled contemporary Asian pariah dogs.
31 Germonpré *et al.* (2009), Pang *et al.* (2009), Savolainen *et al.* (2002), Vilà *et al.* (1997).
32 Boyko *et al.* (2010), Driscoll and Macdonald (2010).
33 Boyko *et al.* (2010), Driscoll and Macdonald (2010).
34 Vilà *et al.* (1997), Wayne *et al.* (2006).
35 Vilà *et al.* (1997, 1999a). Time scales based on presumed mutation rates are not necessarily reliable (Ho *et al.* 2005), as mentioned in Chapter 1.
36 Pang *et al.* (2009).
37 Leonard *et al.* (2002).
38 Pang *et al.* (2009).
39 Pang *et al.* (2009).
40 vonHoldt *et al.* (2010).
41 vonHoldt *et al.* (2010). Scott (1968) had earlier proposed that dogs originated in the Middle East based on morphological similarities between early dogs and indigenous wolves.
42 Verginelli *et al.* (2005).
43 Vilà *et al.* (1997).
44 Gray *et al.* (2010a), Ostrander (2007). The matter remains unsettled in part because the original work (Gray *et al.* 2010a) was challenged. Gray *et al.* (2010b) corrected some errors, but debate on other issues arose (Gray and Wayne 2010, Klütsch and Crapon de Caprona 2010).
45 Ostrander (2007).
46 Lindblad-Toh *et al.* (2005).
47 Gray *et al.* (2009).
48 Germonpré *et al.* (2009).
49 Verginelli *et al.* (2005).
50 Verginelli *et al.* (2005), Vilà *et al.* (1999).
51 Lindblad-Toh *et al.* (2005), Vilà *et al.* (1997).

52 Wolf skeletal material from Pleistocene permafrost in Alaska also revealed unique mtDNA (Leonard *et al.* 2007). These now-extinct wolves were unique genetically and morphologically, and none of the 16 haplotypes recovered from 20 specimens is shared with modern wolves.

53 Garcia (2005).

54 Detry and Cardosa (2010).

55 Benecke (1987).

56 Degerbøl (1961).

57 Verginelli *et al.* (2005).

58 Macintosh (1964; 1975: 91, figure 2).

59 Corbett (1985 and references), Milham and Thompson (1976).

60 Higham *et al.* (1980: 159) wrote: "The size of the prehistoric and modern breeds is indistinguishable statistically. Bones even from the earliest layers correspond with those from modern animals. The shape of the one complete skull is likewise as in the modern dog. The prehistoric Thai breed is considerably smaller than the dingo, but shares with it close similarities in the shape of the jugular process and the mandible with the wolf. They do, however, differ from the wolf in having a relatively short rostrum, broad palate, and small bullae, all widespread symptoms of domestication in the dog. The degree of shortening, however, did not proceed far enough to induce tooth crowding or displacement."

61 Dogs are commonly eaten throughout southeast Asia, and recipes vary by country and region. Cordero-Fernando (1977: 419) quoted a commissioner of health in the Philippines writing in 1905: "The favorite method of preparation was to feed the starving animal with rice until his belly bulged full and round. When he could swallow not one grain more, he was promptly killed and, thus neatly self-stuffed, was roasted and eaten. The undigested rice was esteemed the greatest delicacy of all." A citation for this quote was not provided.

62 Sablin and Khlopachev (2002).

63 Dayan (1994). Remains of a Natufian dog from Shukba Cave in the western Judean hills were mentioned by Bate (1942) without comment.

64 Lawrence (1967).

65 Maher *et al.* (2011).

66 Turnbull and Reed (1974).

67 According to Coon (1951: 44), the oldest of these, consisting of two mandibles and three large teeth, "are undoubtedly *canis* [*sic*] *familiaris*, the domestic dog, and not wolf. The breed was very large and heavy-boned. Levels 4 and 2 [Neolithic] also yield unquestionable dog … Level 15 [Upper Mesolithic] yielded a left maxilla of *canis* [*sic*] *familiaris* with its three incisor teeth in situ."

68 Ralph (1955).

69 Pang *et al.* (2009).

70 Andersone *et al.* (2002), Anonymous (1999), Fain *et al.* (2010), Muñoz-Fuentes *et al.* (2009), Randi and Lucchini (2002), Randi *et al.* (2000), Sharma *et al.* (2004), Vilà *et al.* (2003b).

71 Vilà *et al.* (2003b, 2005).

72 vonHoldt *et al.* (2010).

73 vonHoldt *et al.* (2010 and references).

74 Parker *et al.* (2004), vonHoldt *et al.* (2010). Other seemingly relict breeds might not be old. "Descendants" of the Pharaoh and Ibizan sight hounds, likenesses of which appear on Egyptian tombs dating back more than 5000 years BP, are modern facsimiles developed in recent times from existing breeds and are therefore modern breeds (Boyko *et al.* 2009, Parker *et al.* 2004).

75 Goebel *et al.* (2008).

76 The gene for hairlessness is lethal when homozygous (Cordy-Collins 1994). Consequently, outbred dogs can be hairless or haired, a hairless specimen being identified superficially as a "pure bred" xoloitzcuintle (Wayne *et al.* 2006). In pre-European times the xoloitzcuintle was in domestication at least from Mexico to Peru and perhaps as distant as Paraguay and the Greater Antilles (Allen 1920: 478). Also see Cordy-Collins (1994).

77 Leonard *et al.* (2005).

78 This can be seen by the absence of ancestral New World sequences in modern dogs (Leonard *et al.* 2002: 1614–1615, figures 1 and 2). The figures combine some sequences from Vilà *et al.* (1997, 1999b). See modifications by Wayne *et al.* (2006: 287, figures 19.5 and 19.6).

79 Vilà *et al.* (1999a).

80 Vilà *et al.* (1999a).

81 Leonard *et al.* (2002).

82 Allen (1920: 440) wrote: "The probability therefore is, that the Domestic Dog originated in Asia and was carried by primitive man both east and west into all parts of the inhabited world. That this migration began in late Pleistocene times seems highly probable." See his bibliography for older references.

83 Clutton-Brock (1995).

84 Tome (1854: 29), wrote: "We commenced about the first of July, and continued until November. The wolves and dogs hunting together, sometimes one and sometimes the other obtaining the deer, and if it fell into our hands we always left the wolves their portion to keep them near, for we considered them of great assistance to us in hunting . . . They often aided us to three of four deer in a week. When we . . . had killed a deer, we often stopped to dress it, and left the wolves their portion, and if we had not the fortune to catch one, we would cach [*sic*] fish and leave them, to keep them in our vicinity . . . Frequently when our dogs were chasing a deer the wolves would take it from them, and the dogs would sometimes take one from the wolves in the same manner. The wolves and the dogs would often be in pursuit of the same deer, but when we were near enough, we could generally take it from them."

85 Sablin and Khlopachev (2002: 796, figure 1, top illustration in lateral view).

86 Davis and Valla (1978: 610). See Dayan (1994) for more about Natufian canids.

87 Savolainen *et al.* (2002).

88 Boyko *et al.* (2009), Okumura *et al.* (1996), Pang *et al.* (2009), Vilà *et al.* (1999a), vonHoldt *et al.* (2010), Wayne *et al.* (2006).

89 Olsen and Olsen (1977), Parker *et al.* (2004), Vilà *et al.* (1997, 1999a), Wayne (1993).

90 Wayne *et al.* (2006). Scott (1967, 1968) proposed that domestication was a one-time event based on the curly tails of domestic dogs, which he mistakenly considered evidence of a common ancestor. According to Scott (1967: 378), "this mutation probably occurred early in the history of domestication and was preserved because it was useful as a method of distinguishing wild from domestic animals."

91 Vilà *et al.* (1999a).

92 Vilà *et al.* (2005).

93 Leonard *et al.* (2005).

94 Sharma *et al.* (2004).

95 Sharma *et al.* (2004), Vilà *et al.* (1997).

96 Savolainen *et al.* (2004). Wood Jones (1921) summarized different theories of how the dingo got to Australia, although some thought it had been there all along. He argued convincingly that dingoes had been brought by early seafarers, writing (Wood Jones 1921: 262–263) that the ancestor of modern aboriginal Australians "came with his wife, he came with his dog, and with his dog's wife, and he must have done the journey in a seaworthy boat capable of traversing this unquiet portion of the ocean with his considerable cargo." Neither did Wood Jones doubt that the dingo is a domestic dog and like all others descended from the gray wolf.

97 Savolainen *et al.* (2002). As pointed out by Leonard *et al.* (2005), this statement assumes that ancient and modern Asian dogs constitute a common lineage. They mentioned other qualifying criteria, including data suggesting that levels of diversity past and present might not coincide.

98 Clutton-Brock (1995).

99 Even the scientific literature can be misleading if interpreted incorrectly. Adams *et al.* (2003a: 541), for example, titled one of their papers "Widespread Occurrence of a Domestic Dog Mitochondrial DNA Haplotype in Southeastern US Coyotes." Their use of "widespread occurrence" does not mean "widespread hybridization." It means, in their words, "that a male coyote hybridized with a female dog, and female hybrid offspring successfully integrated into the coyote population." The haplotype now occurs in coyotes from Florida to West Virginia, but the event likely happened one time, long ago, and "does not appear to have substantially affected the coyote's genetic, morphological, or behavioural integrity." Are southeastern coyotes therefore "coydogs?" Not by any reasonable interpretation.

100 Mengel (1971).

101 Mengel (1971).

102 Adams *et al.* (2003a), Kays *et al.* (2010), Lehman *et al.* (1991), Roy *et al.* (1996), Vilà *et al.* (1999b).

103 Roy *et al.* (1994, 1996).
104 Rutledge *et al.* (2010c).
105 vonHoldt *et al.* (2011).
106 Dice (1942).
107 Mengel (1971).
108 Dice (1942: 186).
109 Cook (1952), Pringle (1960).
110 See, for example, Richens and Hughie (1974).
111 Kays *et al.* (2010).
112 Adams *et al.* (2003a).
113 Mengel (1971: 328) defined *coydogs* as "individuals of 50–50 descent – that is, with no backcrossing in their ancestry."
114 Mengel (1971).
115 Severinghaus (1974: 117).
116 Fener *et al.* (2005) traced the chronology of the coyote's movements into New York from southeastern Canada, but never mentioned the eastern coyote specifically.
117 Severinghaus (1974).
118 Silver and Silver (1969: 33). Also see Dice (1942), who described three pups from matings with a female coyote and two hounds. None of the pups, as seen in photographs, resemble coyotes.
119 Dice (1942).
120 In domestic dogs variation in coat color and pattern of growth (e.g. long or short, curly or straight, wiry or soft) is controlled by variants of three genes, *RSPO2*, *FGF5*, and *KRT71* (Cadieu *et al.* 2009).
121 Silver and Silver (1969: 32–34).
122 Iljin (1941, plates 19–21, 23).
123 Reviewed by Trut *et al.* (2009).
124 Allen (1920), Lawrence (1967), Olsen (1974), Riesenfeld and Siegel (1970).
125 Olsen (1974), Olsen and Olsen (1977).
126 Iljin (1941: 385–390), Morey (1986).
127 Iljin (1941: 387–388).
128 Dayan (1994), Morey (1994). Benecke (1987: 33) listed the distinguishing characters. He included the general reduction in body size, which is not necessarily true (Sablin and Khlopachev 2002).
129 Gottelli *et al.* (1994), Iljin (1941: 382–383).
130 Iljin (1941: 383–385).
131 Gottelli *et al.* (1994), Iljin (1941: 363–373).
132 Davis and Valla (1978).
133 Morey (1994).
134 Sablin and Khlopachev (2002 and references).
135 Scott and Fredericson (1951).
136 Saetre *et al.* (2004).
137 Wayne *et al.* (1992). Gray wolf samples came from North America (Canada, United States, Mexico), Europe (Sweden, Finland, Estonia, Italy, Portugal), China, and the Middle East (Israel, Iran).
138 Leonard *et al.* (2002).
139 Vilà and Wayne (1999).
140 Maximilian (1906: 310).
141 Iljin (1941: 360).
142 Young (1944: 207–208).
143 Allen (1920: 446).
144 Coppinger and Coppinger (2001: 49).
145 Zimen (1981: 88–91). Figure 5 of the color plates shows the wolves in harness looking very professional, at least while their picture was being taken.
146 Young (1944: 177).
147 Iljin (1941: 409).
148 Allen (1920: 455).
149 Allen (1920: 446–447).
150 Allen (1920: 449–451).
151 Allen (1920: 454).

152 Wilson (1963: 359).
153 Allen (1920: 451).
154 Andersone *et al.* (2002), Boitani (1992), Ellegren *et al.* (1996), Liberg *et al.* (2005), Randi and Lucchini (2002), Vilà *et al.* (2003a).
155 Blanco *et al.* (1992).
156 Butler (1994).
157 Randi *et al.* (2000), Verardi *et al.* (2006), Vilà and Wayne (1999).
158 Blanco *et al.* (1992), Randi and Lucchini (2002), Randi *et al.* (2000), Vilà and Wayne (1999).
159 Vilà and Wayne (1999).
160 Vilà and Wayne (1999).
161 Roy *et al.* (1994), Vilà and Wayne (1999).
162 Lehman *et al.* (1991).
163 Roy *et al.* (1994).
164 Randi and Lucchini (2002).
165 Vilà and Wayne (1999).
166 Mengel (1971), Randi *et al.* (2000).
167 Mengel (1971).
168 Silver and Silver (1969: 32).
169 Iljin (1941: 405–406).
170 Lehman *et al.* (1991). Captive coydogs raised by Mengel (1971) did not provide paternal care, nor did eastern coyote × dog hybrids (Silver and Silver 1969: 35).
171 Mengel (1971). However, see Gipson (1983) for the capacity of free-ranging pup dogs to survive winter temperatures in interior Alaska despite lack of paternal care.
172 Savolainen *et al.* (2004). Some have speculated that dingoes arose from the Indian pariah dog or semi-domesticated varieties of the Indian wolf (Levy 2009). Genetic analyses of Indian wolves and Indian pariah dogs show neither to be the progenitor (Aggarwal *et al.* 2007).
173 Savolainen *et al.* (2004), Wilton *et al.* (1999).
174 Runstadler *et al.* (2006).
175 van Gelder (1978: 2).
176 Clutton-Brock (1995), Newsome and Corbett (1982). For an earlier summary of the dingo's speculative origin see Macintosh (1975).
177 Jones (2009).
178 Corbett (1985, 1995: 29–48), Daniels and Corbett (2003), Jones (1990), Newsome and Corbett (1982, 1985), Newsome *et al.* (1980), Woodall *et al.* (1996).
179 Jones (2009: 4) pointed out that "while the dingo skull can be regarded as a [taxonomic] type, strictly speaking the domestic dog skull does not represent a specific type, but a subset of types." Moreover, the different equations derived to sort and compare physical characters of dingoes and dogs are "attempting to differentiate two groups of canids that are separate, only at the subspecies level, and both groups have undergone differing degrees of modification by domestication." None of this is likely to work if variation drifts uncertainly along a cline. The investigators themselves seemed unwilling to relinquish morphology to the new genetics. After commenting that current genetic methods of identifying dingoes are probably unreliable, Daniels and Corbett (2003) noted that percentages of hybrids appeared to be increasing in northeastern Victoria. They based this assertion on data from skull morphology, coat pattern and coloration, and other physical factors already demonstrated to be unreliable diagnostic characters.
180 Corbett (1985), Jones (2009), Newsome and Corbett (1982), Newsome *et al.* (1980).
181 Green and Catling (1977).
182 Elledge *et al.* (2008).
183 Corbett (1985), Jones (1990).
184 Jones (1990: 70).
185 Newsome and Corbett (1985), Thomson (1992a).
186 Corbett (1985).
187 Jones (1990).
188 Jones (1990).
189 Newsome and Corbett (1985 and references).
190 Krefft (1866: 2–3). Warrigal was an aboriginal name for the dingo.

191 Jones (1990).
192 Jones (2009). In Victoria's eastern highlands dingo-dogs reportedly produced larger litters than
     dingoes (Catling *et al.* 1992). Whether the two groups could be distinguished is doubtful.

Chapter 3: Visual and tactile communication

1 Palacios *et al.* (2007).
2 Scott and Fredericson (1951). Many definitions of behavior have been proposed, and there is still no
   consensus (Levitis *et al.* 2009).
3 Bekoff (1972), Wiley and Richards (1978).
4 Scott-Phillips (2010).
5 A signal has been defined in semiotics as both a signifier and a "semiotic stimulus" (Nöth 1990: 112),
   and the same logic applies here. The term signal as used in animal behavior is sometimes reserved
   for factors that can be quantified, such as chemical concentrations and sound waves. I extend its use
   to unquantified behaviors defined using only verbal descriptions (e.g. postures expressed during
   dominance behavior).
6 The temptation is to call metaphors ambiguous, but doing so would be inaccurate. A term is
   ambiguous if it has several interpretations each independent of the others. The interpretations of
   a metaphor are not independent but tied to a common literal application (Elgin 1983: 26–27).
7 Elgin (1983: 69).
8 Reddy (1979).
9 Rendall *et al.* (2009: 234, legend to figure 1).
10 Penn and Provinelli (2007: 731) wrote: "After decades of effort ... there is still little consensus on
    whether or not non-human animals understand anything about the unobservable mental states of
    other animals or even what it would mean for a non-verbal animal to understand the concept of
    'mental state'."
11 Csibra (2008).
12 Kovács *et al.* (2010).
13 Cheney and Seyfarth (1990), Cheney *et al.* (1996), Penn and Provinelli (2007).
14 Reddy (1979).
15 Writing about nonhuman primates, Rendall *et al.* (2009: 235) stated: "Thus, although listeners
    sometimes respond to vocalizations '*as if*' they contained semantic information, callers proved to be
    fundamentally unaware of the informational value of their own signals ... These more recent
    findings highlight an informational disconnection between signallers and perceivers and suggest
    they do not share the same representational parity that characterizes human speech."
16 Rendall *et al.* (2009).
17 According to Rendall *et al.* (2009: 236), "either the distinction between the endpoints evaporates, or
    any given signal must be said to exist at multiple locations on the continuum at the same time
    depending on whose perspective is being considered." I agree. Should we call this process "quantum
    signaling?"
18 Tinbergen (1963: 413).
19 Reddy (1979: 305).
20 Schleidt (1973).
21 Fox and Cohen (1977).
22 Fox (1970: 52).
23 Spotte (2006: 24).
24 Smith (1997 and references).
25 Smith (1997: 27).
26 Rendall *et al.* (2009), Scott-Phillips (2008, 2010). Others disagree and saw a viable function for the
    information concept in animal communication (e.g. Carazo and Font 2010; Font and Carazo 2010).
27 Losee (1997).
28 Schleidt (1973).
29 In the system just described, I referred mainly to the direct and automatic (i.e. involuntary) response
    to a signal. The laboratory work of B. F. Skinner was especially interesting because it demonstrated
    how the same principles apply to voluntary behavior. What he termed *operant conditioning* is still

used widely in animal training. In Skinner's experiments, food was the primary signal, eating the primary response, but wedged between the two was a requirement that the animal perform some voluntary act, such as pressing a button. This *secondary response*, R_2, also came to be associated with the primary signal, establishing a sequence comprising two voluntary responses in place of a straightforward signal-response (Scott and Fredericson 1951).

30 Schenkel (1967: 324) defined *submission* "as an impulse and effort of the inferior [subordinate] towards friendly and harmonic social integration."

31 This arrangement was described originally as a linear hierarchy. An "alpha" wolf at the top was followed in the descending social order by a "beta" wolf and finally an "omega" wolf (e.g. Schenkel 1947). Any notion that wolf packs are organized similarly to a "pecking order" seen in barnyard hens is false (Mech 1999; Peterson *et al.* 2002). The terms dominant and subordinate seem more appropriate.

32 Peterson *et al.* (1998). This is not to say that subordinate animals do not also breed on occasion, or that a dominant animal relinquishes breeding in some years.

33 Fox (1975).

34 Schenkel (1967).

35 Fatjó *et al.* (2007: 275), a concept these authors attributed to van Hooff and Wensing (1987).

36 Peterson *et al.* (1984).

37 Rabb *et al.* (1967).

38 Zimen (1975).

39 The earliest use I found of the term *agonistic behavior* was by Scott (1950: 1013, table 1).

40 Scott (1967).

41 From the start, agonistic behavior was defined as including both dominance and submission, as Scott and Fredericson (1951: 273) wrote in context with fighting: "Other common and closely related alternate patterns are escape behavior, defensive behavior, and passivity. It is difficult to consider any of these without the others, and it is with this general group of behavioral adjustments, which may be given the name 'agonistic behavior'." In this context, Berman and Dunbar (1983: 7) incorrectly defined agonism as "aggression directed towards a conspecific." The work of Lockwood (1979) extended the original concept of agonistic behavior as not molded tightly to dominance and was not Lockwood's independent conclusion as implied by van Hooff and Wensing (1987).

42 Scott (1967).

43 Scott (1967: 374).

44 Gartlan (1964: 77) wrote: "The concept of dominance is often associated with, and is in practice generally inseparable from, that of aggression. At this point it should be made clear that dominance, although treated as a terminal concept ... is in fact reducible to more fundamental behaviour components of which aggression is one; in fact dominance is inferred from these more basic behaviour patterns."

45 Ceacero *et al.* (2007).

46 Gartlan (1964: 77).

47 All this and "social stress," the only true dependent variable, has still not been defined adequately and quantified.

48 Scott and Fredericson (1951).

49 Rowell (1974).

50 Scott and Fredericson (1951: 281).

51 Scott and Fredericson (1951).

52 Zimen (1975, 1976).

53 Scott and Fredericson (1951).

54 Zimen (1975).

55 This was mentioned by Scott and Fredericson (1951: 280, footnote) in reference to mice and rats. They attributed the idea to John B. Calhoun.

56 McLeod (1996).

57 Drummond (2006 and references). Also see Gartlan (1964).

58 Rowell (1974).

59 Scott and Fredericson (1951 and references).

60 Sands and Creel (2004 and references).

61 Rowell (1974 and references).

62 Barja *et al.* (2008), Creel (2005), Sands and Creel (2004).
63 Creel (2005).
64 Creel (2005).
65 Creel *et al.* (1996).
66 Fox (1973).
67 Fox (1973).
68 Zimen (1975).
69 Some recognized the distinction between captivity and nature and thought it might be important. Schenkel (1967: 328), for example, noted, "in such [captive] conditions severe fight [*sic*] can occur in species in which only ritualized fighting is observed under natural conditions." Not all investigators showed his prescience. Rabb *et al.* (1967: 310), in their description of wolves at Brookfield Zoo, Chicago, emphasized the "close correspondence to behavior reported in the wild." These animals were siblings, offspring of two mothers and one father and obviously denied any opportunity to outbreed. Whether the original parents were also related was not stated. As discussed by Smith *et al.* (1997), some investigators at the time believed incest in wild wolves might be common (e.g. Peterson *et al.* 1984; Scott 1967). Nonetheless, females were forced to give birth near each other in a concrete block den. There was infanticide, fighting (including group assaults), and intimidation.
70 For lists and discussions of these and similar behaviors (including "ritualized fighting") see Bekoff (1972), Fox (1969a, 1973), Golani and Moran (1983), Goodwin *et al.* (1997), Harrington and Asa (2003), MacDonald and Ginsburg (1981), McLeod (1996), McLeod and Fentress (1997), Mech (1970: 80–95), Schenkel (1947, 1967), Scott (1950), Stahler *et al.* (2002b), van Hooff and Wensing (1987), Zimen (1982). Packard (2003: 41, table 2.2) added additional behaviors, expanding these other *sociograms* into an *ethogram*. Way *et al.* (2006) published an ethogram for captive eastern coyotes.
71 Schenkel (1967: 320, figure 2A).
72 Derix *et al.* (1993) described this behavior (or one similar) as "head/paw on" and evidently directed by males toward females during courtship.
73 Crisler (1958: 90–91).
74 Crisler (1958: 181).
75 Crisler (1958: 181, 250).
76 Fox and Cohen (1977), Mech (1970: 86), Schenkel (1947: 126, figure 45b).
77 Silver and Silver (1969: 23, figure 17). Another interesting behavior of eastern coyotes was males fighting on their hind legs (Silver and Silver 1969: 25, figure 20). Mech (1999) did not consider pin-down to represent dominance behavior in wolves. Also see Mech (1970: 86).
78 Perhaps this behavior is more typical of coyotes. I came across no other such description in the canid literature. Another behavior of eastern coyotes was males fighting on their hind legs (Silver and Silver 1969: 25, figure 20).
79 Murie (1944: 33) called this "hugging," as did Fox and Cohen (1977: 731, footnote). Crisler (1958: 198, 235) mentioned what appears to have been similar behavior but did not name it. Fox and Cohen reserved the term "clasping" to mounting and reproduction.
80 Crisler (1958: 198, 235), Murie (1944: 33).
81 Fatjó *et al.* (2007). Fox and Cohen (1977: 735, table 3) called this (or similar) behavior "licking intention," the equivalent of "tongue-smacking" in primates.
82 Leaver and Reimchen (2008), Schilder and van der Borg (2004).
83 Schenkel (1947, 1967).
84 Derix *et al.* (1993).
85 Mech (1993a).
86 Mech (1988a: 61, 64).
87 Exceptions occur if a strange wolf enters the territory of a resident pack (Mech 1993a) and during mating season (Peterson 1979).
88 Mech (1999). Also see Fox (1973, plate XI, figure 2a), Schenkel (1947: 126, figure 45a; 1967: 322, figure 5A).
89 Schenkel (1947: 118, Fig. 25).
90 Fox and Cohen (1977).
91 Schenkel (1947: 126, figure 46b; 1967: 322, figure 5B).
92 Fox and Cohen (1977).

93 Schenkel (1947: 129, figures 55–57).
94 Fox and Cohen (1977). Also see Fox (1973, plate XI, figure 2b).
95 Fox (1973, plate XI, figure 2c), Schenkel (1967: 324, figure 7).
96 Fox and Cohen (1977). Mech (1970: 86) called this a "fixed stare"; Fox and Cohen (1977: 734, table 2), Harrington and Asa (2003: 90, table 3.7), and Peterson *et al.* (2002) used the term "direct stare." A stare by definition is fixed and direct, making both terms tautologies. Peterson *et al.* (2002) cited Schenkel (1947, 1967) as having described this behavior, but Schenkel (1967) mentioned only the submissive animal turning its gaze away from a dominant.
97 Fox (1970).
98 Fox (1970).
99 Fox (1970).
100 Crisler (1958: 237).
101 Fox (1973, plate XI, figure 2d).
102 Perhaps this last activity transfers aromatic compounds from the subordinate's saliva, activating specific receptors in the dominant's vomeronasal organ and reinforcing submissive status by chemosensory means. Such compounds, if soluble, could enter the vomeronasal organ by means of the incisive duct through the nasal cavity or mouth (Adams and Wiekamp 1984). I hasten to add that this suggestion is entirely speculative and not based on empirical evidence. With a few exceptions (e.g. the coyote), canids seldom display a *flehmen response* in which nonvolatile or low-volatility compounds are supposedly forced to the roof of the mouth by the intake of breath and diagnostic upper lip curl (Adams and Wiekamp 1984).
103 Fatjó *et al.* (2007).
104 Fox (1973, plate X, figure 1b).
105 Fox (1973).
106 Allen (1979: 104), Harrington and Mech (1979), Mech (1988a: 117), Murie (1944: 31–34, 169).
107 Mech (1966: 119–120; 1970: 15).
108 Fox (1973, plate XII, figures 3b–d).
109 Fox (1973, plate XII, figure 3d), Schenkel (1967: 323, figure 6A).
110 Schenkel (1967: 324, figure 7), Fox (1973, plate XI, figure 2c).
111 For example, Darwin (1998), Fox and Cohen (1977), Harrington and Asa (2003), Mech (1970: 68–110), Schenkel (1947, 1967).
112 McLeod (1996); also see Lockwood (1979).
113 Fentress (1967: 349).
114 Hinde (1985).
115 These terms are used in different ways. For example, being moody can also be a trait if moodiness is part of someone's personality.
116 Hinde (1985).
117 Hinde (1985).
118 McLeod (1996). Stand-taut was called "elevated body" in this report.
119 Lockwood (1979).
120 van Hooff and Wensing (1987).
121 Mech (1999: 1198); also see Mech (1970: 71).
122 Mech (1970: 74 and references), Mech (1999).
123 Mech (1970: 70).
124 Mech (1970: 70–71).
125 van Hooff and Wensing (1987).
126 van Hooff and Wensing (1987).
127 Harrington and Asa (2003).
128 Fatjó *et al.* (2007 and references).
129 Fatjó *et al.* (2007).
130 Gartlan (1964: 78) suggested tentatively, "one could justify on grounds of precision alone the removal of basic behaviour patterns such as aggression, mounting, grooming, etc. from the concept complex of dominance."
131 Lockwood (1979: 229).
132 de Waal (1989).
133 Bonanni *et al.* (2010a, 2010b).

134 Rabb *et al.* (1967), Schenkel (1967), Zimen (1975, 1982).

135 de Waal (1989: 244) wrote: "The narrow focus on this theoretical issue has led to dangerous simplifications. Instead of clear-cut winners and losers, we actually observe endless ambivalencies [*sic*], compromises, and a great deal of tolerance among social primates. 'Limited wars' are usually explained on the basis of the risk of incurred damage ... yet this is only the direct physical cost of aggression; we also need to consider the burden aggression places on long-term social relationships. Competitive advantages are often sacrificed for the sake of peace."

136 Bonanni *et al.* (2010a, 2010b) and de Waal (1989) used *formal dominance*, although *formal submission* seems more appropriate considering that unidirectional signaling is initiated by the subordinate animal and then acknowledged or not by its dominant counterpart. Nonetheless, both terms straddle traditional usage of dominance and submission with their hint of aggression just under the surface. All dominance ↔ submission is agonistic, and I see no reason to subdivide it. Furthermore, because the behavior is abbreviated but still acceptable to the other party, it actually appears to be informal, not formal, like discarding your necktie in front of the boss while having a relaxing drink and not being upbraided. Assuming the notion of formal is empty without informal, its counterpart, what repertoire of behaviors would then constitute "informal" dominance and submission among a group of dogs? The answer was just provided but with the terminology reversed. Substituting paying and receiving homage retains the notion of "ritual," behavior observed by Bonanni and co-authors and by de Waal, keeps the incisive distinctions they reported, and partitions the terminology into clearer descriptive units. The fact that ritual of any kind allows shortcuts (taking off your necktie while still acknowledging that the boss is dominant) is simply evidence of dominance ↔ submission having been relaxed for the moment but not changed essentially in character.

137 Bonanni *et al.* (2010b).

138 McLeod (1996 and references). The onset of real fighting is apparently delayed until weaning or beyond (Drummond 2006).

139 McLeod (1996).

140 McLeod (1996).

141 Two of the most intriguing – and flawed – papers I read on the subject of dominance hierarchies in captive wolves require comment. Both concluded that dominance and agonistic behavior are tethered more loosely than previously thought, and although the arguments are intuitively satisfying the methods and supporting data are not.

   The first is Lockwood's 1979 report based on observing 36 Alaskan wolves in 7 groups over 3 years. Lockwood did not state whether he personally collected all the data. If not there should have been a test of observer bias, which is especially important in behavioral experiments. Lockwood used as data a suite of 27 variables describing social interaction. Instead of devising tight definitions of what constitute dominance and submission and testing them as hypotheses, he used factor analysis to mine his data, hoping number-crunching would reveal a pattern. No data or results were provided other than factor loadings, which are scant evidence of anything without explanations in context. Little can be deduced of his pairwise competition tests, which are doubtfully valid anyway because of the "training" factor.

   The second report is that of van Hoof and Wensing (1987). Each year over 5 years two different students collected information for later assessment. The group of wolves during this time was stable. Data were compromised by failure to perform tests of observer bias, which probably accounts for the disparate between-year results (only data from 2 years were used; see p. 223 of their report). The prose and terminology are confusing (e.g. the use of "transitive" to indicate hierarchies that are neither circular nor linear). These authors criticized Lockwood's pairwise comparisons, arguing that the social group should have been assessed as a unit. True, at least some of Lockwood's assessments were pairwise (e.g. food competitions), but it appears that most variables were assessed using all wolves in a group.

   Both experiments were nonetheless creative, and the findings (so far as I can understand them) are interesting but hardly conclusive.

142 For examples of how paired food competition tests have been devised and implemented, seeDrews (1973), Fox (1972a), Scott and Fuller (1965: 155–156), and Silver and Silver (1969: 14–16).

143 Gartlan (1964: 77).

144 Rowell (1974: 136). Rowell's example was about monkeys.

145 Rowell (1974: 138) wrote: "In simplifying the social environment for experimental purposes there is always the risk of removing crucial elements until there is nothing left toward which to direct a [behavioral] functional response. At this point meaningless correlations may be found. Thus experimental findings which cannot be related to observations of behavior under natural conditions must be regarded with suspicion."

146 Rowell (1974: 139 and references).

147 Gartlan (1964).

148 Rowell (1974) pointed this out using primates as examples, but the principle applies generally to other social species.

149 Rowell (1974 and references).

150 Plotnik et al. (1968).

151 Scott (1967).

152 Fatjó et al. (2007).

153 Allen (1979: 103, photograph on p. 119).

154 Leaver and Reimchen (2008).

155 Bonanni et al. (2010b).

156 Schenkel (1947: 98) considered the wolf's tail to be its "most dynamic" visual feature ("Am dynamischsten in optischer Hinsicht ist der Schwanz").

157 Feddersen-Petersen (2000).

158 Bleicher (1963).

159 Goodwin et al. (1997). Fox (1970: 62) wrote, "a number of domesticated breeds of dog have such pendulous ears, bizarre facial markings, pendulous lips and excessive hair that little facial expression can be seen. Others, having been subjected to selective breeding and training, lack normal facial expressions under particular circumstances; many, notably guard dogs, attack with little or no warning. Certainly the wolf's visual signals are more reliable in this respect."

160 Goodwin et al. (1997).

161 Goodwin et al. (1997: 302).

162 Scott (1950).

163 Leaver and Reimchen (2008 and references).

164 Quaranta et al. (2007).

165 Scott (1950, 1967), Scott and Fuller (1965). See in particular the summary of Scott (1950: 1013–1015, table 1).

166 Scott (1967 and references).

167 Goodwin et al. (1997).

168 Corbett (1988).

169 Corbett and Newsome (1975).

170 Corbett (1988: 185).

Chapter 4: Olfactory and vocal communication

1 Buck (2000, 2004), Buck and Axel (1991), Rodriguez (2004).

2 Lesniak et al. (2008).

3 Raymer et al. (1984, 1986 and references in both).

4 Rouquier and Giorgi (2007: 95) actually defined olfaction as "sniffing of chemical compounds permitting the detection of odorants and pheromones." I prefer to separate the physical and physiological responses and think of olfaction as a cellular response. Many of the animals listed by Rouquier and Giorgi (e.g. worms, insects, fishes) do not "sniff" the external environment to deliver air or water to their olfactory receptors.

5 Buck (2000), Keverne (1999), Rodriguez (2004), Rouquier and Giorgi (2007).

6 Keverne (1999), Mombaerts (2004), Rouquier and Giorgi (2007).

7 Kambere and Lane (2007), Rouquier and Giorgi (2007).

8 These genes are sometimes called olfactory receptors or odor receptors.

9 Buck (2000, 2004), Matsunami and Buck (1997).

10 Buck and Axel (1991), Rouquier and Giorgi (2007).

11 Kambere and Lane (2007), Liberles and Buck (2006).

12 Buck (2004), Kambere and Lane (2007), Matsunami and Buck (1997 and references).

13 Grus *et al.* (2005).

14 Kambere and Lane (2007), Keverne (1999), Rodriguez (2004).

15 Two forms of VNO occur in mammals: segregated (rodents, opossums) and uniform (most others including canids). Their anatomical differences were described by Takigami *et al.* (2004).

16 Weiler *et al.* (1999).

17 Meredith (2001), Salazar *et al.* (1992), Takigami *et al.* (2004), Weiler *et al.* (1999).

18 Matsunami and Buck (1997), Rouquier and Giorgi (2007), Spehr *et al.* (2006a).

19 Grus and Zhang (2008 and references), Rouquier and Giorgi (2007), Spehr *et al.* (2006a), Young and Trask (2007).

20 Keverne (1999), Matsunami and Buck (1997), Young and Trask (2007). In reptiles there is evidence that the VNO also serves chemosensory functions not pertaining to pheromones (Halpern and Martínez-Marcos 2003 and references).

21 Matsunami and Buck (1997), Rodriquez (2004).

22 This includes the ability to distinguish between closely related compounds such as indole and skatole, which differ by one methyl group (Sam *et al.* 2001).

23 Spehr *et al.* (2006a).

24 Rodriguez (2005).

25 Adams and Wiekamp (1984).

26 Keverne (1999), Rodriguez (2005).

27 Some authorities, like Doty (2010), deny their existence.

28 Karlson and Lüscher (1959: 55).

29 Ryba and Tirindelli (1997).

30 Mombaerts (2004).

31 Mombaerts (2004) used this convention.

32 Doty (2010).

33 This requirement has continued into the recent literature (e.g. Halpern and Martínez-Marcos 2003, Mombaerts 2004, Young and Trask 2007).

34 Doty (2010: 24).

35 Rouquier and Giorgi (2007). Also see Gilad *et al.* (2004), whose numbers were slightly different.

36 Gilad *et al.* (2004), Rouquier and Giorgi (2007), Young *et al.* (2005). Gilad and co-authors also reported that howler monkeys (*Alouatta* spp.) are the only New World monkeys known to have full trichromatic vision.

37 Dulac and Axel (1995), Halpern and Martínez-Marcos (2003), Rodriguez (2005), Herrada and Dulac (1997), Matsunami and Buck (1997), Ryba and Tirindelli (1997).

38 Keverne (1999).

39 Kambere and Lane (2007), Young and Trask (2007).

40 Roppolo *et al.* (2007).

41 Capello *et al.* (2009).

42 Rouquier and Giorgi (2007), Young and Trask (2007).

43 Takami (2002).

44 Rouquier and Giorgi (2007). Keverne (1999: 719) wrote: "It therefore seems implausible that humans might experience significant behavioral or endocrine regulation by pheromones." Meredith (2001 and references) presented evidence for and against human pheromone detection by whatever VNO tissues remain.

45 Slotnick *et al.* (2010).

46 Young and Trask (2007). Dennis *et al.* (2003) found that the dog VNO expresses several neuronal markers, which suggests at least limited function.

47 Asa *et al.* (1986).

48 Zimen (1981: 132).

49 Grus *et al.* (2005).

50 Grus *et al.* (2005 and references), Halpern and Martínez-Marcos (2003), Keverne (1999 and references).

51 Young *et al.* (2005: 234), however, suggested that "in the process of breeding out certain wild social behaviors (e.g., aggression and dominance) during the domestication of dogs, breeders might have depleted the dog genome of many of its pheromone receptor genes." In their view "it is possible that

entire clusters containing intact V1Rs might have deleted during domestication." Wolves and other wild canids must be tested before domestication can be ruled out completely.

52 Rouquier and Giorgi (2007), Takigami *et al.* (2004), Young *et al.* (2005).

53 In its tame form, the European ferret.

54 Weiler *et al.* (1999 and references).

55 Woodley and Baum (2004).

56 Takami (2002). Ophidian snakes ranked first with the most sophisticated VNS.

57 Grus *et al.* (2005: 5772).

58 Hepper and Wells (2005) showed that tracking dogs can pick up faint scents of footprints and determine their direction. However, the ability of dogs to track specific human odors might be overrated. Brisbin and Austad (1991) showed that a trained tracking dog can distinguish the odor of its trainer's hand from that of a stranger, but not that of its trainer's elbow. Humans possess glands in the hands and feet (Mykytowycz 1972). Therefore, a person's "tracking scent" depends on what part of the body is used for priming dogs to start a search and whether this object is representative of the scent trail laid down.

59 Lesniak *et al.* (2008), Tacher *et al.* (2005).

60 Lesniak *et al.* (2008 and references).

61 Young *et al.* (2005).

62 Rouquier and Giorgi (2007).

63 Mombaerts (2004).

64 Hoon *et al.* (1999).

65 Mombaerts (2004).

66 Powers *et al.* (1990).

67 Gese and Ruff (1997) provided references to similar definitions. Peters and Mech (1975: 628) defined scent-marking simply as "the application of an animal's odor to its environment."

68 Chabot *et al.* (1996).

69 Parsons and Blumstein (2010b), Parsons *et al.* (2007).

70 Parsons and Blumstein (2010a).

71 According to Arnould *et al.* (1998: 571), "these compounds are a cocktail of fatty acids ranging in chain length from C_4 to C_{18} (major constituents of the total extract) mixed with a smaller proportion of neutral compounds."

72 Jorgenson *et al.* (1978).

73 Woolhouse and Morgan (1995).

74 Nolte *et al.* (1994).

75 Rothman and Mech (1979), Schenkel (1947).

76 Rothman and Mech (1979), Schenkel (1947).

77 Gese and Ruff (1997), Rothman and Mech (1979).

78 Gese and Ruff (1997), Jordan *et al.* (1967), Mech (1970), Peters and Mech (1975), Rothman and Mech (1979), Schenkel (1947).

79 Peters and Mech (1975).

80 Gese and Ruff (1997).

81 Schenkel (1947).

82 Bekoff (1979a), Dunbar (1977).

83 Harrington (1981), Mech (1988a: 108).

84 Mech (1977, 1994a and references).

85 Thurber and Peterson (1993).

86 Kleiman (1966: 176).

87 Harrington (1981).

88 Hradecký (1985).

89 Barja Nuñez and Javier de Miguel (2004).

90 Beaver *et al.* (1992).

91 Mech (1970: 72).

92 Scott (1967).

93 According to Doty (2010: 51–52), "In fact, scent marks are hardly ever completely avoided by animals that have not previously encountered the depositor of the mark, and only rarely repel intruders from regions that have been marked … If anything, conspecific scent marks attract conspecifics and lead to increased counter-scenting activities." Also see his references.

94 Gittleman (1991).
95 Sobel *et al*. (1998).
96 This is true at least for dogs trained to detect explosives (Gazit and Terkel 2003).
97 Gittleman (1991).
98 Preti *et al*. (1976), Raymer *et al*. (1985).
99 Asa *et al*. (1985a).
100 Asa *et al*. (1985a).
101 Preti *et al*. (1976). Natynczuk *et al*. (1989) also reported wide variation in the composition of anal gland contents of domestic dogs. For example, trimethylamine, dimethydisulfide, octatriene, and a group of estrogens were the main components of some samples and not present in others.
102 References in Raymer *et al*. (1985).
103 Doty and Dunbar (1974), Preti *et al*. (1976).
104 Mykytowycz (1972).
105 Asa *et al*. (1985a).
106 Asa *et al*. (1985a).
107 Barja *et al*. (2008).
108 Barja *et al*. (2004, 2005, 2008), Peters and Mech (1975), Vilà *et al*. (1994).
109 Barja *et al*. (2005).
110 Barja *et al*. (2004), Vilà *et al*. (1994).
111 Asa *et al*. (1985b), Peters and Mech (1975).
112 Scott and Shackleton (1982).
113 Vernes *et al*. (2001 and references).
114 Iljin (1941: 409), Martins and Valle (1948). For dogs, at 19 weeks according to Berg (1944).
115 Berg (1944).
116 Peters and Mech (1975) considered the average volume of a wolf's urine-mark to be about 5 ml. Also see Rothman and Mech (1979).
117 Asa *et al*. (1985b), Barja Nuñez and Javier de Miguel (2004), Peters and Mech (1975), Rothman and Mech (1979).
118 Asa *et al*. (1985b).
119 Barja Nuñez and Javier de Miguel (2004), Kleiman (1966), Peters and Mech (1975).
120 Berg (1944), Martins and Valle (1948).
121 I was astonished at the detailed descriptions and zeal (not to mention redundancy) with which urination postures have been described in the literature. I would have assumed that everyone has seen a dog urinate on a lawn or against a tree at least once. For reviews of all or some of these postures see Asa *et al*. (1985b, 1986, 1990), Peters and Mech (1975), and Kleiman (1966).
122 In captive wolves, also subordinate males attempting to achieve dominance (Asa *et al*. 1990). Barja Nuñez and Javier de Miguel (2004) reported that both males of a captive group displayed RLU equally.
123 Asa *et al*. (1985b, 1990).
124 Stahler *et al*. (2002a).
125 Martins and Valle (1948).
126 Ranson and Beach (1985).
127 Martins and Valle (1948).
128 Beach (1974).
129 Martins and Valle (1948).
130 Asa *et al*. (1990: 507).
131 Asa *et al*. (1985b, 1990).
132 Asa *et al*. (1985b, 1990), Peters and Mech (1975).
133 Asa *et al*. (1990).
134 Kleiman (1966).
135 Asa *et al*. (1990).
136 Kleiman (1966), Rothman and Mech (1979).
137 Among authors who mentioned "interdigital glands" of canids are Asa *et al*. (1986), Barja Nuñez and Javier de Miguel (2004), Barja *et al*. (2004, 2005), Bekoff (1979b and references), Peters and Mech (1975), and Tembrock (1968). Mykytowycz (1972) implied the presence of scent glands in the paws of dogs.

138 Aoki and Wada (1951) did not mention them. Ground-scratching and deposition of scent by interdigital glands was also been attributed to spotted hyaenas (*Crocuta crocuta*) by Tilson and Henschel (1986), again without cited evidence that hyaenas possess these glands.
139 Sands *et al.* (1977).
140 Mech (1966: 45).
141 Peters and Mech (1975: 632). Also see Rothman and Mech (1979: 750).
142 Peters and Mech (1975).
143 Peters and Mech (1975).
144 Asa *et al.* (1985a), Barrette and Messier (1980).
145 Young (1944: 81).
146 Crisler (1958: 260).
147 Fentress (1967).
148 Fentress (1967).
149 Fox (1970).
150 Fentress (1967).
151 Fox and Cohen (1977: 743, table 6) presented this in a table without explanation.
152 Crisler (1958: 259).
153 Silver and Silver (1969: 21).
154 Crisler (1958: 165, 259), Silver and Silver (1969: 21).
155 Fox and Cohen (1977).
156 Fox (1970: 60); also see Zimen (1981: 132).
157 Ryon *et al.* (1986).
158 Peterson *et al.* (1981) described the surgical procedure.
159 Hart and Haugen (1971).
160 Asa *et al.* (1985a).
161 Asa *et al.* (1986).
162 Gipson (1983).
163 Fentress (1967).
164 Fox (1970).
165 Fox (1970).
166 Mech (1988a: 107).
167 Parmelee (1964: 5).
168 Peters and Mech (1975).
169 Peters and Mech (1975: 634).
170 Mech (1988a: 108).
171 Mech (1970: 159–160).
172 Peters and Mech (1975: 634).
173 Peters and Mech (1975).
174 Benhamou (1989).
175 Asa *et al.* (1986).
176 Asa *et al.* (1986: 273).
177 Seyfarth and Cheney (2003).
178 Hirsch (1986: 18).
179 The lone exception might be the chimpanzee, in which theory of mind experiments have produced mixed results (Seyfarth and Cheney 2003 and references).
180 Seyfarth and Cheney (2003). Even the notion that information is transmitted in vocal signals is a contentious point among animal behaviorists (Seyfarth and Cheney 2003 and references), as it should be. In Chapter 3 I argued that signals are unable to "contain" anything.
181 Yin (2002 and references).
182 Shelley and Blumstein (2005).
183 Shelley and Blumstein (2005 and references).
184 McNay (2002), Scott (1967).
185 Tembrock (1976).
186 Dugatkin *et al.* (2003), Shelley and Blumstein (2005).
187 Cohen and Fox (1976: 90) stated that "canid vocal communication is essentially an 'emotional language', or sound repertoire of emotional reactions and intentions comparable to the

intentionality expressed in non-vocal body postures and facial expressions." Theirs would be a reasonable assessment were "intention" and "intentionality" removed.

188 Tembrock (1976).
189 Seyfarth and Cheney (2003).
190 Faragó *et al.* (2010). I substituted "interpretant" for their "referent."
191 Slocombe and Zuberbühler (2005).
192 Slocombe and Zuberbühler (2005).
193 Seyfarth and Cheney (2003).
194 As Yin (2002: 191) wrote: "It follows that if barking in dogs has specific functions, then the acoustical parameters of dog barks should vary predictably with context, and researchers should be able to classify barks into context-specific subtypes."
195 Newton-Fisher *et al.* (1993). Also see Ohl (1996). For a list of 12 vocalizations having onomato-poeic designations see Cohen and Fox (1976: 78); Schassburger (1993) listed 11 along with numerous combinations.
196 Cohen and Fox (1976). Also see Frommolt *et al.* (1988), Harrington and Asa (2003).
197 How these sounds are identified, named, and categorized is largely a matter of opinion. For examples of taxonomies see Bleicher (1963), Cohen and Fox (1976), Coscia *et al.* (1991), Feddersen-Petersen (2000), Fox and Cohen (1977), Ohl (1996), Tembrock (1976).
198 Schassburger (1993: 10).
199 Cohen and Fox (1976).
200 Schassburger (1993: 56).
201 Riede and Fitch (1999).
202 According to Durbin (1998: 200), when made between animals the dhole's whistle-call is "a repetitive ... medium amplitude, whine-like sound, ranging in dominant frequency from 553–936 Hz and often containing harmonics." The call is uttered by lifting the muzzle and projecting the call through the semi-closed mouth.
203 Palacios *et al.* (2007).
204 Yin and McCowan (2004) claimed the contrary, that the fundamental frequency is an acoustical feature that discriminates among individual vocalizations including the barks of domestic dogs.
205 Rendall *et al.* (2009: 236).
206 The "dog-appeasing pheromone" (DAP), a commercial product reputed to reduce or eliminate undesirable behaviors of pet dogs (e.g. barking, urinating and defecating indoors, noise phobia, separation anxiety), is an unspecified formulation, and current efforts to test its effectiveness have not met basic empirical stands of quality (Frank *et al.* 2010). If the active ingredient used in experiments evaluated by Frank and co-authors was *p*-hydroxybenzoate (the so-called "dog pheromone") a reason for its failure could be low flow response; that is, an influent nasal air flow too low to induce neural stimulation. Tests of this sort are essentially bioassays, or measures of dosage vs. response, with the response depending on (1) the nature of the substance, (2) its concentration in the entrained air, and (3) the flow rate into the nasal passages of air spiked with a predetermined concentration of odorant.
207 Wiley and Richards (1978 and references).
208 Yin and McCowan (2004 and reference).
209 Male songbirds are under strong selection to produce repetitive signals that seem acoustically distinctive against the songs of male conspecifics (Rendall *et al.* 2009).
210 Scott (1964).
211 Faragó *et al.* (2010 and references).
212 Feddersen-Petersen (2000), Taylor *et al.* (2009), Yin and McCowan (2004).
213 Faragó *et al.* (2010 and references).
214 Faragó *et al.* (2010 and references).
215 Faragó *et al.* (2010).
216 Nagel (1974).
217 Seyfarth and Cheney (2003). I substituted "influential value" for their "functional value."
218 Morton (1977: 855).
219 Morton (1977: 855–856).
220 August and Anderson (1987) used published data from 76 low-frequency (aggressive) and 75 high-frequency (appeasing or friendly) sounds from 50 species of mammals to test Morton's hypothesis indirectly.

221 Coscia *et al.* (1991).
222 Silver and Silver (1969: 21).
223 Harrington (1987).
224 Crisler (1958: 268), Coscia *et al.* (1991), Fentress (1967), Mech (1970: 95).
225 Silver and Silver (1969: 18, 21).
226 Fentress (1967).
227 Tembrock (1976).
228 Ognev (1931: 149).
229 Crisler (1958: 179) wrote: "Neither in sound, way of delivering nor intent was it like a dog sound. The utterance was extraordinarily interesting and pleasing. It was long and varied, inflected expressively, a hoarse mellow wowing."
230 See Morton (1977: 857–858, tables 1 and 2) for species comparisons of aggressive and nonaggressive sounds.
231 Darwin (1998: 122, footnote).
232 Lord *et al.* (2009).
233 Riede and Fitch (1999). The high-frequency whining that often accompanies submission is more tonal and narrowband (Riede and Fitch 1999 and references).
234 Taylor *et al.* (2010).
235 Schassburger (1993: 42).
236 Cohen and Fox (1976), Tembrock (1976).
237 Riede and Fitch (1999).
238 Crisler (1958: 151). A female wolf owned by the Crislers was especially impressive at controlling its vocalizations. According to Crisler (1958: 151) she "ululated, drawing her tongue up and down in her mouth like a trombone slide. Sometimes on a long note she held the tip of her tongue curled against the roof of her mouth. She shaped her notes with her cheeks, retracting them for plangency, or holding the sound in with them for horn notes." Wolves have a remarkable repertoire of sounds. What most of them signify is anyone's guess. Crisler (1958: 149) divided wolves' vocal communications into four kinds: "The famous howls, of which there are many kinds. Next, a whole range of expressive little 'you-and-me' noises, protesting or cheerful. Third, the ... short, unemotional communications of fact that we called simply 'speaking.' And fourth, long, fervently passionate 'talking.'"
        Sometimes the emotional attributions associated with wolf howls get out of hand. Stanwell-Fletcher (1942: 147) reported hearing a wolf "bewail her loneliness ... Not loud, but soft and mournful came the lament, and it was easy to imagine that this wolf had lost her mate and was alone in the world, with only memories of a happy past and of litters of frisky young pups at her side." Stanwell-Fletcher never confirmed whether this wolf was even female.
239 Riede and Fitch (1999).
240 Lord *et al.* (2009: 362, table 2). In addition to canids, mammals that bark include other carnivorans, some deer, primates, and rodents.
241 Domestic dogs bark in many contexts. According to Cohen and Fox (1976: 90) these include "greeting, play-soliciting, threat, defense, care soliciting, distress, contact-seeking, or during group vocalizations." The street dogs of Istanbul at the turn of the twentieth century were said to bark even while eating (Brummett 1995 and references).
242 Pongrácz *et al.* (2010).
243 Scott (1964), Tembrock (1968, 1976).
244 Tembrock (1976).
245 Cohen and Fox (1976), Fox (1971b: 184).
246 Cohen and Fox (1976).
247 Tembrock (1976).
248 Lord *et al.* (2009) based their barking-mobbing hypothesis on a detailed evaluation of the literature, which is both thorough and intriguing. However, without empirical support their argument is unconvincing. The putative link of barking with mobbing behavior is based on the undemonstrated premise that barking dogs are conflicted about whether to attack or run away, a situation especially applicable in urban areas where confinement in small spaces could heighten the effect. Barking in all canids might retain elements of conflict (Tembrock 1976). Lord *et al.* (2009: 365) claimed that a long-term experiment with foxes at a Siberian fur farm has shown that

animals bred explicitly for tameness "exhibited a significantly increased tendency to bark, compared with non-selected animals." This is incorrect and a weak argument even if true. The report they cited did not mention barking at all, stating only that "the vocal repertoire of foxes changes under domestication" and that some of the calls resemble those of dogs (Trut 1999: 168). Moreover, tameness has been defined as the *absence* of conflict behavior (Scott and Fredericson (1951: 275). If selecting for it has reduced *flight distance* in these foxes while at the same time increasing their inclination to bark, it seems antithetic to then label barking as ambivalent behavior.

249 Cohen and Fox (1976).

250 Pongrácz *et al.* (2010), Yin (2002).

251 Fox (1971b: 184).

252 Cohen and Fox (1976: 91) suggested that barking in domestic dogs might represent a behavioral "hypertrophy" of domestication. Taylor *et al.* (2009: 905) defined *hypertrophied traits* as "behaviours that have become generalized outside their original function as a byproduct of the relaxed selection associated with domestication, often resulting in a loss of functionality." Their definition makes synonyms of the terms trait and behavior.

253 Cohen and Fox (1976).

254 Feddersen-Petersen (2000).

255 The "silver fox" is a gray color morph of the red fox and not a different species.

256 Trut (1999).

257 Gogoleva *et al.* (2008).

258 Yin (2002), Yin and McCowan (2004).

259 Also called *isolation-barks*. Analogous in function to *contact-call*, as when an animal is separated from its group or a young animal from its mother (Yin and McCowan 2004).

260 Cohen and Fox (1976: 80) painted with too broad a brush in claiming that all categories of sound (e.g. barks, howls) made by canids are both species- and context-specific: "No variations in occurrence of sound types in individuals of the same species were ever recorded in different contexts i.e. sound types and context specificity was evident for each species studied."

261 Scott (1967).

262 Mech (1966: 66).

263 Cheney *et al.* (1996).

264 This hypothesis was proposed by Pongrácz *et al.* (2010). I merely simplified the name used to describe it.

265 Nesbitt (1975 and references).

266 Pongrácz *et al.* (2010).

267 Daniels and Bekoff (1989a).

268 Macdonald and Carr (1995).

269 Causey and Cude (1980) in reference to the free-ranging dogs described by Scott and Causey (1973).

270 Causey and Cude (1980).

271 Darwin (1897: 27–28).

272 Allen (1920: 492).

273 Fentress (1967), Scott (1964).

274 Feddersen-Petersen (2000).

275 Yin (2002), Yin and McCowan (2004).

276 Maros *et al.* (2008).

277 Maros *et al.* (2008), Pongrácz *et al.* (2010).

278 Maros *et al.* (2008).

279 Molnár *et al.* (2009).

280 As an older report by (Cohen and Fox 1976: 90) suggested, "this contextual variety [of barks] indicates that the sound itself may not always convey specific information, but rather, attracts the attention of the receiver. The more specific information to follow would then be received through other sensory channels (visual and/or olfactory). These cues would then identify the 'meaning' of the accompanying barks."

281 Fentress (1967: 343, legend to figure 1), Mech (1970: 136–137; 1988a: 58), Murie (1944: 46). Four hand-reared Iranian pups never howled even at 6 months (Joslin 1982). They were transferred to a

US facility and housed next to North American wolves, but they howled only when prompted by their neighbors or human imitators, never on their own. Iranian wolves in the wild also seemed disinclined to vocalize, and howling was considered rare.

282 Silver and Silver (1969: 22).
283 Joslin (1967).
284 Palacios *et al.* (2007).
285 Crisler (1958: 151).
286 Mech (1970: 102), Palacios *et al.* (2007), Theberge and Falls (1967), Tooze *et al.* (1990).
287 Joslin (1967), Theberge and Falls (1967), Tembrock (1976).
288 Young (1944: 78 and references).
289 Mech (1966: 66; 1970: 100–101), Rutter and Pimlott (1968: 136), Theberge and Falls (1967).
290 Joslin (1967), Harrington (1987), Harrington and Mech (1979, 1983).
291 Joslin (1967), Harrington (1987), Harrington and Mech (1979, 1983), Mech (1970: 102).
292 Yin and McCowan (2004 and references).
293 Palacios *et al.* (2007). Durbin (1998) could assign 90% of whistle-calls to the correct dhole.
294 Cohen and Fox (1976: 90).
295 Seyfarth and Cheney (2003).
296 Wiley and Richards (1978: 88).
297 Harrington and Mech (1979 and references).
298 Estimated maximum range 9.6–11.2 km (Harrington and Mech 1979: 243). Also see Joslin (1967), who estimated 6.5 km.
299 Henshaw and Stephenson (1974).
300 Yin and McCowan (2004). Wolf howls contain fundamental frequencies of 150–780 *Hertz* (*Hz*) and as many as 12 harmonic overtones (Theberge and Falls 1967).
301 Theberge and Falls (1967).
302 Theberge and Falls (1967).
303 Tooze *et al.* (1990).
304 Wiley and Richards (1978).
305 Wiley and Richards (1978).
306 Schleidt (1973).
307 Wiley and Richards (1978).
308 Wiley and Richards (1978 and references).
309 Theberge and Falls (1967).
310 Wiley and Richards (1978: 78).
311 Wiley and Richards (1978: 91) proposed that a sender, in producing a signal that degraded during transmission, might allow the receiver to judge its distance. Otherwise, the receiver is forced to approach the sender to determine its location, and if a signal "included information [*sic*] about the distance of the signaler, a receiver could avoid the signaler without risking an interaction." To force rejection of the null hypothesis a sound must therefore degrade in predictable fashion with distance from the source. The howls of wolves are often prolonged, and any consistent patterns of degradation could be examined objectively. If such patterns exist, determining if they have relevance to listening wolves is much more difficult. A starting place is searching for features of degradation in signals that correlate with expected spacing of senders and receivers (Schleidt 1973).
312 Harrington and Mech (1979).
313 Crisler (1958), Joslin (1982), Lehner (1978), Jordan *et al.* (1967), Joslin (1967), Harrington (1989), Harrington and Mech (1979, 1983), McCarley (1975), Palacios *et al.* (2007), Silver and Silver (1969: frontis), Theberge and Falls (1967), Tome (1854: 38). Also see Harrington (1987).
314 Mech (1966: 67 and references).
315 Young (1944: 79).
316 Crisler (1958), Joslin (1982), Theberge and Falls (1967), Schassburger (1993), Silver and Silver (1969, frontis), Zimen (1981: 72–73, 242, 257, 274, color figure 1).
317 Cohen and Fox (1976), Rabb *et al.* (1967), Silver and Silver (1969: 22).
318 Fentress (1967), Silver and Silver (1969: 22).
319 Harrington (1989).

320 Crisler (1958: 151) wrote: "Wolves love a howl. When it is started, they instantly seek contact with one another, troop together, fur to fur. Some wolves ... love to sing more than the others do and will run from any distance, panting and bright-eyed, to join in, uttering as they near, fervent little wows, jaws wide, hardly able to wait to sing."

321 Crisler (1958: 151).

322 Harrington (1989: 126). The dhole's chorus-howls might be similar in this respect (Durbin 1998).

323 Maynard Smith (1979: 482).

324 Maynard Smith (1979).

325 Maynard Smith (1979: 483).

326 Joslin (1967: 281–282).

327 Harrington and Mech (1979), Peters and Mech (1975).

328 Location within the territory, however, has no bearing on response (Harrington and Mech 1983).

329 Joslin (1967), Theberge and Falls (1967).

330 Harrington and Mech (1979).

331 Harrington and Mech (1979).

332 Harrington (1987).

333 Harrington and Mech (1979: 234) also listed a third possibility: "They [the pack howled to] should reply, for separated wolves frequently respond to the howls of fellow pack members." However, this is not different from the second possibility; that is, under the conditions set forth no group should respond unless a pack member is missing.

334 I assume Harrington and Mech (1979: 245) meant strange conspecifics because of this speculation: "In every case where a lone female approached, only one person had howled. Thus it is possible that the females were investigating the howler, perhaps looking for a potential mate or the remains of a nearby kill."

335 Theberge and Falls (1967).

336 Theberge and Falls (1967).

337 Cohen and Fox (1976).

338 Iljin (1941: 408).

339 Fentress (1967).

340 Theberge and Falls (1967).

341 Mech (1988a: 58).

342 Iljin (1941: 408).

Chapter 5: Space

1 Burt (1943: 351).

2 Territoriality has been used in many contexts (Maher and Lott 1995 and references).

3 van Ballenberghe et al. (1975).

4 Mech et al. (1998: 75).

5 Mech (1966: 50).

6 Olson (1938a).

7 Harrington and Mech (1979), van Ballenberghe et al. (1975).

8 Messier (1985b).

9 Pulliainen (1965: 246).

10 Cowan (1947), Olson (1938b).

11 Cowan (1947). Whether either home range constitutes a seasonally defended territory was not stated. I assumed the space occupied from spring through autumn is a territory.

12 Walton et al. (2001).

13 The areas of these ranges are enormous. However, straight-line distances from the farthest location on the winter range to the den sites (Chapter 8) averaged 508 km during one winter and 265 km the next (Walton et al. (2001).

14 Ballard et al. (1998).

15 Ballard et al. (1997).

16 Heard and Williams (1992), Kuyt (1962), Stephenson and James (1982).

17 Thompson (1952).

18 Stebler (1944).
19 Smith *et al.* (1997).
20 Fuller (1989a).
21 Smith *et al.* (1997).
22 Murie (1944: 42). I assumed this to be a circle.
23 Young (1944: 81). These "runways," as Young called them, were estimated as "an irregular circle, the diameter of which may be between 20 and 60 miles." Young's definition is vague (an "irregular circle"). He also referred to it as a "hunting route ... a travelway giving access to the territory of a given pair or family" (Young 1944: 81). I think he meant the periphery of a territory and not simply a network of paths through the territory.
24 Boitani (1992).
25 Burkholder (1959), calculated as a rectangle.
26 Stahler *et al.* (2002a).
27 Lehman *et al.* (1992).
28 Hayes and Harestad (2000a).
29 Hayes and Harestad (2000a), Hayes *et al.* (2000).
30 Mech (1966: 50).
31 Thompson (1952).
32 van Ballenberghe *et al.* (1975).
33 Burkholder (1959).
34 Peterson *et al.* (1984).
35 Peterson *et al.* (1984).
36 Peterson *et al.* (1984).
37 Barja *et al.* (2004), Brown and Lanning (1954), de Vos (1949), Dunne (1939), Mech (1966: 50, 1970: 152–159), Ognev (1931: 142), Olson (1938b), Pulliainen (1965, 1982), Thompson (1952), Vilà *et al.* (1994).
38 de Vos (1950).
39 Mech (1966: 50–51, 53, 57).
40 Olson (1938b), van Ballenberghe *et al.* (1975).
41 Fritts and Mech (1981).
42 Burkholder (1959).
43 Murie (1944: 108–109).
44 Cowan (1947).
45 Scott and Shackleton (1982).
46 Pulliainen (1982).
47 Boitani (1982).
48 Young (1944: 304).
49 Burkholder (1959), Cowan (1947), Dunne (1939), Ognev (1931: 150), Pulliainen (1982), Stanwell-Fletcher (1942).
50 Dunne (1939).
51 Hayes and Harestad (2000a).
52 Hayes and Harestad (2000a).
53 Fuller (1989a), Hayes and Harestad (2000a).
54 Hayes and Harestad (2000a). Pack size in southwestern Québec, however, correlated directly with prey density (Messier 1985b).
55 Mech (1977).
56 Peterson and Page (1988).
57 Bibikov (1982), Fritts and Mech (1981), Hayes and Harestad (2000a), Pulliainen (1982), Rausch (1967), vonHoldt (2008).
58 Hayes and Harestad (2000a).
59 Fritts and Mech (1981).
60 Compared to the mean of the previous 3 years (Mech 1977).
61 Rausch (1967).
62 vonHoldt *et al.* (2008).
63 Hayes and Harestad (2000a).
64 Pulliainen (1982).
65 Mech (1977).

66 Allen (1979: 1) believed that wolves colonized Isle Royale early in February 1949. Coyotes had preceded them, arriving about the same time as the moose 40 years earlier and disappearing after wolves became permanent residents. Red foxes have been present since the 1920s.

67 Peterson and Page (1988 and references). My description of events are from this source.

68 Peterson and Page (1988: 97).

69 Messier (1994).

70 Peterson and Page (1988).

71 Ballard *et al.* (1987).

72 Mech (1977). Peterson and Page (1988: 97), who had monitored this series of events on Isle Royale, wrote: "It is clear that the only natural limits to wolf density are those ultimately imposed by food supply. Social behavior, however, responsive to variation in food supply, was the key proximate regulator of wolf density."

73 Thurber and Peterson (1993).

74 According to Peterson and Page (1988: 97), "by 1986, even the spatial organization of the population was similar, with a large, dominant pack inhabiting the southwestern two-thirds of the island and a smaller pack resident on the remainder. We interpret this as a response to similar levels of food availability, as the moose population numbered 600–1,000 and was increasing during both periods."

75 Fritts and Mech (1981), Mech (1994a), Stahler *et al.* (2002a).

76 Fritts and Mech (1981), Mech (1977), Meier *et al.* (1995), Peterson and Page (1988), Peterson *et al.* (1998).

77 Ballard *et al.* (1987), Kunkel *et al.* (2004), Mech (1994a), Peterson and Page (1988).

78 Mech (1994a).

79 Ballard *et al.* (1987), Fritts and Mech (1981), Jordan *et al.* (1967), Mahrenke (1971), Mech (1993a, 2000), Mills *et al.* (2008), Murie (1944: 43–44), Peterson *et al.* (1998), van Ballenberghe and Erickson (1973).

80 Allen (1979: 262), Mech (1966: 87, 91).

81 Fritts and Mech (1981).

82 Allen (1979: 99), Jordan *et al.* (1967).

83 Messier (1985b).

84 Cowan (1947).

85 Cowan (1947), Crisler (1958: 251).

86 Peters and Mech (1975).

87 Mech *et al.* (1998: 49, 81–82), Meier *et al.* (1995).

88 Ballard *et al.* (1997).

89 Mech (1977).

90 Fritts and Mech (1981).

91 Messier (1985b).

92 Messier (1985b).

93 Fritts and Mech (1981), van Ballenberghe (1983a).

94 Lehman *et al.* (1992).

95 Messier (1985b).

96 Fritts and Mech (1981), Gese and Mech (1991), Lehman *et al.* (1992).

97 Lehman *et al.* (1992).

98 Kokko and Lundberg (2001).

99 Kokko and Lundberg (2001: 198).

100 Mech (1970: 38).

101 Lehman *et al.* (1992).

102 Ballard *et al.* (1987).

103 Meier *et al.* (1995).

104 Meier *et al.* (1995).

105 Hayes and Harestad (2000b), Thurber and Peterson (1993).

106 Meier *et al.* (1995).

107 Ognev (1931: 143).

108 Rausch (1967).

109 Ballard *et al.* (1997).

110 Jordan *et al.* (1967).
111 Cowan (1947).
112 Olson (1938b).
113 Mech (1977).
114 Hayes and Harestad (2000a and references).
115 Mech (1970: 40).
116 Rausch (1967).
117 Fritts and Mech (1981).
118 van Ballenberghe *et al.* (1975), vonHoldt *et al.* (2008).
119 Ballard *et al.* (1998), Forbes and Theberge (1995). A few studies in the 1980s reported direct correlations (e.g. Ballard *et al.* 1987; Messier 1985b; Peterson *et al.* 1984), but later observations showed either weak associations or none (Ballard *et al.* 1998; Fuller 1989a; Hayes *et al.* 2000; Thurber and Peterson 1993). Also see Ballard *et al.* (1997), Mech *et al.* (1998: 78–80), Potvin (1987).
120 Ballard *et al.* (1987, 1997) and Peterson *et al.* (1984) relied on VHF telemetry; the later work used satellite telemetry (Ballard *et al.* 1998).
121 Mech *et al.* (1998: 79 and references).
122 Mech (1970: 41).
123 Cowan (1947).
124 Mech (1970: 42, 218).
125 Thurber and Peterson (1993).
126 Murie (1944: 45).
127 Fritts and Mech (1981).
128 Mech (1970: 44, 1988a), Mech and Boitani (2003), Murie (1944: 24, 44–45), vonHoldt *et al.* (2008), Young (1944: 120).
129 Information in this paragraph and the next is from vonHoldt *et al.* (2008).
130 Also see Fritts and Mech (1981), Mech and Hertel (1983), Stahler *et al.* (2002a).
131 vonHoldt *et al.* (2008).
132 Rothman and Mech (1979).
133 Lehman *et al.* (1992), Meier *et al.* (1995).
134 This is a composite definition. See Mech and Boitani (2003) and vonHoldt *et al.* (2008).
135 Ballard *et al.* (1983).
136 Hayes and Harestad (2000a).
137 Meier *et al.* (1995).
138 Meier *et al.* (1995).
139 Theuerkauf *et al.* (2003).
140 Jordan *et al.* (1967).
141 Burkholder (1959).
142 Oosenbrug and Carbyn (1982).
143 Jordan *et al.* (1967), Mech (1966: 40–43, 60).
144 Much of this section is based on Wolff (1997).
145 Bergerud and Elliott (1998).
146 Wolff (1997 and references). Inbreeding was once thought to be common in wolves (e.g. Peters and Mech 1975; Peterson *et al.* 1984), but the data were based on observations of captive animals (Rabb *et al.* 1967).
147 Wolff (1993).
148 Lambs of Dall's sheep are precocial. When only a day or two old, and "so small that they can walk erect under their mothers, [they can] clamber up cliffs so precipitous that even the mothers can scarcely find footing" (Murie 1944: 89). They also have astonishing speed and endurance from the start, able to run along with their mothers over long distances. Caribou calves are weaned and subsisting on vegetation within a month (Murie 1944: 158).
149 Wolff (1997).
150 Broom *et al.* (2009), Legge (1996).
151 Hayes and Harestad (2000b), Messier (1994), Messier and Crête (1984, 1985). Ecologists distinguish between *population limitation* and *population regulation*, considering that to be limiting a predator's effect on its prey is additive (i.e. another source of mortality). According to Dale *et al.*

(1994: 644), regulation maintains prey numbers at a given level requiring "a density-dependent feedback mechanism, i.e. the limiting effect must increase when prey numbers increase." Wolves appear able to regulate moose density in North American single prey–single predator systems except on Isle Royale (Messier 1991), probably because it is an insular system.

152 Bergerud and Elliott (1998), Fuller (1989a), Messier (1994), van Ballenberghe *et al.* (1975).
153 Bergerud and Elliott (1998).
154 Wolff (1997: 3 and references).
155 Wolf (1997).
156 Kojola *et al.* (2006), but see Boyd and Pletscher (1999).
157 Messier (1985b), Peterson and Page (1988).
158 Hayes and Harestad (2000a).
159 Gese and Mech (1991).
160 Fritts and Mech (1981).
161 Kuyt (1962).
162 Mech (1977), Messier (1985a).
163 Boyd and Pletscher (1999).
164 Messier (1985b).
165 Fuller (1989a), Mech (1977), Messier (1985b).
166 Boyd and Pletscher (1999), Kojola *et al.* (2006), Messier (1985b), Peterson *et al.* (1984), Smith *et al.* (2010).
167 Berg and Kuehn (1982).
168 Mills *et al.* (2008).
169 In that time, according to Ciucci *et al.* (2009: 1304), "wolf M15 traveled across 2 national, 5 regional, and several provincial administrative units, and went as close as 0.8–5 km to large towns such as Cuneo and Genoa. The wolf navigated several potential barriers, including 4 fenced 4-lane highways (traffic volumes in Jul-Sep ranging 49,928–143,081 vehicles/day ...), several main railways, and many state, provincial, and local paved roads."
170 Merrill and Mech (2000).
171 Pulliainen (1965).
172 Pulliainen (1982).
173 Dawes *et al.* (1986).
174 Boyd and Pletscher (1999), Kojola *et al.* (2006).
175 Boyd and Pletscher (1999), Messier (1985a), Wydeven *et al.* (1995: 150, table 3).
176 Wabakken *et al.* (2007).
177 Linnell *et al.* (2005), Pulliainen (1965).
178 Ognev (1931: 135 and references).
179 Ognev (1931: 135).
180 Dawes *et al.* (1986).
181 Hutt (2003).
182 Ballard *et al.* (1987), Fritts and Mech (1981), Gese and Mech (1991), Hayes and Harestad (2000a), Mech (1987).
183 Kojola *et al.* (2006), Gese and Mech (1991).
184 Mech *et al.* (1998: 48).
185 Mech *et al.* (1998: 116).
186 Hayes and Harestad (2000a), Rothman and Mech (1979).
187 Ballard *et al.* (1987), Messier (1985b), Peterson and Page (1988).
188 Fuller (1989a), Jordan *et al.* (1967).
189 Gese and Mech (1991), Messier (1985a).
190 Ballard *et al.* (1987, 1997), Fritts and Mech (1981), Fuller (1989a), Peterson *et al.* (1984).
191 Ballard *et al.* (1987).
192 Fuller (1989a).
193 Kojola *et al.* (2006).
194 Gese and Mech (1991). Others reported sex bias in dispersal (Gese and Mech 1991 and references).
195 Gese and Mech (1991).
196 Fritts and Mech (1981).
197 Hayes and Harestad (2000a).

198 Fritts and Mech (1981).
199 Ballard *et al.* (1997).
200 Meier *et al.* (1995).
201 Ballard *et al.* (1987).
202 Ballard *et al.* (1987).
203 Ballard *et al.* (1987). Mech *et al.* (1998: 48–49) reported the average straight-line distance dispersed by Denali wolves to be 133 km, the maximum distance nearly 700 km.
204 Ballard *et al.* (1997).
205 Mech *et al.* (1998: 91–92, 119).
206 Stahler *et al.* (2002a).
207 Peterson *et al.* (1984).
208 Fritts and Mech (1981).
209 Peterson *et al.* (1984), van Ballenberghe (1983a).
210 Just 5 of 20 dispersals from January through May were permanent on the Kenai Peninsula (Peterson *et al.* 1984).
211 Boyd and Pletscher (1999).
212 Fuller (1989a), Gese and Mech (1991), Hayes and Harestad (2000a), Messier (1985a), Stephenson and James (1982), Wabakken *et al.* (2007), Walton *et al.* (2001).
213 Gese and Mech (1991).
214 Fuller (1989a).
215 Messier (1985a: 243).
216 Ballard *et al.* (1987), Fritts and Mech (1981), Gese and Mech (1991), Hayes and Harestad (2000a).
217 Gese and Mech (1991).
218 Kojola *et al.* (2006).
219 Boyd and Pletscher (1999).
220 Gese and Mech (1991).
221 van Ballenberghe *et al.* (1975).
222 Fritts and Mech (1981).
223 Lehman *et al.* (1992).
224 This might not be true when a population is in flux. Reproductive tracts of 89 adults and two-year-old Alaskan wolves collected from mid-March through the end of April showed that 89% were pregnant (Rausch 1967). Some of these populations were still being exploited by aerial bounty hunters, which could account in part for the high rate of pregnancy.
225 Packard *et al.* (1985), Mech (1970: 320–322).
226 Malcolm and Martin (1982).
227 Sillero-Zubiri *et al.* (1996).
228 Rausch (1967).
229 Fritts and Mech (1981), Mech (1977).
230 Corbett (1988), Medjo and Mech (1976), Packard *et al.* (1985), Rabb *et al.* (1967), vonHoldt *et al.* (2008).
231 Corbett (1988), Gier (1957), McLeod (1990 and references), Mech (1966: 90), Paquet *et al.* (1982), Rabb *et al.* (1967), Silver and Silver (1969: 21). Paulraj *et al.* (1992) reported infanticide in captive dholes. The unusually high incidence of infanticide reported in some captive coyote studies (Gier 1957) might be explained by their generally less social nature than wolves and dogs and greater susceptibility to stress while attempting to rear young in the presence of humans.
232 McLeod (1990), Packard (2003: 59). Mech (1988a: 33) could cite no incidences of wild wolves killing their pups after dens had been disturbed by humans.
233 Lions make an interesting comparison. Lion prides do not have dominance hierarchies. Females defend the territory against females, but they must also guard against infanticide by males, not other females (Legge 1996 and references).
234 Mech (1999).
235 Mech (1999).
236 Mech (1999).
237 Frame *et al.* (1979). Fox (1984: 87) claimed this to be true based on a film *The Innocent Killers* by Hugo and Jane van Lawick-Goodall. I found no mention of it in their book of the same title.
238 Corbett (1988).

239 Mech (1977), Peters and Mech (1975).

240 Someone else used this phrase first, but I was unable to find the reference.

241 Young (1944: 73) wrote: "The urine carries a strong and, to wolves apparently, an identifying odor for each individual. Field observations that urine taken from a strange wolf and exposed on a runway [territorial boundary or path inside the territory] causes the greatest excitement to the wolf or group of wolves using that run. Much scratching and kicking up of dirt, and often excessive deposits of excreta, are to be noted when such urine is applied to the scent posts. The great interest led to the use of urine as a lure in trapping wolves." He continued (Young 1944: 81), "As wolves pass over their runways, they stop at these posts, invariably voiding urine, and often feces as well."

242 Asa *et al.* (1990), Mech (1999 and references), Peters and Mech (1975), Peterson and Page (1988).

243 Peterson and Page (1988).

244 Fritts and Mech (1981).

245 Fritts and Mech (1981), Peters and Mech (1975), Rothman and Mech (1979).

246 Asa *et al.* (1990), Mech (1995a, 1999), Peterson *et al.* (2002), Rothman and Mech (1979).

247 Mech (1988a: 107–108), Fritts and Mech (1981).

248 Mech (1988a: 107–108).

249 In this case, over-marking serves a different function than it does between members of a mated pair during courtship (Chapter 7).

250 Briscoe *et al.* (2002).

251 Rothman and Mech (1979).

252 The random walk is a simple model described by $X_2 = X_{t-1} + e_t$, where X_t = the value in time period t, X_{t-1} = the value in time period t – 1, and e_t = the value of the error term in time period t (i.e. noise). Because a random walk is defined in terms of first differences the relationship can be expressed as $X_t - X_{t-1} = e_t$. Briscoe *et al.* (2002) described a system of spatial movements based on the number of urine-marks, their production (which depends on those marked previously), and incorporating some reasonable assumptions (e.g. urine-marks decay at a constant rate, wolves mark at a constant rate but mark more often when urine-marks of a stranger are encountered).

253 Lewis and Murray (1993), Lewis *et al.* (1997), White *et al.* (1996).

254 Loew and Fraser (1977: 101).

255 Loew and Fraser (1977: 103)

256 Causey and Cude (1980), Nesbitt (1975). The term feral, with regard to dogs, also means not socialized to humans (Daniels and Bekoff 1989a, 1989b), although this property could include most strays. Daniels and Bekoff (1989c) briefly reviewed other suggested qualities and argued that the feral state is ontogenetic rather than evolutionary and therefore not domestication in reverse, or "de-domestication."

257 Daniels and Bekoff (1989a), Scott and Causey (1973).

258 Causey and Cude (1980), Gipson (1983), Nesbitt (1975).

259 Causey and Cude (1980), Daniels and Bekoff (1989a).

260 Scott and Causey (1973).

261 Daniels and Bekoff (1989c: 87–88).

262 Boitani and Ciucci (1995), Daniels and Bekoff (1989c).

263 Scott and Causey (1973) referred to rural dogs in this category as free-ranging, meaning they did not travel in a pack and were intermediate in aggressiveness between feral and owned dogs when live-trapped. According to Blanco *et al.* (1992), dogs that might actually be feral dogs are sometimes classified as strays. In my opinion, such instances would be rare.

264 Beck (1973), Berman and Dunbar (1983).

265 Boitani and Ciucci (1995 and references). See Daniels and Bekoff (1989c) for an evolutionary perspective on feralization.

266 Rubin and Beck (1982).

267 Bonanni *et al.* (2010a: 982) studied strays outside Rome: "With very few exceptions, dogs were not socialized to humans although they were dependent on humans for food provisioning."

268 Daniels (1983a).

269 Berman and Dunbar (1983).

270 Rubin and Beck (1982).

271 Rubin and Beck (1982).

272 Rubin and Beck (1982).
273 Fox *et al.* (1975), Nesbitt (1975).
274 Oppenheimer and Oppenheimer (1975).
275 Choudhuri *et al.* (1984).
276 Berman and Dunbar (1983), Causey and Cude (1980), Choudhuri *et al.* (1984), Daniels (1983a), Daniels and Bekoff (1989a), Nesbitt (1975), Scott and Causey (1973).
277 Oppenheimer and Oppenheimer (1975).
278 Beck (1973), Causey and Cude (1980), Kruuk and Snell (1981), Nesbitt (1975), Scott and Causey (1973). Free-ranging owned dogs are also likely to be most active early in the morning (Rubin and Beck 1982), perhaps because their owners release them at this time.
279 Boitani (1992).
280 Berman and Dunbar (1983), Choudhuri *et al.* (1984), Fox *et al.* (1975), Oppenheimer and Oppenheimer (1975).
281 Fox *et al.* (1975), Oppenheimer and Oppenheimer (1975).
282 Oppenheimer and Oppenheimer (1975), Scott and Causey (1973).
283 Daniels (1983a).
284 Thomson (1992b, 1992c).
285 Thomson (1992a, 1992b).
286 Beck (1973).
287 Scott and Causey (1973).
288 Nesbitt (1975).
289 Nesbitt (1975).
290 Ortolani *et al.* (2009).
291 Allen (1979: 258).
292 Beck (1971, 1973), Fox *et al.* (1975). Oppenheimer and Oppenheimer (1975: 90), in a report on free-ranging dogs from a town 40 km north of Calcutta, make the intriguing statement, "toward the end of December, males begin to restrict their movements to their normal home range and strange males are no longer tolerated." Nothing more is said on the subject; no data are given. Are these dogs really territorial in the breeding season?
293 Harrington and Mech (1979 and references).
294 Harrington and Mech (1979).
295 Berman and Dunbar (1983).
296 Daniels (1983a).
297 Boitani and Ciucci (1995), Causey and Cude (1980), Daniels and Bekoff (1989b), Macdonald and Carr (1995), Nesbitt (1975), Scott and Causey (1973).
298 Beck (1973: 32–33).
299 Fox *et al.* (1975).
300 Fox *et al.* (1975; statement only, no data).
301 Fox *et al.* (1975).
302 Beck (1971), Fox *et al.* (1975), Macdonald and Carr (1995).
303 Daniels (1983a).
304 Fox *et al.* (1975).
305 Berman and Dunbar (1983).
306 Berman and Dunbar (1983).
307 Ortolani *et al.* (2009).
308 Thomson (1992d).
309 Daniels (1983a).
310 Daniels (1983a).
311 Daniels (1983a).
312 Daniels (1983a).
313 Rubin and Beck (1982).
314 Choudhuri *et al.* (1984).
315 Scott (1967).
316 Daniels (1983a).
317 Boitani (1992), Choudhuri *et al.* (1984), Font (1987), Ghosh *et al.* (1984), Macdonald and Carr (1995).

318 Choudhuri *et al.* (1984), Font (1987).
319 Choudhuri *et al.* (1984), Macdonald and Carr (1995).
320 Daniels and Bekoff (1989b).
321 Daniels and Bekoff (1989a).
322 Daniels and Bekoff (1989a).
323 Macdonald and Carr (1995).
324 Macdonald and Carr (1995).
325 Rubin and Beck (1982).
326 Hopkins *et al.* (1976).
327 Daniels and Bekoff (1989b).
328 Rubin and Beck (1982: 166).
329 Ortolani *et al.* (2009).
330 Beck (1973, 1975), Choudhuri *et al.* (1984), Fox *et al.* (1975), Macdonald and Carr (1995), Pal (2003), Pal *et al.* (1998), Rubin and Beck (1982). The three dogs observed by Fox and co-authors also visited a park. Inclusion of the park expanded the home range to about 61 ha.
331 Gipson (1983).
332 Nesbitt (1975).
333 Causey and Cude (1980).
334 Scott and Causey (1973).
335 Daniels (1983a).
336 Daniels and Bekoff (1989a).
337 Choudhuri *et al.* (1984).
338 Choudhuri *et al.* (1984), Daniels and Bekoff (1989b), Pal (2003), Pal *et al.* (1998).
339 Sternthal (2010).
340 Description is based on Beck (1971, 1973).
341 Marlowe (2004).
342 Drastic reduction in home range size seems typical of adopted dogs. For example, see Daniels and Bekoff (1989a).
343 Boitani and Ciucci (1995). I disagree with Bonanni *et al.* (2010a, 2010b) that unowned free-ranging dogs form true packs. Their statement (Bonanni *et al.* 2010b: 982) that such groups "are highly cooperative in conflicts against conspecifics" contradicts their own observations clearly indicating reluctance by some members to participate in aggressive displays against rivals (Bonanni *et al.* 2010a).
344 Jordan *et al.* (1967).
345 Messier and Barrette (1982).
346 Thomson (1992d).
347 Robley *et al.* (2010).
348 Thomson (1992d).
349 Robertshaw and Harden (1986), Vernes *et al.* (2001).
350 Thomson *et al.* (1992).
351 Green and Catling (1977).
352 Thomson (1992d).
353 Thomson *et al.* (1992).
354 Thomson (1992d).
355 Harden (1985).
356 Robley *et al.* (2010).
357 Green and Catling (1977).
358 Catling *et al.* (1992) and Claridge *et al.* (2009), for example, referred consistently to home ranges of dingoes without mentioning territories. Robley *et al.* (2010) and Thomson (1992d) used both terms. Some of the other literature is equally confusing. Bekoff and Wells (1981: 795), for example, defined coyote packs as "groups ... consisting of about three to eight individuals occupying a defined home range and defending a territory."
359 Thomson (1992a: 516) commented on "the defence of territories" by dingoes in the Fortescue River region then said no more, citing Thomson (1992d). During this lengthy investigation dingoes were trapped, radio-collared, and monitored from the air. Thomson (1992d) presented plots of areas occupied over time by different groups, stating that dingoes belonging to the same

group had overlapping home ranges all confined within the boundaries of a stable territory that was more or less exclusive of other groups. Thus a home range was apparently one of several overlapping spaces confined within the fixed boundaries of a larger territory. Thomson (1992d: 545) defined a territory as "an area utilised by a pack over a long period (>8 months) [and] represented a group home range." He gave no evidence that any of these spaces was ever *defended* against other dingoes. The classic definition of a territory as a defended space was instead redefined as a stable mosaic of home ranges occupied by dingoes known to each other that existed longer than 8 months. On the basis of this and other information from the same study I conclude that Fortescue River dingoes occupied home ranges (which can also have long-term stable boundaries) but not territories.

360 Claridge *et al.* (2009).
361 Thomson (1992d: 551). The fallacy of presumption. *Premise*: A territory is a space having long-term stable boundaries. *Inference*: Spaces occupied by dingoes have long-term stable boundaries. *Conclusion*: Dingoes occupy territories. Although logically (formally) valid both the premise and conclusion of this argument are false. The premise is false because home ranges can also have long-term stable boundaries (i.e. home range and territory are not synonyms).
362 Mech *et al.* (1998: 49, 81–84), Meier *et al.* (1995).
363 Peterson and Page (1988).
364 Fritts and Mech (1981), Mech (1994a).
365 vonHoldt *et al.* (2008).
366 Once in nine observed encounters (Thomson 1992d).
367 Thomson (1992d: 558) wrote: "A social rank order ... was evident in the packs, although the fact that it was impossible to individually recognize all pack members during all sightings precluded the clear identification of hierarchies." To reinforce the presumed existence of an unseen rank order Thomson cited Corbett (1988), which was a study of captive – not wild – dingoes.
368 Thomson (1992d).
369 Bowen (1981).
370 Meggitt (1965).
371 Meggitt (1965).
372 Macintosh (1975: 99) went on to state, "admittedly, at night one may have the occasional experience of being apparently surrounded by 10 to 20 dingoes about half a mile away arranged in a circle around one's camp fire and holding a howling concert."
373 Corbett (1995: 89, table 6.1).
374 Robley *et al.* (2010).
375 Corbett and Newsome (1975).
376 Mech (1970: 38–39).
377 Corbett and Newsome (1975: 373).
378 Thomson *et al.* (1992).
379 Corbett and Newsome (1975).
380 Thomson (1992d).
381 Newsome *et al.* (1983b).

Chapter 6: Foraging

1 van Lawick-Goodall (1971).
2 Murie (1944: 29, 42).
3 Barja (2009: 152) argued that wolves are facultative foragers and not opportunists "because a facultative specialist may change from a key food item when other profitable prey is available." I fail to see the distinction if facultative is given the usual meaning of adaptable and not obligatory. The term "facultative specialist" therefore seems oxymoronic. As shown later in this chapter, wolves indeed make prey choices, and in multiple-prey habitats are often reluctant to switch from a favored prey species even when doing so seems in their best interest.
4 Carbone *et al.* (1999).
5 Fuller and Keith (1980), Peterson *et al.* (1984).

6 Canids living in colder climates have higher mass-adjusted BMRs than those inhabiting hot deserts. Wolves of 35 kg in temperate zones have a BMR of 3872 kJ/day, for those living in deserts (20 kg) the rate is 2411 kJ/day; for dingoes of 18 kg living in temperate locations the rate is 3487 kJ/day (Careau et al. 2007).

7 Jordan et al. (1967), Mech (1966: 60; 1970: 218), Murie (1944: 45), Rodman (1981), Zimen (1976).

8 Allen (1979: 126).

9 Creel (1997). Schmidt and Mech (1997) refuted this notion.

10 For example, adult males are responsible for most ungulate kills in southcentral Alaska (Ballard et al. 1987).

11 Fritts and Mech (1981), Jordan et al. (1967), Messier (1985b), Ognev (1931: 146).

12 Fritts and Mech (1981), Harrington et al. (1983 and references), Mech (1988a: 118), Schmidt and Mech (1997).

13 Ballard et al. (1987).

14 Packer and Ruttan (1988).

15 Stephenson and James (1982).

16 Allen (1979: 262), Fritts and Mech (1981), Peterson et al. (1984), Rothman and Mech (1979), van Ballenberghe et al. (1975).

17 Thurber and Peterson (1993).

18 Fritts and Mech (1981 and references).

19 Fritts and Mech (1981).

20 Mech (1970: 183).

21 Thurber and Peterson (1993).

22 Schmidt and Mech (1997).

23 Ballard et al. (1997).

24 Messier (1994).

25 Messier (1985b).

26 Howe et al. (1912).

27 Kreeger et al. (1997), Mech et al. (1984).

28 Young (1944: 121). Coyotes also gorge. The stomach of a 15-kg coyote killed in Québec contained 3.7 kg of deer meat, equivalent to one-quarter its body mass (Larivière and Crête 1993).

29 Hayes et al. (2000).

30 Ballard et al. (1987).

31 Mech (1966: 77–78, 163).

32 Messier (1985b).

33 Mech (1970: 43).

34 Cowan (1947). An adult female mule deer is about 70 kg.

35 Mech (1966: 78).

36 Mech (1966: 78 and references).

37 Burkholder (1959).

38 Mech (1966: 79).

39 Bjärvall and Isakson (1982).

40 Messier and Crête (1985).

41 Ballard et al. (1987, 1997), Fuller and Keith (1980).

42 Oosenbrug and Carbyn (1982). An adult male bison can be 570 kg, an adult female 420 kg (Oosenbrug and Carbyn 1982 and references).

43 Ballard et al. (1987), Messier and Crête (1985).

44 Ballard et al. (1997).

45 Ballard et al. (1987).

46 Mech (1994b).

47 Stanwell-Fletcher (1942).

48 Mech (1966: 51).

49 Burkholder (1959).

50 Burkholder (1959).

51 Pulliainen (1965).

52 Dale et al. (1995).

53 Mech (1992). The remainder of 2% was classified as "other."

54 Peterson and Page (1988).
55 Dale *et al.* (1994, 1995). This factor is sometimes defined as the proportion of prey killed daily (Hayes *et al.* 2000, Messier 1994).
56 Messier (1994).
57 Lundberg and Fryxell (1995), Messier (1994), Pimlott (1967). Some of the terminology can be confusing. Jost *et al.* (2005: 809), for example, defined functional response as "number of prey eaten per predator per unit of time." This is also the kill rate. The *total response* (product of kill rate × numerical response) might show the rate of predation in density-dependent models at low prey densities and the inverse at high prey densities (Fryxell *et al.* 1988; Messier 1994; Messier and Crête 1985).
58 Dale *et al.* (1994). Population limitation, defined in Chapter 5, refers to the depressive effect of a predator on the population of a prey species; in population regulation (also defined in Chapter 5) those depressive effects are associated with density-dependent population processes and can actually stop population growth (Messier and Crête 1985).
59 Bandyopadhyay and Chattopadhyay (2005).
60 Bandyopadhyay and Chattopadhyay (2005).
61 Kuang and Beretta (1998).
62 For mathematical treatment of prey/predator ratio-dependent models, see Bandyopadhyay and Chattopadhyay (2005) and Kuang and Beretta (1998).
63 Jost *et al.* (2005 and references), Lundberg and Fryxell (1995 and references). The modeling of prey–predator relationships comprises a large and controversial literature, and I mention it only briefly. Messier (1994) wrote that ratio-dependent models are poor predictors of wolf predation by not integrating the kill rate. Others disagreed. Bandyopadhyay and Chattopadhyay (2005: 915) wrote: "Actually prey-dependent and ratio-dependent models are extremes or limiting cases; prey-dependent models are based on the daily energy balance of predators; on the other hand ratio-dependent models presuppose that prey are easy to find and that predator dynamics are, in essence, governed by direct density dependence, with prey densities determining the sizes of defended territories." Whether these assumptions can withstand testing in the field remains to be seen.
64 Bandyopadhyay and Chattopadhyay (2005).
65 Kuang and Beretta (1998).
66 Jost *et al.* (2005), Vucetich *et al.* (2002).
67 Jost *et al.* (2005).
68 Ballard *et al.* (1997), Dale *et al.* (1994), Hayes *et al.* (2000), Jost *et al.* (2005), Thurber and Peterson (1993).
69 Hayes *et al.* (2000).
70 Ballard *et al.* (1997), but see Messier (1994) who examined several published reports and found no independent effect of pack size on kill rate. Pack size in African wild dogs correlates directly with foraging time, size of prey that can be captured, and capture probability, and negatively with chase distance (Rasmussen *et al.* 2008). Net energy uptake is most efficient for a pack of five.
71 Hayes and Harestad (2000b).
72 Hayes *et al.* (2000).
73 Dale *et al.* (1995), Peterson *et al.* (1984), Stanwell-Fletcher (1942). Allen (1979: 133) made an important point when stating that "wolves and other predators kill *vulnerable* individuals in a prey population, but this does not always mean weak or diseased."
74 Snow depth is not the only factor. A healthy moose in deep crusted snow is vulnerable (Bjärvall and Isakson 1982). Places where snow is deep with a frozen surface crust favor wolves, which are able to walk on it (Bibikov 1982; Peterson 1977: 48–49). A wolf's foot-loading is much lighter than an ungulate's, or 89–114 g/cm^2 compared with 368–1204 g/cm^2 for a moose (Peterson 1977: 48 and references; Pulliainen 1982 and references). Snow that is light and deep without a surface crust favors the prey (Ognev 1931: 141). Mech (1970: 227–228) discounted this, although without evidence, pointing out that a wolf might be able to walk on a hard surface crust but would surely break through when bounding after prey, speculating that surface crusts able to withstand a bounding wolf could also support a deer.
75 Hayes and Harestad (2000a), Hayes *et al.* (2000), Thurber and Peterson (1993), Schmidt and Mech (1997).

76 What might be true of wolves does not necessarily apply to African wild dogs. Loners and pairs on the Serengeti were never seen to attack wildebeest (*Connochaetes taurinus*), and packs consisting of 4 or more were the most successful hunters (Fanshawe and FitzGibbon 1993).

77 Jordan *et al.* (1967).

78 Hayes *et al.* (2000: 53). For similar findings see Dale *et al.* (1995) and Messier and Crête (1985).

79 Dale *et al.* (1995).

80 Walton *et al.* (2001).

81 Kunkel *et al.* (2004).

82 A pack of African wild dogs might split into smaller groups, each in pursuit of a different animal in a herd and not always reuniting near the hunt's culmination to focus on a single animal (Fanshawe and FitzGibbon 1993).

83 Dale *et al.* (1995).

84 Ballard *et al.* (1997).

85 Dunne (1939), Frijlink (1977).

86 van Ballenberghe (1983a).

87 Kunkel *et al.* (2004).

88 Fritts and Mech (1981), van Ballenberghe *et al.* (1975), Mech (1966: 145–151 and references), Weaver *et al.* (1992).

89 Mech (1966: 146).

90 Allen (1979: 104), Mech (1966: 151).

91 Hayes *et al.* (2000).

92 Ballard *et al.* (1997).

93 Peterson *et al.* (1984).

94 Peterson *et al.* (1984).

95 Burkholder (1959).

96 Hayes *et al.* (2000).

97 Cowan (1947).

98 Gittleman (1985).

99 Murie (1944: 55–57).

100 Ethiopian wolves, for example, prey on small game (rodents almost exclusively), and cooperative hunting is unnecessary (Sillero-Zubiri *et al.* 1996). Reports of wolves on the Arabian peninsula described them foraging alone or in pairs (Mendelssohn 1982 and references), probably because the prey organisms are small and dispersed.

101 Murie (1944: 57).

102 Peterson *et al.* (1984).

103 Thompson (1952).

104 Fuller (1989a).

105 Cowan (1947).

106 Murie (1944: 53, table 2).

107 Murie (1944: 52–59).

108 Murie (1944: 55).

109 Olson (1938b). Also see van Ballenberghe *et al.* (1975).

110 Fritts and Mech (1981).

111 Cowan (1947), Young (1944: 105).

112 Reference in Schmidt and Mech (1997).

113 Pasitschniak-Arts *et al.* (1988).

114 Gray (1970).

115 Mech and Frenzel (1969).

116 Murie (1944: 144).

117 Burkholder (1959).

118 Crisler (1956). African wild dogs, like tundra wolves, hunt in packs in open country. Pack size did not diminish the time required to conclude a hunt, and loners killed gazelles in the same amount of time it took a pack (Fanshawe and FitzGibbon 1993). Even near the end of a chase when a gazelle started zig-zagging, loners gained on the prey as rapidly as packs. Thomson's gazelles are small, however. Success when wildebeest were the prey depended on pack size. Groups of four or more were the most efficient, and here cooperation became evident. In this context African wild dogs are similar to coyotes (Bowen 1981).

119 Murie (1944: 156).
120 Bibikov (1982).
121 MacFarlane (1905: 693) wrote that "a single wolf will go among any number of Eskimo dogs and carry one off from among them without the others attempting an attack."
122 Gipson (1983).
123 Anonymous (2010b), Hopkins (2010), Mech and Goyal (1995), van Ballenberghe *et al.* (1975), Wydeven *et al.* (1999).
124 van Ballenberghe *et al.* (1975).
125 Fritts and Paul (1989).
126 Vos (2000).
127 Boitani and Ciucci (1995).
128 For predation on dogs by wolves in other parts of eastern Europe and Asia see Pulliainen (1967 and references). Large carnivorans in Africa also prey on dogs. According to Butler *et al.* (2004), free-ranging dogs in Zimbabwe are sometimes killed and eaten by leopards (*Panthera pardus*), lions, and spotted hyaenas. Several dogs sent by their owners to chase away adult male chacma baboons (*Papio ursinus*) were killed.
129 Boitani (1982).
130 Barja (2009).
131 Andersone *et al.* (2002).
132 Blanco *et al.* (1992).
133 Gula (2008).
134 Dawes *et al.* (1986 and references).
135 Tener (1954).
136 Bibikov (1982).
137 Ognev (1931: 142, 148–149).
138 Joslin (1982).
139 Pulliainen (1965).
140 Young (1944: 274–275).
141 Gipson and Ballard (1998: 737).
142 Gipson (1983).
143 Gipson and Ballard (1998).
144 Murie (1944: 59).
145 Mech *et al.* (1998: 91).
146 Miller *et al.* (1985).
147 Harper (1955: 11, 66).
148 Bjärvall and Nilsson (1976).
149 Eide and Ballard (1982).
150 Ballard *et al.* (1997).
151 Dale *et al.* (1995).
152 Ognev (1931: 147).
153 Ognev (1931: 149).
154 Barja (2009 and references).
155 Bibikov (1982).
156 Gipson and Ballard (1998).
157 Seton (1962: 2).
158 Gipson and Ballard (1998).
159 Gipson and Ballard (1998).
160 Boitani (1982).
161 Fritts and Mech (1981).
162 Fritts and Mech (1981).
163 Mech (1970: 56, 1988a: 54).
164 Theuerkauf *et al.* (2003).
165 Kolenosky and Johnston (1967).
166 Boitani (1982), Kolenosky (1972), Scott and Shackleton (1982).
167 Harrington and Mech (1982), Mech (1966: 53), Theuerkauf *et al.* (2003).
168 Scott and Shackleton (1982).

169 Mech (1970: 151 and references).
170 Mech (1988a).
171 Murie (1944: 31).
172 Theuerkauf *et al.* (2003).
173 Harrington and Mech (1982).
174 According to Boitani (1982: 163), these wolves "move toward urban centers, valleys and areas inhabited by man in search of food. They move surely and carefully between houses, avoiding lights and noises when crossing roads and entering towns."
175 Allen (1979: 117, 119).
176 Crisler (1958: 289).
177 Mech (1970: 199).
178 Bjärvall and Isakson (1982).
179 Quay (1959).
180 Chapman (1985).
181 Wood *et al.* (2010).
182 Janicki *et al.* (2003: 34).
183 Some doubt that interdigital secretions can be left as scent-marks because the gland is located on the dorsal surface where it would not come into direct contact with the ground (Atoji *et al.* 1988 and references; Parillo and Diverio 2009 and references).
184 Atoji *et al.* (1988), Brundin and Andersson (1979), Brundin *et al.* (1978), Carroll (2001), Chapman (1985), Gassett *et al.* (1996), Janicki *et al.* (2003), Parillo and Diverio (2009), Wood *et al.* (1995). The roe deer has interdigital pockets only on the hind feet (Janicki *et al.* 2003).
185 Pferd (1987: 131 and references).
186 Alexy *et al.* (2003).
187 Quay (1959).
188 Brownlee *et al.* (1969), Miller *et al.* (1998), Sawyer *et al.* (1993).
189 Carroll (2001 and references).
190 Brownlee *et al.* (1969). Lawson *et al.* (2000) found that odors varied not just by species of deer but also by individual. Each individual's odor remains stable over time, its concentration perhaps modified and modulated by bacteria, and sufficiently consistent to be a possible "signature." Cues to age, sex, and reproductive status are possibilities too. Also see Sawyer *et al.* (1993).
191 Müller-Schwarze *et al.* (1984).
192 Miller *et al.* (1998).
193 Ballard *et al.* (1997), Hayes *et al.* (2000), Thurber and Peterson (1993).
194 Oosenbrug and Carbyn (1982).
195 Jordan *et al.* (1967), Stiehl and Trautwein (1991), Theuerkauf *et al.* (2003).
196 Hayes *et al.* (2000), Thurber and Peterson (1993).
197 Hyaenas were present at 85.5% of African wild dog hunts on the Serengeti and posed an important source of food loss except when prey items were small and could be consumed quickly (Fanshawe and FitzGibbon 1993). Low numbers of hyaenas and large packs of dogs gave some advantage to the dogs, which could usually fend off the hyaenas until satiated. However, even large packs lost carcasses to large groups of hyaenas.
198 Mech (1966: 159; 1970: 279, 287), Harrington (1978).
199 Harrington (1978).
200 Bjärvall and Isakson (1982), Frijlink (1977).
201 Frijlink (1977).
202 Allen (1979: 358).
203 Hayes *et al.* (2000).
204 Pulliainen (1965).
205 Arjo and Pletscher (1999), Arjo *et al.* (2002), Atwood (2006), Atwood and Gese (2010), Berger and Gese (2007), Gipson and Ballard (1998).
206 Arjo and Pletscher (1999), Atwood and Gese (2010).
207 Gipson and Ballard (1998).
208 Crabtree and Sheldon (1999).
209 Berger and Gese (2007).
210 Atwood (2006), Atwood and Gese (2010).

211 Switalski (2003).
212 Atwood (2006).
213 Wilmers *et al.* (2003).
214 Ballard (1982).
215 Ballard (1982: 76) described the interactions: "Initially, three wolves were observed equally spaced around the bear. One of the wolves attempted to nip the bear in the rump. The bear made several charges at the wolves which were approaching to within 3–5 m. The wolves easily outmaneuvered the bear and three of the wolves appeared to keep the bear away from the kill as a fourth wolf fed on it."
216 Pulliainen (1965).
217 The pre-hunt description is based mainly on Allen (1979: 269–270), Mech (2000), and Murie (1944: 31–34).
218 A hunt is a momentous event, and the excitement does not subside when it ends. Fentress (1967) remarked that his captive wolf ate with more enthusiasm and ingested larger amounts of food after killing a small animal.
219 Murie (1944: 32).
220 Mech (2000: 260) wrote: "After that, the two would arise and go off again, but sometimes they would repeat this behavior a few times. Eventually the pair would leave the area, and after 5 to 30 minutes the female often returned alone … apparently having sufficiently motivated the male well enough to trust that he was actually continuing on."
221 Mech (1988a: 102). African wild dogs use a similar method of stalking (Fanshawe and FitzGibbon 1993).
222 Mech (1988a: 102, 105).
223 Tener (1954).
224 Tener (1954).
225 According to Mech (1988a: 102) about 20 musk oxen are necessary to form a complete circle with the calves in the middle of the herd. Smaller groups can form only semicircles or lines, which allows wolves more opportunity to attack from the rear and avoid the heavy horns. Tener (1954: 18) saw an unsuccessful stalk of 14 musk oxen on Ellesmere Island by a pair of wolves and wrote: "Occasionally one of the wolves circled the herd and then returned to lie down. Eventually 10 of the musk-oxen lay down, while four remained standing facing the wolves. The calf in the herd kept close to the cows, grazing near the resting adults until the white wolf suddenly dashed around the four standing adults and toward the calf that was now outside the group of animals lying down. The calf immediately ran to the centre of the herd and all the musk-oxen rose to their feet. The one adult bull charged the wolf in an attempt to gore it but the wolf nimbly turned aside and trotted off to its mate."
226 Murie (1944: 29, 169).
227 Murie (1944: 165).
228 Cowan (1947), Mech (1966: 126–127). Cowan (1947) gave an account of a cow elk that survived being cornered by seven wolves.
229 Mech (1966: 125).
230 Mech *et al.* (1998: 112–113).
231 Crisler (1956; 1958: 106), Harper (1955: 65), Mech (1966: 121).
232 Mech (1966: 144).
233 Peterson *et al.* (1984).
234 Bibikov (1982).
235 Bjärvall and Isakson (1982).
236 Murie (1944: 100–143, 163–175).
237 Mech (1988a: 88).
238 Summarized in Mech (1988a: 99–100).
239 Mech (1966: 119, 121). Contrary to myth, wolves do not "hamstring" ungulates as a means of bringing them down (Allen 1979: 95; Cowan 1947; Mech 1966: 136; 1970: 204–205, 245). Crisler (1958: bottom photo facing p. 79) depicted a husky grasping a slow-running caribou by the lower right hind leg and labeled it hamstringing in the figure legend. She described this hunt briefly on p. 278, but later recanted that actual hamstringing had occurred (Allen 1979: 95–96, 448). Corbett (1995: 114) claimed that dingoes hamstring fleeing kangaroos but without citing a source. No

mention of hamstringing has appeared in necropsy reports of kangaroos killed by dingoes (e.g. Shepherd 1981).

240 Allen (1979: 122–123), Mech (1966: 126).

241 Mech (1988a: 113). African wild dogs employ the same method when hunting wildebeest. One dog usually grabs the wildebeest by the nose to immobilize it while the rest of the pack disembowels it (Fanshawe and FitzGibbon 1993). To bring down an elk, wolves seize the throat or flank near the abdomen (Cowan 1947).

242 Pferd (1987: 130–132 and references).

243 Cowan (1947: 159).

244 Crisler (1958: 98–109).

245 Allen (1979: 127). Some ungulates seem aware of this. Dall's sheep being watched by wolves walked slowly until near the safety of cliffs before breaking into a run (Murie 1944: 101).

246 Lyons et al. (1982) put it like this: "It is not necessary that the participants 'know' they are cooperating; each may be responding without regard for the partner, to stimuli in a manner that has produced reinforcement previously. The net result, however, is still cooperative in that both animals' responses were necessary, and both participants received 'pay-offs' for their actions."

247 Murie (1944: 165–166), Crisler (1956).

248 Wright (1960).

249 Crisler (1958: 256), Murie (1944: 166–167).

250 Crisler (1956), Garrott et al. (2007), Mech (1966: 121, 124 and references), Murie (1944: 165–167), Wright (1960).

251 Crisler (1956).

252 Murie (1944: 166–167).

253 Crisler (1956), Mech (1966: 121–122), Mech et al. (1998: 108), Murie (1944: 54, 165–166), Fuller and Keith (1980), Carbyn (1983), Wright et al. (2006 and references).

254 Sokolov et al. (1990: 125).

255 Murie (1944: 111–126).

256 Olson (1938b: 335).

257 Wright et al. (2006). Similar results were obtained at Canada's Riding Mountain National Park (Carbyn 1983).

258 Rausch (1967).

259 Murie (1944:186).

260 Stanwell-Fletcher (1942).

261 Peterson and Page (1988).

262 Mech and Nelson (1989).

263 Frijlink (1977).

264 Savile and Oliver (1964).

265 MacFarlane (1905: 693).

266 Ballard (1982).

267 Ballard et al. (1987).

268 Mech (1988a: 112–113).

269 Mech (1988a: 113).

270 Fritts and Mech (1981).

271 Mech (1966: 79).

272 Mech (1988a: 115).

273 Burkholder (1959: 10) wrote: "Rather, a spirit of co-operation and play seemed to be the theme. There was much tugging at the meat. Once a tug-of-war ensued between a grey and a black wolf, but here again the pattern was playful rather than antagonistic."

274 Mech (1988a: 115), Mech et al. (1999).

275 Mech (1988a: 117).

276 Johnson (1921).

277 Pulliainen (1965).

278 Harper (1955: 64–65).

279 Cowan (1947).

280 Fritts and Mech (1981), van Ballenberghe et al. (1975).

281 van Ballenberghe *et al.* (1975).

282 van Ballenberghe *et al.* (1975).

283 Quoted reference in Ognev (1931: 149).

284 Rausch (1967).

285 Fritts and Mech (1981), van Ballenberghe *et al.* (1975).

286 van Ballenberghe and Erickson (1973).

287 van Ballenberghe (1983a).

288 Jordan *et al.* (1967).

289 Frijlink (1977).

290 Ognev (1931: 149) wrote: "A wounded wolf which happens to fall among a wolf pack is torn to pieces mercilessly by its fellows. If it succeeds in escaping from the ruthless attackers they locate it by its trail of blood, and consequently certain death awaits the unfortunate individual."

291 Boitani (1992), Theuerkauf *et al.* (2003 and references).

292 Fuller and Keith (1981), Henshaw and Stephenson (1974), Mech and Hertel (1983), Mech *et al.* (1999), Murie (1944: 59), van Ballenberghe *et al.* (1975).

293 Boitani (1982).

294 Barja (2009).

295 Mendelssohn (1982).

296 Barja (2009), Bibikov (1982), Boitani (1982), Pulliainen (1965).

297 Mech (1988a: 115), Murie (1944: 59–60).

298 Mech (1988a: 115) wrote, "at times individuals would rip out great chunks, such as lungs, and steal off to cache them. Generally they would head out for several hundred feet, where the other wolves would not see them." These comments are speculative.

299 The social Siberian jay (*Perisoreus infaustus*) caches food selfishly and without evidence of kinship sharing (Ekman *et al.* 1996).

300 McNamara *et al.* (1990).

301 Mech (1970: 190; 1988a: 115), Murie (1944: 60).

302 Mech *et al.* (1998: 118).

303 Mech (1988a: 115).

304 Mech *et al.* (1998: 148).

305 Harriman and Berger (1986).

306 Burkholder (1959).

307 Forbes (1989).

308 Fritts and Mech (1981 and references), van Ballenberghe *et al.* (1975).

309 Hayes and Harestad (2000b), Hayes *et al.* (2000).

310 Dale *et al.* (1995).

311 Murie (1944: 63, table 2).

312 Garrott *et al.* (2007).

313 Ease of capture was once considered the factor affecting choice of prey in multiple-prey habitats as reviewed by Mech (1970: 246–263).

314 Fritts and Mech (1981 and references), Garrott *et al.* (2007), van Ballenberghe *et al.* (1975).

315 Kunkel *et al.* (2004).

316 Garrott *et al.* (2007).

317 Dale *et al.* (1995).

318 Bjärvall and Isakson (1982).

319 Geffen *et al.* (2004), Pilot *et al.* (2006).

320 Carmichael *et al.* (2001), Musiani *et al.* (2007).

321 Muñoz-Fuentes *et al.* (2009).

322 Vilà *et al.* (1999b).

323 Gomerčič *et al.* (2010 and references).

324 Pilot *et al.* (2006). The use of mitochondrial and nuclear DNA analyses can produce different results. As Pilot *et al.* (2006: 4545) noted, male-biased dispersal can cause "male-biased gene flow [implying] low introgression of mtDNA haplotypes from neighbouring populations, and therefore greater structuring in mtDNA as compared with nuclear markers." In addition, mtDNA is more sensitive to genetic drift than nuclear DNA. Both males and females are known to disperse long distances (Chapter 5), but male-biased dispersal in European wolves has been noted (Flagstad *et al.* 2003, Wabakken *et al.* 2001).

325 Pilot *et al.* (2006).
326 Geffen *et al.* (2004).
327 Dawes *et al.* (1986: 129).
328 Dawes *et al.* (1986 and references).
329 Dawes *et al.* (1986 and references).
330 Riewe (1975).
331 Bibikov (1982).
332 Milakovic and Parker (2011).
333 Milakovic and Parker (2011).
334 Darimont *et al.* (2008).
335 Milakovic and Parker (2011 and references).
336 Watts *et al.* (2010).
337 Banfield (1954 and reference).
338 Ballard *et al.* (1997), Stephenson and James (1982).
339 Ballard *et al.* (1997).
340 Kuyt (1962), Musiani *et al.* (2007), Parker (1973), Walton *et al.* (2001).
341 Musiani *et al.* (2007).
342 Heard and Williams (1992 and references).
343 Critchell-Bullock (1930: 209) wrote: "By November 11th [1924] all the wolves had apparently gone north ... On the 20th, however, they were numerous again, moving in the middle of the caribou which were and had been numerous. With the disappearance of the caribou on the 22nd the wolves also departed ... From March 16th to 20th [of 1925] wolves were numerous again. Once again apparently heading the caribou movement, at least certainly not in rear of it. By the 31st, all the fur was on the move and between that date and April 3rd wolves and foxes passed in hundreds travelling northwards. The wolves, more often than not, were in packs of from three to five. Then until the 8th wolves were not seen, but with the great eastward movement of the caribou at that time they again commenced to pass."
344 Musiani *et al.* (2007).
345 Carmichael *et al.* (2001), Geffen *et al.* (2004), Musiani *et al.* (2007), Pilot *et al.* (2006).
346 Pulliainen (1965).
347 Forbes and Theberge (1995).
348 Packer and Ruttan (1988) built their models using data from 60 species, but wolves were not included.
349 Spong and Creel (2004).
350 Mech (1966: 60).
351 A male wolf in a pack observed by Murie seemed debilitated, although well fed. Murie (1944: 28) named it Grandpa and wrote, "he moved as though he were old and a little stiff. Sometimes he had sore feet which made him limp." Whether this animal lived as a scrounger is unknown.
352 Packer and Ruttan (1988: 167) wrote, "if the nth individual cheats [scrounges] rather than cooperates, then on the average he receives $(n-1)/n$ as much food as if he had cooperated. [If $n = 2$] the cheater [scrounger] receives only half as much as a cooperator, but as n becomes large, $(n-1)/n$ approaches one. Thus, as group size increases, the cheater [scrounger] could receive almost as much from feeding from companions' kills as he would from his own without incurring any costs of hunting."
353 Marlowe (2004 and references).
354 Higashi and Yamamura (1993) pointed out these discrepancies and developed an interesting model for predicting group size and assessing its determinants.
355 Thurber and Peterson (1993).
356 Hayes *et al.* (2000), Thurber and Peterson (1993).
357 Packer and Ruttan (1988).
358 Packer *et al.* (1990).
359 Packard *et al.* (1983).
360 Packard *et al.* (1983), Schmidt and Mech (1997).
361 Bergerud and Elliot (1998), Hayes and Harestad (2000a).
362 Harrington *et al.* (1983), Hayes and Harestad (2000a).
363 Hayes and Harestad (2000a).

364 Thurber and Peterson (1993).
365 Messier (1985a).
366 Fritts and Mech (1981).
367 Thurber and Peterson (1993).
368 Allen (1979: 162).
369 Scott and Causey (1973).
370 Corbett (1989).
371 Nesbitt (1975).
372 Gipson and Sealander (1976: 251, table 1).
373 Fox *et al.* (1975).
374 Fox *et al.* (1975).
375 Fox *et al.* (1975).
376 Boitani (1992), Coppinger and Coppinger (2001), Oppenheimer and Oppenheimer (1975).
377 Choudhuri *et al.* (1984).
378 Allen (2010), Daniels (1987), Marsack and Campbell (1990), Thomson (1992c), Whitehouse (1977).
379 Causey and Cude (1980), Scott and Causey (1973: 261, table 7).
380 Gipson (1983).
381 Nesbitt (1975).
382 Causey and Cude (1980), Nesbitt (1975), Scott and Causey (1973).
383 Comment by Phillip [*sic*] Gipson in Denny (1974: 289).
384 Murie (1944: 186–187).
385 Butler *et al.* (2004).
386 Boggess *et al.* (1978), Gipson (1983).
387 Nesbitt (1975).
388 Boitani (1992).
389 Macdonald and Carr (1995).
390 Ryabov (1979).
391 Street (1962: 402) wrote: "As early as 1526, [Jean and Raoul] Parmentier observed that packs of wild dogs limited the cattle numbers by preying on the calves. A report to Philip II in 1561 contained a statement to the same effect. Raising of large dogs to hunt wild cattle, dogs that often escaped to breed with their wild cousins, exacerbated the problem of predation." The Parmentier brothers were French corsairs who traveled along the coast of Hispaniola in 1526 (Street 1962 and references).
392 Bibikov (1982 and references).
393 Bibikov (1982 and references).
394 Bibikov (1982).
395 Mendelssohn (1982).
396 Mendelssohn (1982).
397 Kamler *et al.* (2003).
398 Campos *et al.* (2007).
399 Gipson (1983).
400 Scott and Causey (1973).
401 Macdonald and Carr (1995).
402 Beaver *et al.* (1992).
403 Dugatkin *et al.* (2003).
404 Marlowe (2004).
405 Those observed in northwestern Australia were traveling 69% of the time (Thomson 1992b).
406 Robley *et al.* (2010).
407 Harden (1985).
408 Harden (1985).
409 Corbett and Newsome (1975).
410 Thomson (1992c).
411 Marsack and Campbell (1990).
412 Vernes *et al.* (2001).
413 Short *et al.* (2002). Adults in some parts of Australia are larger. Males average 18.9 kg, females 15.2 kg in northwestern Australia (Thomson 1992a); males are 17.4 kg, females 15.2 kg at

Kapalga, Northern Territory (see Corbett 1985 for this last region, other regions in Australia, and parts of southeast Asia).

414 Green and Catling (1977), Harden (1985), Johnson *et al.* (2007), Thomson (1992a).

415 Moss and Croft (1999).

416 Bino (1996), Corbett (1995: 102–124), Newsome *et al.* (1983b).

417 Marsack and Campbell (1990).

418 Green and Catling (1977).

419 Corbett and Newsome (1987).

420 Newsome *et al.* (1983b).

421 This is conservative. The carcass of an adult elk contains 68% edible matter (Wilmers *et al.* 2003).

422 Vernes *et al.* (2001).

423 See, for example, Corbett (1985: 345, table 1), Mitchell and Banks (2005: 585–586, tables 1 and 2), Newsome *et al.* (1983a: 479, table 1; 1983b: 351, table 1), Pavey *et al.* (2008: 679, table 2), Robertshaw and Harden (1985: 41, table 1), Vernes *et al.* (2001: 342, table 1), Whitehouse (1977: 146, table 1).

424 Corbett and Newsome (1987).

425 Corbett and Newsome (1987).

426 Corbett and Newsome (1987) reported a functional response, but did not incorporate an actual kill rate (prey killed per unit of time).

427 Thomson (1992c).

428 Pavey *et al.* (2008).

429 Gittleman (1985).

430 Corbett and Newsome (1987).

431 Newsome *et al.* (1983b).

432 Robertshaw and Harden (1986).

433 Newsome *et al.* (1983a).

434 *Australian dingoes*: Corbett (1989: 345, table 1) listed prey identified in dingo scats. For lists of dietary items found in stomachs and scats see Marsack and Campbell (1990: 354: table 5). Whitehouse (1977: 146, table 1) gave an extensive list of dingo stomach contents that included remnants of at least 14 species of mammals. Robertshaw and Harden (1986: 162, appendix 1) listed animal remains identified in dingo scats from northeastern New South Wales including 26 species of mammals. *New Guinea dingoes* (provisional species list without quantification): Bino (1996: 45, table 1).

435 Whitehouse (1977).

436 Marsack and Campbell (1990).

437 Van Vuren and Thomson (1982).

438 Robertshaw and Harden (1986). The data can sometimes be misleading in terms of prey size. In southeastern Australia, for example, the percentage of "large mammals" in the diet increased during the time young kangaroos and wallabies were leaving the pouch and vulnerable (Newsome *et al.* 1983b and references).

439 Robertshaw and Harden (1986).

440 Robertshaw and Harden (1985) recorded 7 prey items comprising 74.4% of the total number; Whitehouse (1977) recorded 5 prey items making up 86.2%.

441 Marsack and Campbell (1990).

442 Allen (2010).

443 Robertshaw and Harden (1986: 154).

444 Corbett and Newsome (1987). Recent references still report dingoes as incapable of killing large prey animals except in groups (e.g. Glen *et al.* 2007).

445 Bourke *et al.* (2008).

446 Shepherd (1981: 257) wrote: "Extensive bite wounds were always present, either over neck and thorax ... or throat ... or both. These were deep penetrating wounds accompanied by subcutaneous and intramuscular haemorrhage and oedema. They often penetrated major organs (trachea, oesophagus, lungs and major blood vessels) or caused fractures to ribs ... scapula ... or vertebrae ... Thoracic punctures often resulted in pronounced bloodstained subcutaneous emphysema in the region of the thorax and neck ... congestion or haemorrhage in the lungs, and free blood in the thorax." Twenty-seven kangaroo kills examined by Marsack and Campbell

(1990: 353) were in similar condition: "The attacks resulted in some puncture wounds but most damage was subcutaneous. Bites resulted in severe bruising and tearing of underlying muscle."

447 Thomson (1992c).

448 Corbett (1995: 113–114) described dingoes hunting kangaroos in the Fortescue River region but did not cite a source. His claim that groups are far more successful than loners is not supported by any data I found.

449 Newsome *et al.* (1983b).

450 Marsack and Campbell (1990).

451 According to Thomson (1992c) these results supported the hypothesis that group foraging increases efficiency, which would seem to be refuted by his own data. They certainly do not justify a general statement that dingoes in groups hunt kangaroos more successfully than loners (Purcell 2010).

452 Marsack and Campbell (1990).

453 Marsack and Campbell (1990: 356).

454 Corbett and Newsome (1975).

455 From an unpublished manuscript by A.Y. Hassell in the Mitchell Library, Sydney, quoted by Meggitt (1965: 12). The kangaroo "hopped first one way, then another, while the two dogs which were of a beautiful golden sable colour, seemed to be acting on a settled plan. They kept heading the kangaroo off as it ran. At last it could hop no longer, so stood with its back to a big tree and tried to fight off its enemies with its feet, but they were too wary to go too close. One would lie down some distance away, while the other worried and snapped at the kangaroo. When it was tired, the one lying down took its place ... At last the dog caught the kangaroo off its guard, and made a spring at its neck; in a second the other dog rushed up and attacked on the other side and the poor beast was pulled struggling to the ground, and in a few moments was dead. I think the combat must have lasted quite half an hour."

456 Marsack and Campbell (1990).

457 Thomson (1992d).

458 Corbett and Newsome (1975). A comparison by location was not provided.

459 Levy (2009).

460 Meggitt (1965: 20) wrote: "Indeed, if, as often happened, a cunning dingo became known as a great killer of stock, local graziers contributed a relatively large sum of prize money to go to the man who destroyed the beast. This practice, which persists today, attracted many skilled trappers and riflemen to the area."

461 Short *et al.* (2002), Thomson (1992c and references).

462 Shepherd (1981). Marsack and Campbell (1990) reported surplus killing of kangaroos in the Nullarbor.

463 Newsome *et al.* (1983b).

464 Short *et al.* (2002 and references).

465 Green and Catling (1977).

466 Short *et al.* (2002 and references).

467 Levy (2009).

468 Marsack and Campbell (1990).

469 Levy (2009).

470 Johnson *et al.* (2007).

471 Letnic *et al.* (2009).

472 Letnic *et al.* (2009).

473 Johnson *et al.* (2007), Letnic *et al.* (2009).

474 Letnic and Koch (2010).

Chapter 7: Courtship and conception

1 Asa (1996), Asa and Valdespino (1998), Verstegen-Onclin and Verstegen (2008).

2 Concannon *et al.* (1977b).

3 Rausch (1967).

4 For additional information on breeding season by location see Mech (1970: 117, table 12).

5 Rabb *et al.* (1967), Seal *et al.* (1979).

6 Cowan (1947).

7 Murie (1944).

8 Ballard *et al.* (1991).

9 Ballard *et al.* (1987), Mech (1993b).

10 Mech (1966: 69), Rausch (1967).

11 Lentfer and Sanders (1973).

12 Fritts and Mech (1981).

13 Mech and Goyal (1995), Mills *et al.* (2008).

14 Seal *et al.* (1979).

15 Riley and McBride (1975).

16 Silver and Silver (1969: 8).

17 Mendelssohn (1982).

18 Theuerkauf *et al.* (2003).

19 Pulliainen (1965).

20 Ognev (1931: 143).

21 Ognev (1931: 145).

22 Young (1944: 95).

23 Asa *et al.* (1990: 502) defined puberty in captive Great Lakes wolves as "first ovulation, inferred from sustained serum progesterone concentrations of greater than 2 ng/ml through at least three samples following observed estrus, sanguinous discharge, or increased estradiol." Also see Asa *et al.* (1986).

24 Asa (1996), Asa and Valdespino (1998), Asa *et al.* (1990), Lentfer and Sanders (1973), Mech *et al.* (1998: 47), Ognev (1931: 143), Pulliainen (1965), Rausch (1967), Zimen (1976).

25 Cowan (1947), Murie (1944: 17), Rabb *et al.* (1967).

26 Mech *et al.* (1998: 47).

27 Seal *et al.* (1979).

28 Gese and Mech (1991).

29 Some (e.g. Asa 1996; Asa and Valdespino 1998) prefer *monestrum* and *polyestrum* to monestrus and polyestrus, which makes sense only if the older terms proestrum, estrum, and diestrum (e.g. Evans and Cole 1931) are then substituted for proestrus, estrus, and diestrus.

30 Asa (1996), Asa and Valdespino (1998), de Gier *et al.* (2006), Concannon (1993), Concannon *et al.* (1993), Rehm *et al.* (2007), Verstegen *et al.* (1997), Wildt *et al.* (1979). Jöchle and Andersen (1977: 114) used monestrous incorrectly as "exhibiting estrus only once annually in a distinct season." A distinct season is not required of monestrus, as demonstrated by the domestic dog. What distinguishes monestrous species from those that are *polyestrous* is the anestrous stage and the reproductive cycle not being interrupted by pregnancy. The cyclic stages in *polyestrus* are proestrus, estrus, and diestrus, and the cycle is interrupted by pregnancy. In the view of Jöchle and Andersen (1977) the domestic dog fits neither category, although dogs are clearly monestrous.

31 Asa *et al.* (1986).

32 Catling *et al.* (1992), Taha *et al.* (1981).

33 Taha *et al.* (1981).

34 Asa *et al.* (1987), de Gier *et al.* (2006), Evans and Cole (1931), Holst and Phemister (1974), Jöchle and Andersen (1977), Phemister *et al.* (1973), Seal *et al.* (1979), Verstegen *et al.* (1997), Wildt *et al.* (1978, 1982).

35 Rehm *et al.* (2007 and references).

36 de Gier *et al.* (2006), Wildt *et al.* (1978).

37 Concannon *et al.* (1989), Evans and Cole (1931), Goodwin *et al.* (1979), Holst and Phemister (1974), Jöchle and Andersen (1977), Onclin *et al.* (2002), Wildt *et al.* (1978).

38 Seal *et al.* (1979). Asa and Valdespino (1998) and Asa *et al.* (1986) stated that proestrus in the wolf lasts about 6 weeks, but provided no data.

39 Asa *et al.* (1986), Seal *et al.* (1979), Young (1944: 84, 95).

40 Kennelly and Johns (1976).

41 Silver and Silver (1969: 26).

42 Proestrous bleeding in the dog is a result of *diapedesis*; menstrual bleeding by human females is caused by hemorrhage. Menstruation takes place at the end of a reproductive cycle (i.e. at

termination of the luteal phase) when estrogen and progesterone are at their lowest levels. Proestrous bleeding in canids is the reverse, a response to increasing concentrations of estrogen. Studies in the mid-1840s concluded correctly that the bloody discharge of proestrous dogs correlated directly with ovulation. Unfortunately, the same knowledge was then extended to humans. According to Jöchle and Andersen (1977) "this erroneous interpretation from observations in the dog had serious consequences in human medicine and early attempts at birth control, as the concept of ovulation during the menses remained in the literature for almost three quarters of a century." Such a serious oversight could explain why people who practice the "rhythm method" of birth control are commonly referred to as "parents" even today.

43 Zimen (1981: 132).
44 Zimen (1975).
45 Beach (1974).
46 Ghosh *et al.* (1984).
47 Beach and Gilmore (1949).
48 Whitten *et al.* (1980).
49 Raymer *et al.* (1984).
50 Woolhouse and Morgan (1995).
51 Raymer *et al.* (1984) found isopentyl methyl sulfide and aliphatic ketones associated with intact males and acetophenome to be characteristic of intact females and castrated males. Isopentyl methyl sulfide in intact males fluctuates seasonally, spiking in March after the breeding season. Some compounds – methyl propyl sulfide, 4-methyl-3-heptanone, 3,5-dimethyl-2-decanone, 3,5,7-trimethyl-2-decanone – were brought to normal concentrations in castrated males treated with testosterone, and it was speculated that these and similar compounds might be important in chemical communication.
52 Raymer *et al.* (1986).
53 Beach and Merari (1968).
54 Beach and Gilmore (1949).
55 Doty and Dunbar (1974).
56 Beach and Gilmore (1949).
57 Schultz *et al.* (1985 and references).
58 Lydell and Doty (1972).
59 Lydell and Doty (1972: 205).
60 Batchelor *et al.* (1972).
61 Raymer *et al.* (1986).
62 Schultz *et al.* (1985).
63 Goodwin *et al.* (1979).
64 Kruse and Howard (1983).
65 Schultz *et al.* (1988).
66 Schultz *et al.* (1985).
67 Isopentenyl methyl sulfide and other compounds in red fox urine are manufactured as egg-based repellants and deterrents against brush-tailed opossums in Australia (Woolhouse and Morgan 1995).
68 Seal *et al.* (1979).
69 Raymer *et al.* (1986).
70 Silver and Silver (1969: 31).
71 Gier (1957).
72 Kooistra *et al.* (1999 and references).
73 Onclin *et al.* (2002).
74 Kooistra *et al.* (1999).
75 Holst and Phemister (1975), Phemister *et al.* (1973), Wildt *et al.* (1979).
76 Beach and Merari (1968), Concannon *et al.* (1977a).
77 Kooistra *et al.* (1999).
78 The fact that ovulation occurs near the start of estrus instead of near the end is unusual. (Holst and Phemister 1971).
79 Concannon *et al.* (1975).
80 Rehm *et al.* (2007).
81 Concannon *et al.* (1977a).
82 Concannon *et al.* (1977a).

83 Asa *et al.* (1990), Wildt *et al.* (1979).

84 Concannon *et al.* (1977a, 1979a), de Gier *et al.* (2006), Onclin *et al.* (2002), Wildt *et al.* (1979).

85 Rehm *et al.* (2007).

86 Olson *et al.* (1984a, 1984b, 1989).

87 Concannon and Castracane (1985).

88 Concannon and Castracane (1985), Olson *et al.* (1989).

89 Concannon and Castracane (1985).

90 Rehm *et al.* (2007). Wildt *et al.* (1979) suggested that androstenedione arose from the follicles, and Olson *et al.* (1984a) saw increases in testosterone during the follicular phase.

91 Wildt *et al.* (1978).

92 Concannon *et al.* (1989), Evans and Cole (1931), Holst and Phemister (1971, 1974), Jöchle and Andersen (1977), Kooistra *et al.* (1999), Onclin *et al.* (2002).

93 Kooistra and Okkens (2002).

94 Asa and Valdespino (1998), Asa *et al.* (1986), Seal *et al.* (1979). I found no information for length of estrus in eastern coyotes.

95 Kennelly and Johns (1976).

96 Holst and Phemister (1971), Jöchle and Andersen (1977), Olson *et al.* (1984a), Rehm *et al.* (2007).

97 Concannon *et al.* (1975, 1979a, 1979b), Wildt *et al.* (1979).

98 Concannon *et al.* (1989), Rehm *et al.* (2007).

99 Concannon *et al.* (1989).

100 Concannon *et al.* (1993) considered ovulation in the domestic dog to commence 1–2 days after progesterone rises above 1 ng/mL and 62–64 days before parturition.

101 Wildt *et al.* (1978).

102 Asa *et al.* (1987) set the limit as 2 ng/mL for wolves, Verstegen *et al.* (1997) at 1 ng/mL for dogs.

103 Phemister *et al.* (1973).

104 Rehm *et al.* (2007).

105 van Haaften *et al.* (1994).

106 Concannon *et al.* (1993).

107 de Gier *et al.* (2006), Wildt *et al.* (1978).

108 de Gier *et al.* (2006) summarized the disparate findings on this point. According to Wildt *et al.* (1979), the surge in estradiol-17β prior to ovulation triggers the pre-ovulatory LH surge, although Concannon (1993) and Concannon *et al.* (1979a) found a decrease in estradiol-17β. Onclin *et al.* (2002) saw estradiol-17β peak 1–2 days before the LH surge.

109 Concannon *et al.* (1979a). However, de Gier *et al.* (2006: 1355) explained the sequential surges of estradiol-17β and LH differently, suggesting that "the increase in plasma estradiol-17βacts via positive feedback on GnRH [see Chapter 8], and hence LH secretion, to cause the pre-ovulatory LH surge." Concannon's group showed that estradiol-17β administered to ovariectomized female dogs induced a peak in LH only after treatment was stopped, indicating that estradiol-17β has a negative feedback on LH release. Thus dogs without ovaries might not react like intact dogs in anestrus or proestrus when estradiol-17β is used to induce an LH surge.

110 de Gier *et al.* (2006).

111 Concannon *et al.* (1975), de Gier *et al.* (2006).

112 Onclin *et al.* (2002).

113 Evans and Cole (1931), Holst and Phemister (1971).

114 Onclin *et al.* (2002).

115 Concannon (1980), Concannon *et al.* (1977a).

116 Concannon *et al.* (1989).

117 Concannon (1980), de Gier *et al.* (2006), Evans and Cole (1931), Jöchle and Andersen (1977). Estrus in rodents (and perhaps most opossums) is induced; that is, a male in breeding condition must be present to release putative pheromones that stimulate the female's VNO receptors (Chapter 4). Estrus in carnivorans and primates (including humans) is spontaneous, not induced, and occurs more or less regularly whether a male is present or not. Spontaneous ovulators might not need reproductive pheromones, which could account for their generally atrophied VNOs. However, this is speculation. Asa *et al.* (2007) reported that estrus, ovulation (or both) might be induced in the island fox (*Urocyon littoralis*). DeMatteo *et al.* (2006) gave evidence that the presence of males shortened the intervals between estrus in captive bush dogs (*Speothos venaticus*).

118 Holst and Phemister (1971), Phemister *et al.* (1973).
119 Concannon *et al.* (1989). Also see Holst and Phemister (1971).
120 Phemister *et al.* (1973).
121 Concannon *et al.* (1989).
122 Concannon *et al.* (1989: 12) based this "on the assumption that oocyte maturation occurs 2 days after ovulation (Day 4) and that unfertilized oocytes rapidly degenerate after Day 7 or 8."
123 Phemister *et al.* (1973). Inconsistent use of terms has been part of the problem of defining when fertilization occurs. Phemister *et al.* (1973: 80) wrote: "By substituting 'fertilization' for 'ovulation' in most reports which claim late ovulation . . . the results . . . would be compatible with ovulation in early estrus."
124 Jöchle and Andersen (1977).
125 Doak *et al.* (1967), Holst and Phemister (1974).
126 Evans (1933).
127 Concannon *et al.* (1989), Kooistra *et al.* (1999). Both proestrus and estrus can also be recognized by taking vaginal smears and monitoring the change in cell type. Using this method the onset of *cytological proestrus* has been defined as the day on which >90% of cells are of the *superficial* (cornified) *cell type* and *cytological estrus* as the fourth day after this (Fernandes *et al.* 1987). Also see Evans and Cole (1931), Holst and Phemister (1971), Phemister *et al.* (1973). Gestation can be estimated from the first day of mating, first day of refusal of the female to be mounted, and first day when a vaginal smear contains predominantly noncornified epithelial cells (Holst and Phemister 1971).
128 Holst and Phemister (1974, 1975).
129 Onclin *et al.* (2002).
130 Phemister *et al.* (1973).
131 Holst and Phemister (1974).
132 Beach and LeBoeuf [*sic*] (1967).
133 Concannon *et al.* (1975, 1989), Holst and Phemister (1971), Wildt *et al.* (1978).
134 Holst and Phemister (1971).
135 de Gier *et al.* (2006).
136 Phemister *et al.* (1973).
137 Medjo and Mech (1976), Seal *et al.* (1979).
138 Asa *et al.* (1987).
139 Evans and Cole (1931), Scott (1950, 1967).
140 Concannon *et al.* (1993).
141 Evans and Cole (1931).
142 Christie and Bell (1971).
143 Seal *et al.* (1979).
144 Engle (1946).
145 Christie and Bell (1971).
146 Daniels (1983b: 370) wrote, "equating promiscuous breeding with indiscriminate breeding is a premature simplification of a complex system."
147 Beach and LeBoeuf [*sic*] (1967).
148 Beach and LeBoeuf [*sic*] (1967: 547).
149 Pal (2003).
150 Female wolves unwilling to mate sit down with their tails between their legs (Mech 1970: 113).
151 Le Boeuf (1967).
152 Also see Evans and Cole (1931).
153 Beach (1970).
154 Beach (1970: 146).
155 Le Boeuf (1967).
156 The following comments are based on Le Boeuf (1967: 285–286).
157 Pal (2003). Pal (2010), without justification, changed these categories to: pups (birth to 3 months), adolescents (3–12 months), adults (1–7 years), and old adults (>7 years). I use his earlier system. Scott and Fuller (1965: 108) considered the "juvenile" period to begin at 12 weeks and extend past 6 months.
158 Engle (1946).

159 Oppenheimer and Oppenheimer (1975).
160 Boitani (1992), Macdonald and Carr (1995).
161 Pal (2005).
162 Pal (2003), Pal *et al.* (1998).
163 Daniels and Bekoff (1989b).
164 Asa *et al.* (1990 and reference).
165 Boitani (1992) made this claim, but without data.
166 Daniels (1983b: 367) described these associations as "mainly localized, short-lived phenomena, that did not permanently alter the social organization in an area." He used to assess male hierarchies the proportion of attacks initiated and received within an estrous group.
167 Daniels (1983b: 371).
168 Daniels (1983b), Pal (2003, 2005).
169 Daniels (1983b).
170 Daniels (1983b).
171 Ghosh *et al.* (1984).
172 Pal (2003).
173 Pal (2003). Also see Ghosh *et al.* (1984).
174 Daniels (1983b).
175 Qvarnström and Forsgren (1998), Rodríquez-Muñoz *et al.* (2010).
176 Daniels (1983b).
177 Information is mainly from Corbett (1995: 35–39).
178 Jones and Stevens (1988).
179 Thomson (1992b: 519) wrote: "Levels and scent-marking (raised-leg urination and ground-scratching), howling and general activity increased over the 2–3 months prior to the mating period, suggesting that dingoes may have a long pro-oestrus (1–2 months)." No supporting data were provided.
180 Kleiman (1968).
181 Personal communication in Thomson (1992b: 528).
182 Kleiman (1968).
183 Giraldeau and Caraco (1993: 435–436).
184 Allen (1979: 265).
185 Mech and Knick (1978).
186 Zimen (1981: 133).
187 Dunbar and Buehler (1980).
188 Peters and Mech (1975), Rothman and Mech (1979).
189 Asa and Valdespino (1998), Asa *et al.* (1986, 1990), Mech and Knick (1978), Rothman and Mech (1979).
190 Hradecký (1985).
191 Asa *et al.* (1986).
192 Packard *et al.* (1985), Rabb *et al.* (1967), Zimen (1975, 1976).
193 Silver and Silver (1969: 17).
194 See, for example, Lentfer and Sanders (1973).
195 Packard (2003).
196 Zimen (1981: 132).
197 Lack of interest in courtship by the dominant male and allowing a subordinate male to mate with the dominant female has been reported elsewhere in captive wolves (Kleiman 1968; Woolpy 1968).
198 Zimen (1981: 133).
199 Zimen (1981: 134).
200 Asa *et al.* (1986), Packard *et al.* (1985), Seal *et al.* (1979).
201 Sands and Creel (2004).
202 Packard *et al.* (1983: 79).
203 Packard *et al.* (1983 and references).
204 Sands and Creel (2004).
205 Murie (1944: 44).
206 Ognev (1931: 144).
207 Murie (1944).

208 Woolpy (1968). Rabb *et al.* (1967) mentioned these behaviors briefly.

209 Critchell-Bullock (1930). A case of a male coyote × female red fox captive mating has been documented. The pair was observed copulating, and two male pups were later born that soon died (van Gelder (1977).

210 Packard (2003: 41, bottom of table 2.2) gave a brief sociogram of wolf courtship behaviors.

211 Packard *et al.* (1985).

212 Testosterone response refers to the relative spike in blood concentration of testosterone following injections of gonadotropin-releasing hormone (Chapter 8). Application of this hormone assesses a male's state of reproductive readiness in canids and other social mammals (e.g. Illius *et al.* 1983) and often serves to confirm its social status. Results in this case showed dominant male wolves to have a more pronounced response (i.e. higher spiking blood testosterone concentrations) than subordinates. All the males (adults and adolescents) had responses exceeding 110 ng/mL during the 4-week breeding season (Packard *et al.* 1985). Testicular enlargement also occurred during this period, which is expected in sexually mature canids.

213 Packard *et al.* (1985).

214 Rabb *et al.* (1967 and references).

215 vonHoldt *et al.* (2008: 252).

216 Rutledge *et al.* (2010a).

217 vonHoldt *et al.* (2008), Jankovic *et al.* (2010).

218 Boehm and Zufall (2006).

219 Thornhill *et al.* (2003 and references).

220 Spehr *et al.* (2006b and references).

221 This has been demonstrated conclusively using murine MHC class I peptide ligands, which are nonvolatile molecules usually nine amino acid residues long (Spehr *et al.* 2006b). The mouse MOE can detect these peptides at concentrations near the vanishing point (10^{-11} M).

222 Spehr *et al.* (2006b: 1963). Emphasis added.

223 Ellegren *et al.* (1996), Kojola *et al.* (2006), Liberg *et al.* (2005), vonHoldt *et al.* (2008).

224 Meier *et al.* (1995).

225 Mech *et al.* (1998: 98–99), Smith *et al.* (1997), vonHoldt *et al.* (2008).

226 According to Fox (1973: 291), "the chance of brother × sister mating is normally reduced by the social dynamics within the pack as well as by different rates of sexual maturation."

227 Ellegren (1999), Vilà *et al.* (2003a).

228 Liberg *et al.* (2005).

229 Ellegren (1999).

230 Vilà *et al.* (2003a) asserted that this wolf's genes "saved" the Scandinavian population, but Liberg *et al.* (2005: 3) saw the situation differently: "Our interpretation is that before this male arrived there was no population but just a strongly inbred family."

231 Kojola *et al.* (2006).

232 Kalinowski *et al.* (1999).

233 The dwarf mongoose (*Helogale parvula*), a pack-living carnivoran on African savannas, consistently inbreeds without evidence of inbreeding depression (Keane *et al.* 1996).

234 Peterson *et al.* (1998).

235 Räikkönen *et al.* (2006). Congenital defects in the Scandinavian population include malformations of the vertebrae.

236 Laikre and Ryman (1991). Highly inbred wolves tended to die sooner than outbred captive wolves (29.1 months compared with 60.9 months) even when juvenile mortality was excluded. Litter size was also smaller than in less inbred wolves (5.5 compared with 3.3 pups).

237 For early histories of wolves in Yellowstone National Park see Kay (1995), Schullery and Whittlesey (1995).

238 Young (1944: 120).

239 vonHoldt *et al.* (2008).

240 Aspi *et al.* (2006), vonHoldt *et al.* (2008).

241 Laikre and Ryman (1991), Liberg *et al.* (2005), Packard *et al.* (1985), Smith *et al.* (1997).

242 Peterson *et al.* (1998), Smith *et al.* (1997). Isle Royale in Lake Superior is about 25 km from mainland Ontario. Prior to the current warming trend ice bridges formed periodically, and wolves crossed at least once to colonize the island in the late 1940s. The population has been isolated

since. Why no wolves immigrated later is puzzling. About the same time, de Vos (1950: 171) wrote: "Mr. J. Cross saw a wolf pack from the air, several years ago, approximately south of Sibley, halfway between the peninsula [Sibley Peninsula, Ontario] and Isle Royale. This indicates that it may not be out of the question that wolves will visit Isle Royale some winter in the future." Perhaps the wolves seen by Mr. Cross were the original founders.

243 Packard *et al.* (1985).

Chapter 8: Reproduction and parenting

1 Broad *et al.* (2006: 2200).

2 Holst and Phemister (1974).

3 *Metestrus* also appears in the literature, usually as a synonym of diestrus (Concannon *et al.* 1975, 1989; Evans and Cole 1931; Holst and Phemister 1974; Jöchle and Andersen 1977). The term is ambiguous and often used loosely. Olson *et al.* (1989: 27) gave an abbreviated history of it. As Holst and Phemister (1974: 401) discussed, other investigators have omitted diestrus completely and defined metestrus as the brief interval of 3–5 days "following ovulation when the corpora lutea are organizing and progesterone secretion is increasing." This is curious because the corpus luteum forms late in proestrus and continues into estrus (Holst and Phemister 1974; Olson *et al.* 1989; Rehm *et al.* 2007). The estrous stage thus proceeds smoothly into diestrus with no intervention requiring another arbitrary break in the reproductive cycle. Consequently, I incorporate the function of "metestrus" into late estrus rather than treating it as a separate stage and consider the term itself to be a synonym of diestrus.

4 Concannon (2009); up to 90 days according to Evans and Cole (1931).

5 Jöchle and Andersen (1977).

6 Rehm *et al.* (2007).

7 Rehm *et al.* (2007).

8 de Gier *et al.* (2006).

9 Wildt *et al.* (1978).

10 Concannon *et al.* (1975).

11 Gobello *et al.* (2001), Kooistra *et al.* (1999).

12 Asa (1996), Gobello *et al.* (2001), Okkens *et al.* (1997), Tsutsui *et al.* (2007).

13 Gobello *et al.* (2001 and references).

14 In one study, 77% of first refusals by females to be mounted occurred within days 1–5 of actual diestrus as determined by cytology (Holst and Phemister 1974). The start of diestrus is identified when cells shift abruptly from a cornified to a noncornified epithelium during which superficial (cornified) cell types (Chapter 7) are replaced by small intermediate and *parabasal cells* (Holst and Phemister 1974).

15 Olson *et al.* (1989).

16 Onclin *et al.* (2002).

17 Onclin *et al.* (2002).

18 Concannon *et al.* (1975, 1977b, 1978), Olson *et al.* (1989).

19 Concannon *et al.* (1989), Olson *et al.* (1989).

20 Concannon *et al.* (1977b), Olson *et al.* (1989), Verstegen-Onclin and Verstegen (2008). Placental gonadotropin might also be important for maintenance of early pregnancy and could account partly for the rise in plasma progesterone (Concannon *et al.* 1975, 1977b). *Hypophysectomy* (surgical removal of the pituitary gland) causes dogs to abort at 5–7 weeks of gestation (Concannon 1980 and references). Progesterone attenuates much more slowly in pseudopregnant dogs (84 days compared with 65 days for dogs that are pregnant), and the normal progression of diestrus depends heavily on secretion of gonadotropins by the pituitary (Concannon 1980).

21 Because LH can increase in both pregnant and pseudopregnant females late in diestrus, the slow decline of progesterone is unlikely to be caused by insufficient LH production (Olson *et al.* 1984b, 1989). Also see Concannon *et al.* (1977b).

22 Verstegen-Onclin and Verstegen (2008).

23 Concannon *et al.* (1975, 1989). After recalculating their 1975 data to account for changes in plasma volume during diestrus, Concannon and co-authors reported that the drop to <2 ng/mL begins 36–48 h prepartum (Concannon *et al.* 1977b).

24 Concannon *et al.* (1989). The long-lived corpus luteum could account for monestrus. By the time it disintegrates the "seasonal window" for ovarian recrudescence has closed (Asa and Valdespino 1998).

25 Concannon *et al.* (1975).

26 Concannon *et al.* (1975, 1978), Fernandes *et al.* (1987: 807, figure 2b), Olson *et al.* (1989).

27 Concannon *et al.* (1989).

28 Concannon *et al.* (1977b).

29 Concannon (1980).

30 Olson *et al.* (1984b).

31 Holst and Phemister (1971), Jöchle and Andersen (1977).

32 Concannon *et al.* (1977b).

33 Concannon *et al.* (1977b).

34 Jöchle and Andersen (1977 and reference), Verstegen-Onclin and Verstegen (2008).

35 Jöchle and Andersen (1977).

36 Verstegen-Onclin and Verstegen (2008).

37 Concannon *et al.* (1989), Kooistra and Okkens (2002).

38 Concannon (2009).

39 Verstegen-Onclin and Verstegen (2008).

40 Kreeger *et al.* (1991 and references).

41 Kreeger *et al.* (1991 and reference).

42 Fuller (1956), Scott (1967); Scott and Fuller (1965: 50, 67, 279).

43 Concannon (2009).

44 Asa *et al.* (1987).

45 Kreeger *et al.* (1991).

46 Concannon (2009).

47 Arnason *et al.* (2007).

48 Asa *et al.* (1987).

49 Asa *et al.* (1987).

50 Concannon *et al.* (1978, 1989).

51 Okkens *et al.* (1997).

52 Fernandes *et al.* (1987).

53 Concannon *et al.* (1978), Kooistra and Okkens (2002), Rehm *et al.* (2007).

54 Olson *et al.* (1989).

55 Kreeger *et al.* (1991).

56 Concannon *et al.* (1977b, 1978), Jöchle and Andersen (1977).

57 Concannon *et al.* (1977b, 1987).

58 Concannon *et al.* (1977b).

59 Onclin *et al.* (2002).

60 Brown (1936), Lentfer and Sanders (1973), Ognev (1931: 145), Scott (1967), Seal *et al.* (1979), Woolpy (1968), Young (1944: 95).

61 Concannon *et al.* (1989).

62 Information is mainly from Corbett (1995: 39–40). Baverstock and Green (1977) gave the dingo's average gestation as 63 days.

63 Chambers (1992), Silver and Silver (1969: 8).

64 Holst and Phemister (1974).

65 Concannon *et al.* (1989).

66 Holst and Phemister (1974).

67 Concannon *et al.* (1989 and references).

68 Concannon *et al.* (1977b).

69 Romsos *et al.* (1981).

70 Brand Miller and Colagiuri (1994 and references).

71 Concannon *et al.* (1989).

72 Peaker (1995: 190).

73 The baseline itself is arbitrary too: <1.0 ng/mL (Rehm *et al.* 2007), <3 ng/mL (Kooistra *et al.* 1999).

74 Concannon (2009).

75 Asa (1996).

76 Concannon *et al.* (1989, 1993), Rehm *et al.* (2007). Reviewed by Okkens and Kooistra (2006).
77 Okkens and Kooistra (2006).
78 Christie and Bell (1971).
79 van Haaften *et al.* (1994).
80 Jöchle and Andersen (1977).
81 Verstegen *et al.* (1997).
82 Kooistra *et al.* (1999).
83 van Haaften *et al.* (1994).
84 Kooistra *et al.* (1999).
85 Verstegen *et al.* (1997).
86 Kooistra *et al.* (1999) reported nearly constant but distinct pulses in LH and FSH in pseudopregnant dogs during diestrus and anestrus. The concordance of their pulses was interpreted as evidence that gonadotropin is the only hypothalamic releasing hormone for both LH and FSH.
87 Onclin *et al.* (2002).
88 de Gier *et al.* (2006), Kooistra *et al.* (1999).
89 Kooistra *et al.* (1999).
90 Verstegen *et al.* (1997). As might be expected injecting anestrous dogs with GnRH stimulates a rapid dosage-dependent rise in plasma LH (van Haaften *et al.* 1994).
91 Verstegen *et al.* (1997).
92 Mech *et al.* (1998: 47), Packard *et al.* (1983).
93 Smith *et al.* (1997).
94 Ballard *et al.* (1991).
95 Harrington and Mech (1982).
96 Ballard *et al.* (1991).
97 Ballard *et al.* (1991).
98 van Ballenberghe *et al.* (1975).
99 Murie (1944: 29).
100 Hayes and Harestad (2000a).
101 Hayes and Baer (1992), Mills *et al.* (2008).
102 As Ballard (1982: 75) described the scene, "when the bears stopped running, one wolf typically crouched and approached the sow. The sow would charge the approaching wolf at which time the other wolf would charge and chase the yearling cubs, causing the sow to charge the second intruding wolf. On one occasion the wolves treed all three cubs. The wolves appeared to press their charge when the bears' direction of movement was toward the wolves' den, <2 km away ... These activities lasted 15 minutes and covered 0.6 km."
103 Peak concentrations (about 20 ng/mL) are sustained in dog plasma for 25–30 days after the LH spike; at 50–80 days following the LH spike progesterone has dropped to <1 ng/mL (Rehm *et al.* 2007).
104 Ryon (1977).
105 As described by Ryon (1977: 87), "digging initially consisted of alternate scraping by the forepaws, but backward movements of both forelimbs increased as the tunnel deepened. The tunnel and end chamber were widened by swiping movements of one forepaw, during which the animal would sometimes lay [*sic*] on its side or back ... When a pile of earth had been knocked from the wall or ceiling, the animal pushed it backwards with the side of a forelimb, and then removed it by normal digging movement."
106 Ballard *et al.* (1987), Fritts and Mech (1981).
107 Ognev (1931: 144), Pulliainen (1965). In Murie's time (Murie 1944: 21), all known wolf dens in Denali had originally belonged to foxes.
108 Fuller (1989b), Joslin (1967), Ognev (1931: 144), Pulliainen (1965).
109 Young (1944: 99).
110 Scott and Shackleton (1982).
111 Ognev (1931: 144).
112 Kaartinen *et al.* (2010).
113 Mech *et al.* (1998: 47, 103–104).
114 Mech *et al.* (1998: 89).
115 Cowan (1947), Mech (1970: 119–121).
116 Jordan *et al.* (1967).

117 The description of dens is a blend of information from Cowan (1947: 156–157), Jordan *et al.* (1967), Joslin (1967), Mech (1970: 119–122), Murie (1944: 18–19), and Young (1944: 97–98). Cowan (1947) reported that a wolf (or wolves) in the Canadian Rockies had started digging a den in a beaver dam but abandoned it.

118 Joslin (1967), Scott and Shackleton (1982).

119 Jordan *et al.* (1967).

120 Cowan (1947).

121 Murie (1944: 19, 22).

122 Mech (1988a: 92), Murie (1944: 18–19, 39).

123 McLoughlin *et al.* (2004).

124 Mech (1988a: 92).

125 Heard and Williams (1992).

126 Mech (1993b).

127 Mech *et al.* (1998: 104).

128 Mech (2000).

129 Silver and Silver (1969: 20).

130 Ballard *et al.* (1987), Fritts and Mech (1981), Young (1944: 103).

131 Mech (1988a: 88). Also see Peters and Mech (1975), van Ballenberghe *et al.* (1975).

132 Murie (1944: 25).

133 van Ballenberghe *et al.* (1975 and references).

134 Mech (1970: 146–148, 152), Messier (1985b).

135 Joslin (1967).

136 Kolenosky and Johnston (1967) called these locations "resting sites"; to Young (1944: 103) they were "loafing spots." "Homesite" (see Kolenosky and Johnston 1967) has been used to include both den and rendezvous sites (Harrington and Mech 1982, Mills *et al.* 2008, Joslin 1967, Potvin *et al.* 2004). Fritts and Mech (1981) distinguished between dens and homesites and used homesite as a synonym of rendezvous site. The term should be avoided because of this inconsistent usage.

137 Joslin (1967).

138 Scott and Shackleton (1982).

139 Ausband *et al.* (2010).

140 Ballard *et al.* (1987).

141 Kolenosky and Johnston (1967).

142 Kolenosky and Johnston (1967).

143 Mech (1970: 56), Murie (1944).

144 Messier (1985b).

145 Harrington and Mech (1982).

146 Mech (1988a).

147 van Ballenberghe *et al.* (1975).

148 Fritts and Mech (1981), van Ballenberghe *et al.* (1975), Mech *et al.* (1998: 104).

149 van Ballenberghe *et al.* (1975).

150 Ballard *et al.* (1987).

151 Some pups lag behind others in growth, and not all reach full size by winter. A pup in SNF was 9.1 kg on 12 October 1971, another 32.7 kg on 28 October (van Ballenberghe and Mech 1975). By December pups and adults are nearly the same size (van Ballenberghe *et al.* (1975).

152 Fritts and Mech (1981).

153 Darwin (1897: 28).

154 Bibikov (1982 and references).

155 Gipson (1983), Macdonald and Carr (1995), Nesbitt (1975).

156 Puja *et al.* (2005).

157 Boitani and Ciucci (1995).

158 Daniels and Bekoff (1989b).

159 Scott and Causey (1973), Gipson (1983). Macdonald and Carr (1995: 210) called these places "base camps."

160 Scott and Causey (1973).

161 Information is mainly from Corbett (1995: 41–42). Also see Corbett and Newsome (1975).

162 Thomson (1992b).

163 Thomson (1992b: 523).
164 Thomson (1992d).
165 Lentfer and Sanders (1973).
166 Mech (1988b).
167 Ausband *et al.* (2009).
168 Ausband *et al.* (2009).
169 Crandall (1964: 271), Mech (1988b), Young (1944: 179).
170 Boitani (1982).
171 Gipson and Ballard (1998 and references).
172 Hayes and Harestad (2000a).
173 Rausch (1967), Scott (1967).
174 Rausch (1967).
175 Ballard *et al.* (1987).
176 Hayes and Harestad (2000a).
177 Cowan (1947), Mech (1970: 118–119, table 13), Young (1944: 96).
178 Fritts and Mech (1981).
179 Fuller (1989a).
180 Ognev (1931: 145 and references).
181 Young (1944: 96).
182 Mech (1977).
183 Mills *et al.* (2008).
184 Kerr *et al.* (2004).
185 Kokko and Ekman (2002).
186 Hayes and Harestad (2000a).
187 Gipson and Ballard (1998).
188 Gipson and Ballard (1998), Mech and Nelson (1989).
189 Ballard (1982), Murie (1944: 30, 45).
190 Peterson *et al.* (1984).
191 Ballard *et al.* (1987).
192 Murie (1944: 39–40).
193 van Ballenberghe (1983b).
194 Mech *et al.* (1998: 47, 91, 96, table 4.6), Meier *et al.* (1995).
195 Stahler *et al.* (2002a).
196 vonHoldt *et al.* (2008).
197 Paquet *et al.* (1982 and references).
198 Paquet *et al.* (1982), Rabb *et al.* (1967).
199 Woolpy (1968).
200 Jordan *et al.* (1967).
201 Hayes and Harestad (2000a).
202 Fritts and Mech (1981).
203 Boyd and Jimenez (1994), Stephenson and James (1982).
204 Scott (1967).
205 Malm (1995), Scott (1967).
206 Frank and Frank (1982b).
207 Ognev (1931: 146).
208 Silver and Silver (1969: 12).
209 Ognev (1931: 146).
210 Joslin (1967).
211 Mech (1988a: 60), Mech *et al.* (1999), Murie (1944: 31).
212 Crisler (1958: 226).
213 MacDonald and Ginsburg (1981).
214 Mech *et al.* (1999).
215 Mech (2000), Mech *et al.* (1999).
216 Mech (2000).
217 Fentress and Ryon (1982). Theirs is a complete report of solicitation and regurgitation in a group of captive wolves.

218 Mech (1988a: 60), Mech *et al.* (1999).

219 Kreeger *et al.* (1991). Observations of one captive colony (Fentress and Ryon 1982: 257) showed that "*every* adult wolf feeds other wolves during breeding and pup care seasons. Pups are fed by, but never feed, other animals. Yearlings [adolescents] tend to be intermediate in that they are both fed by adults, and also feed pups. Mothers almost always solicit, and are fed by, other adults. In contrast, barren adult females were never fed, and rarely solicited feeding. Only occasionally do females who have unsuccessful pregnancies solicit or get fed. With the exception of one animal, we have never observed adult males to be fed."

220 Stevens and Stephens (2002: 393).

221 Stevens and Stephens (2002).

222 Stevens and Stephens (2002 and references).

223 Mech (1988a: 60).

224 Mech (1988a: 60).

225 Mech (1988a: 60), Mech *et al.* (1999). For observations of distributed regurgitations by captive wolves see Fentress and Ryon (1982).

226 Ballard *et al.* (1991).

227 Iljin (1941: 407).

228 Concannon *et al.* (1989), Whitney (1971: 110).

229 Daniels and Bekoff (1989b), Pal (2005).

230 Daniels and Bekoff (1989b), Ivanter and Sedova (2008), Pal (2003, 2005).

231 Corbett (1995: 40, table 3.4).

232 Scott (1968).

233 Pal (2005).

234 Daniels and Bekoff (1989b).

235 Pal (2005).

236 Pal (2003).

237 Pal (2005).

238 Daniels and Bekoff (1989b), Oppenheimer and Oppenheimer (1975), Scott and Causey (1973).

239 Pal (2005).

240 Boitani and Ciucci (1995). In contrast, Gipson (1983) reported the survival of free-ranging pups in interior Alaska to be high with almost no recruitment from the nearby population of owned dogs.

241 Macdonald and Carr (1995).

242 Gipson (1983), Macdonald and Carr (1995).

243 Mengel (1971).

244 Gipson (1983).

245 An Australian cattle dog named Bluey herded cattle and sheep for almost 20 years and then retired. He died in 1939 at age 29 years, 5 months. An Australian mongrel died in 1984 at a reported 32 years, 3 days, but its age was incompletely documented. A collie called Bramble in Wales recently turned 27. The source of this information is a website (Anonymous 2011). Among pet dogs mutts generally outlive pure breeds (Patronek *et al.* 1997), and small dogs outlive large ones (Li *et al.* 1996) despite their higher metabolic rates (Speakman *et al.* 2003). An analysis of 77 American Kennel Club breeds comprising 700 dogs assessed the effects of height, body mass, and breed on longevity. Only body mass exerted a significant effect, and the association was negative: on average, little dogs live longer than big ones (Greer *et al.* 2007). Also see Deeb and Wolf (1994).

246 Beck (1973: 36), Daniels and Bekoff (1989b).

247 Fiorello *et al.* (2006).

248 Boitani and Ciucci (1995).

249 Macdonald and Carr (1995), Nesbitt (1975).

250 Corbett and Newsome (1975), Malm (1995), Scott (1967).

251 Pal (2005).

252 Thomson (1992b).

253 Malm (1995).

254 Elliot and King (1960).

255 Frank and Frank (1982a).

256 Boitani and Ciucci (1995).

257 Pal (2003, 2005).
258 Pal (2005).
259 Macdonald and Carr (1995).
260 Nesbitt (1975).
261 Macdonald and Carr (1995).
262 Pal (2003).
263 Thomson (1992b).
264 Thomson (1992b).
265 Scott (1950, 1968).
266 Miller (1977).
267 Lickliter and Ness (1990: 214).
268 Miller (1977).
269 Crosses are easy to identify. They look mottled, having some of the dark feathers of mallards while retaining much of the white of mallards.
270 Murie (1944: 29).
271 Dugatkin et al. (2003).
272 Sherman (1980).
273 Kerr et al. (2004).
274 Riedman (1982).
275 Mech et al. (1999).
276 Murie (1944: 30–31).
277 Silver and Silver (1969: 12, 20).
278 Dugatkin et al. (2003 and references).
279 Hamilton (1963, 1964).
280 Riedman (1982).
281 Riedman (1982).
282 West et al. (2002).
283 Armitage (1987).
284 Asa (1996: 144) made the point that "a subordinate that is deferring reproduction shares on average as many genes with its siblings as it would with its own offspring." Although true, presuming no loss in direct fitness by staying home to be a helper is false.
285 Armitage (1987) and references.
286 Riedman (1982).
287 Hayes and Harestad (2000a).
288 Ghiselin (1974: 143).
289 Griffin and West (2002).
290 Magrath and Yezerinac (1997).
291 Kokko et al. (2001 and references).
292 Heinsohn and Legge (1999: 56).
293 Spong and Creel (2004), West et al. (2001). Ghiselin (1974: 25) discounted altruism as a factor in selection. "In nature, only that which in a sense benefits an individual will be selected. It follows that an organism never does anything for the good of the species. A species is something that an organism uses. The economy of nature is altogether individualistic, and 'altruism' is a metaphysical delusion."
294 Clutton-Brock et al. (2000, 2001).
295 Clutton-Brock et al. (2000).
296 Grafen (1990 and references).
297 Hare and Murie (1996).
298 Wilkinson (1985).
299 Hepper (1994).
300 Broad et al. (2006).
301 Dunbar et al. (1981).
302 Corbett (1995: 97–98).
303 Corbett and Newsome (1975).
304 Asa and Valdespino (1998). Some pseudopregnant dogs lactate (Jöchle and Andersen 1977; Okkens et al. 1997), and lactation in general can be prolonged by administering prolactin (Jöchle and Andersen 1977 and references).

305 Crisler (1958: 225–226, 230–239).
306 Hepper (1994).
307 King (1954).
308 Think of it as a putative kind of "breed familiarity." This hypothesis could be tested easily by replicating the experiment just described in parallel with one in which newborn pups are fostered between breeds and later exposed to strangers of both sexes and breeds.
309 Clutton-Brock *et al.* (1998).
310 Armitage (1987).
311 Hoogland (1985).
312 Kokko and Lundberg (2001 and references).
313 Armitage (1987).
314 The mechanism of limited dispersal is thought to facilitate cooperation in some social animals by keeping kin nearby. However, it would also heighten competition among kin brought about by the increase in population resulting from altruism (Gardner and West 2006 and references). This probably does not apply to wolves, which often disperse great distances and seem not to respect kinship at territorial boundaries.
315 Rodman (1981).
316 Kerr *et al.* (2004).
317 Griffin and West (2002), West *et al.* (2001, 2002). Queller (1994) gave an equation (a modification of Hamilton's inequality) demonstrating the results of competition among relatives: $r = \sum(p_y - \overline{p})/\sum(p_x - \overline{p})$, where r = relatedness, $\overline{p}$ = population frequency of the altruist allele, p_x = frequency of the allele in helpers carrying out altruism, and p_y = frequency of the allele in the beneficiaries. Thus Hamilton's rule is correct if relatedness to the beneficiary of altruistic behavior (r) is measured based on those in competition with the beneficiaries and not the global population; in other words, the relatedness coefficient, r, is a ratio of genetic similarity and the population mean (Griffin and West 2002).
318 Pusey and Packer (1987).
319 Spong and Creel (2004: 325) wrote, "degree of relatedness did not affect the decision [of lions] to approach simulated intrusions, nor did it affect the behaviour during approaches. The decision to approach was instead affected by position within the territory."
320 Schenkel (1967). Schenkel's observations were made on captive wolves, but in this context they apply to wild wolves too.
321 Meier *et al.* (1995).
322 Griffin and West (2002).
323 Widdig *et al.* (2002).
324 Meier *et al.* (1995).
325 Merrill and Mech (2000).
326 Mills *et al.* (2008).
327 Mech and Seal (1987).
328 Fritts and Mech (1981).
329 Mech *et al.* (1998: 97).
330 Mech *et al.* (1998: 98). Also see Lehman *et al.* (1992) and Meier *et al.* (1995).
331 Gaston (1978).
332 An exception is the planktonic larva of the colonial ascidian *Botryllus schosseri* (Grosberg and Quinn 1986). Grafen was criticized for the narrow scope of his definitions (Barnard 1991 and references), but this is how hypotheses are strengthened and made more falsifiable.
333 Grafen (1990).
334 Barnard (1991: 311).
335 Also see Jamieson and Craig (1987).
336 Ghiselin (1997).
337 Grafen (1990: 45).
338 Chapais *et al.* (1997, 2001).
339 Silk *et al.* (2006).
340 Ceacero *et al.* (2007).
341 Kokko *et al.* (2001).

342 The situation is different in animals that queue waiting for opportunities to breed (see text) and among human foragers. People can keep track of who has given them food, recalling previous gifts and their historical contexts and calculating the resultant obligations. Foraging societies are based on debts remembered by both parties that calls for reciprocity (Marlowe 2004).

343 Wiley and Rabenold (1984: 618).

344 Harrington and Mech (1982).

345 Harrington and Mech (1982: 104).

346 Messier (1985b).

347 Mech *et al.* (1999).

348 Mech (1988a: 71).

349 Prairie dogs are social ground-dwelling squirrels. A South Dakota colony of black-tailed prairie dogs (*Cynomys ludovicianus*) studied by Hoogland (1985) had existed at least 35 years with sequential generations occupying the same burrows. The colony spread over 6.6 ha and contained an average of 133 adults and adolescents.

350 Wiley and Rabenold (1984).

351 Queues possibly exist in captive groups. Even then an assumption must be made that terms like alpha, beta, and so forth mean to the wolves what we think they mean to us.

352 Fox (1975).

353 Harrington *et al.* (1983).

354 This arrangement was called "'payment' for the right to remain" by Gaston (1978: 1095); Kokko *et al.* (2001: 187) termed it "payment of rent."

355 Heinsohn and Legge (1999).

356 Ghiselin (1974: 143).

357 Mech *et al.* (1999).

358 Kokko and Lundberg (2001).

359 Kokko and Ekman (2002 and references), Kokko and Lundberg (2001). How saturation and other ecological constraints affect dispersal of wolves has yet to be quantified. The ongoing studies in Yellowstone should eventually provide answers.

360 Wiley and Rabenold (1984).

361 Johnson and Gaines (1990).

362 Wiley and Rabenold (1984).

363 Kokko and Ekman (2002).

364 Wiley and Rabenold (1984).

365 Kokko and Ekman (2002).

366 Kokko and Lundberg (2001).

367 Boyd and Jimenez (1994).

368 Hayes and Harestad (2000a).

369 Mills *et al.* (2008).

370 Harrington *et al.* (1983).

371 Mech (2000).

372 Mech (1988a: 27).

373 Mech (2000: 261), citing observations in Mech (1995b), wrote: "I once watched the breeding pair leave three [adolescents] at their rendezvous site and travel 9.5 km away, where the male then dug up a cached Muskox calf shoulder and delivered it to the breeding female. She consumed it and immediately returned to the [adolescents] and regurgitated to them."

374 Harrington *et al.* (1983), Peterson *et al.* (1984). Inferences drawn from straightforward correlation between group size and reproductive success are seldom informative. As stated by Jamieson and Craig (1987: 93), "analyses of costs/benefits and reproductive success can only potentially show that provisioning behavior by helpers can positively affect reproductive output of communal groups. They provide a limited explanation of the evolutionary origin or variable expression of such behavior seen in the communal breeding context." Consequently, a report claiming to have shown how helper effects increase the lifetime fitness of red wolves (Sparkman *et al.* 2011) was actually a test of survivorship based on pack size. The authors admitted that helping behavior in red wolves had not yet been documented. Lacking field observations they performed an analysis of data collected previously on social groups. Helpers were defined as nonbreeding offspring from

previous years, their influence assessed by whether or not they were members of the different packs. I followed the circular trail back to its origin and could only conclude that some of these wolves performed no helping function because they were absent. Nothing specific was required of those present, evidently confirming Woody Allen's rubric that most of life is just showing up.

375 Rabb *et al.* (1967: 310).
376 Ghiselin (1974: 247).
377 Ghiselin (1974: 41).
378 Jamieson and Craig (1987).
379 Frank and Frank (1982a).
380 Fox (1969c).
381 Payne (1977).
382 Payne (1977).
383 Rothstein (1982 and references).
384 Jamieson and Craig (1987: 80).
385 Boland *et al.* (1997).
386 Jamieson and Craig (1987).
387 Jamieson and Craig (1987: 92).
388 Crisler (1958: 288).
389 Packard *et al.* (1985).
390 Magrath and Yezerinac (1997).
391 Murie (1944: 31).
392 Maynard Smith (1974, 1979).
393 Johnson and Gaines (1990).
394 Dispersal has been modeled often (Johnson and Gaines 1990). I discuss the diploid part of a deterministic model in which v^* depends solely on surviving dispersal (Hamilton and May 1977). Later efforts have become more stochastic, mathematically rigorous, and in my opinion realistic with availability of increased computing power.

Chapter 9: Socialization

1 Ghiselin (1997).
2 Daniels and Bekoff (1989c: 83).
3 Daniels and Bekoff (1989c).
4 Scott (1968). The lone exception seems to be the domestic cat.
5 My summary of socialization is based on Fentress (1967), Freedman *et al.* (1961), Scott (1958, 1962, 1964, 1967), Scott and Fuller (1965: 84–150), Scott and Marston (1950).
6 Scott (1962: 949–950).
7 Scott and Fuller (1965: 84–88), Scott and Marston (1950).
8 Scott (1968).
9 A neonate rat emits the pheromone dodecyl propionate from its preputial glands which, after being imbibed by the mother's vomeronasal organ (Chapter 4), prompts her to lick the young's anogenital area, keeping it free of urine and feces (Brouette-Lahlou *et al.* 1999). No similar stimulant has been found in canids.
10 Fox (1972b).
11 Ackerman *et al.* (2010).
12 Bleicher (1963).
13 Scott (1967).
14 Jensen and Ederstrom (1955).
15 Scott (1958).
16 Scott (1958).
17 Brodbeck (1954), Scott (1958).
18 Gazzano *et al.* (2008).
19 Scott (1968).
20 Mech (1970: 49, 1988a: 58), Scott (1967).
21 Bleicher (1963).

22 Bleicher (1963) suggested that a sound described as a groan seems different and could serve as a distress signal, attracting a mother dog if her pup was out of sight. This too is conjecture.

23 Wells and Hepper (2006) demonstrated prenatal chemosensory learning in dogs. If confirmed, neonates are capable of olfaction and taste.

24 In the words of Scott (1967: 375), "the modification of neonatal behavior by experience may leave adult behavior unchanged." Scott (1958: 47) had earlier written, "we would expect and have found that it would be extremely difficult to produce psychological trauma upon very young puppies, and that any future effects on their behavior produced at this time would have to be made by physiological or anatomical injury."

25 Scott (1964).

26 As Scott (1964: 165) wrote, "this challenges one of the older and simpler concepts of behavioral development, namely that development is a sort of unfolding or unflowering and that consequently everything that happens at one stage of development leads to something else. The general course of development in the puppy suggests that certain lines of behavioral development may lead nowhere except that they are necessary for neonatal survival, and that they are abandoned at a later age."

27 Gácsi et al. (2005), Topál et al. (2005).

28 Scott and Fuller (1965: 89–101), Scott and Marston (1950).

29 Ballard et al. (1987 and references), Mech (1970: 143, table 17; 1993b), Murie (1944: 46), Ryon (1977). A litter of captive pups appeared at the den's entrance at 24 days (Ryon 1977).

30 Scott (1967).

31 Scott (1968).

32 Scott (1958).

33 Scott (1958).

34 Silver and Silver (1969: 9).

35 Ryon (1977).

36 Bleicher (1963).

37 Mech (1988a: 58).

38 Fox (1970: 55) used the term face-lick.

39 Freedman et al. (1961), Scott (1958, 1962, 1964, 1967), Scott and Fuller (1965: 117–150), Scott and Marston (1950). Belyaev et al. (1985: 359) wrote: "It is during this time [critical stage] that species-identification of the young animal is established and, in particular, the mechanisms of social defensive behaviour are functionally organized, and the behavioural phenotype is most easily amenable to modification."

40 Scott and Fuller (1965: 111, 117–129).

41 Silver and Silver (1969: 12–14).

42 Some canids show sex preferences for humans depending on whether they were raised by men or women. Coyote pups raised by a woman thereafter preferred women to men (Snow 1967). Sex preference was also shown by a hand-raised female wolf (Silver and Silver 1969: 29). An animal reared by a woman might be more amenable to handling by an unknown woman than a man who is a stranger.

43 Mech (1988a: 58).

44 Bleicher (1963), Ohl (1996), Scott (1964).

45 Coscia et al. (1991).

46 Bleicher (1963).

47 Fox (1970).

48 Fox (1970: 56) stated that the ears are flattened during a submissive approach, but they can also be folded.

49 Fox (1970: 58).

50 Bekoff (1972: 417).

51 Burghardt (2005: 45–82) reviewed some of the better ones and pointed out their flaws.

52 Martin and Caro (1985: 65).

53 Scott (1964).

54 Scott (1958).

55 Fentress (1967) reported that a wolf he raised did not follow scent trails until 14 weeks old.

56 Packard et al. (1992).

57 Fentress (1967).

58 Scott (1964).
59 Fentress (1967), Murie (1944: 47–50).
60 Bleicher (1963).
61 Woolpy and Ginsburg (1967: 359).
62 Fox (1969c).
63 MacDonald and Ginsburg (1981). These wolves were isolated at times just beyond the critical period.
64 MacDonald and Ginsburg (1981: 159) wrote that the wolves "exhibited substantially normal behavior within hours of exposure to social experience with the other restricted animals, and without the need of 'therapy' from normally reared wolves or from chronologically younger 'pacemakers.' The deprived animals, when exposed to each other, were their own 'therapists.' They may be considered comparable to younger 'pacemakers' in the sense that they were all deprived of normal social experience."
65 Rabb et al. (1967), Zimen (1981).
66 MacDonald and Ginsburg (1981: 157).
67 That was the situation thousands of years ago and remains true today despite all the available information about wolf behavior and modern training methods. Wolves and wolfdogs make dangerous pets, and their use for this purpose should be outlawed. As of 1994 there were about 2000 wild wolves in the lower 48 US, but an estimated 100 000 in captivity and another 400 000 crosses (Hope 1994). Wolves in nature are timid in the presence of humans unless habituated by being fed, which increases the danger of being bitten (McNay 2002). There is almost no chance of being attacked by a wild wolf not habituated to humans (McNay 2002). Captive wolves are different, and crossing a wolf with a large ferocious breed of dog produces offspring that can be exceptionally dangerous.
68 Ballard et al. (1997).
69 The age at which male dogs start to RLU varies widely: 22–50 weeks in one study of 10 beagles with a mean of 38.8 weeks (Ranson and Beach (1985).
70 Peterson and Page (1988).
71 Ballard et al. (1987), Mech (1995b).
72 Zimen (1975: 340).
73 Fox (1971a).
74 Fox (1971a).
75 Zimen (1975).
76 Mech (1995b).
77 Gácsi et al. (2001).
78 Fentress (1967).
79 Bekoff (1972: 417) after Tinbergen (1963).
80 Ghiselin (1974: 259). Bekoff (1972: 424), for example, wrote, "play is a very productive activity, in so far as it allows the developing organism to realize behavioral potentialities essential for normal behavioral development and adult life."
81 Ghiselin (1974: 260).
82 Bekoff (1972: 418).
83 Ghiselin (1974: 258–261).
84 Crisler (1958: 260).
85 Ghiselin (1974: 261). Others have suggested this too (Bekoff 1972 and references).
86 Bekoff (1972 and references).
87 Bleicher (1963).
88 Bekoff (1972 and references).
89 Fox et al. (1975).
90 Goodwin et al. (1997).
91 Bekoff (1974), Silver and Silver (1969).
92 Mech (1966: 68).
93 Mech (1966: 120).
94 Mech (1966: 68), Murie (1944: 31–34).
95 Specifically, Murie (1944: 31–32) wrote: "But as I looked back from the river bar ... I saw the two blacks and the two gray males assembled on the skyline, wagging their tails and frisking together.

There they all howled, and while they howled the gray female galloped up from the den 100 yards and joined them. She was greeted with energetic tail wagging and general good feeling. Then ... five muzzles pointed skyward. Their howling floated softly across the tundra. Then abruptly the assemblage broke up. The mother returned to the den to assume her vigil and four wolves trotted eastward into the dusk."

96 Crisler (1958), Murie (1944).
97 Mech (1970: 47), Woolpy and Ginsburg (1967).
98 Murie (1944: 43–44).
99 Stahler *et al.* (2002a).
100 Ballard (1982: 76).
101 Crisler (1958: 91) described it like this: "We crouched, elbows to sides, and flipped forearms sidewise. A wolf reads the lowering of your elevation as friendliness."
102 See Bekoff (1972: 426, fig. 4).
103 Fox (1970).
104 Bekoff (1974).
105 Mech (1970: 199).
106 Murie (1944: 56).
107 Koler-Matznick (2002: 99) wrote: "With careful conditioning using modern methods, wolves can be tamed ... but not trained to follow commands reliably. Although they respect limits on inter-individual conduct, wolves resist human direction of their activities and inhibition training ... This is why there are no wolf acts in circuses."
108 Gipson and Ballard (1998).
109 Allen (1979: 16).
110 Woolpy and Ginsburg (1967).
111 Woolpy (1968).
112 Ognev (1931: 152).
113 Iljin (1941: 409) wrote that wolves could be trained to pull sleds and obey other commands: "Moreover, the experiments we carried out at the Moscow Zoopark demonstrated the possibility of training and taming pure wolves born in captivity or caught wild (both as puppies or as adult animals). Our collaborators taught old wolves to obey the command 'run', 'here', 'slowly', 'quietly', 'back', 'don't' (No), 'hop', etc."
114 Woolpy and Ginsburg (1967).
115 Woolpy and Ginsburg (1967).
116 Topál *et al.* (2005).
117 Woolpy and Ginsburg (1967: 361).
118 Elliot and King (1960).
119 Scott (1962).
120 Frank and Frank (1988).
121 Scott (1962 and references).
122 Scott (1962 and references).
123 Scott (1962: 950).
124 Parmelee (1964: 8).
125 Parmelee (1964: 9) wrote: "By the time we were half way to camp it was pitch dark. I was hungry and sore and not thinking about much of anything else when Stu discreetly told me to glance backwards. Following close in my footsteps was the big she-wolf, her nose touching the ptarmigans as they swayed back and forth. Incredible as it surely is, we several times had to drive that wolf off with snowballs for fear that we would lose our specimens!"
126 Murie (1944: 47) described the scene: "On August 11, at 7 o'clock in the evening, the wolf pup was heard whining softly. On looking out I saw the black female only a few yards from the pup. The following evening at 8 o'clock I heard the pup whining again and saw the black female with it. She traveled slowly and reluctantly up the slope, looking back repeatedly. The pup tried to follow and when it reached the end of the chain, kept jumping forward to be away."
127 Crisler (1958: 224).
128 Murie (1944: 33).
129 Mech (1970: 45).
130 Mech (1970: 47).

131 Woolpy and Ginsburg (1967).
132 Mech (1970: 47).
133 Mendelssohn (1982).
134 Description based on Mech (1995b).
135 Murie (1944: 30–31).
136 Frank and Frank (1982a).
137 McLeod (1996: 113).
138 Fentress (1967: 346–347).
139 Murie (1944: 47).
140 Fentress (1967).
141 Crisler (1958: 153).
142 Mech (1970: 6). This event was described briefly by Mech and Frenzel (1969).
143 Palmer and Custance (2008). Attachment has been defined in many ways. For some of these see Topál et al. (1998).
144 Prato-Previde et al. (2003), Gácsi et al. (2001 and references).
145 Hepper (1994). Mekosh-Rosenbaum et al. (1994) performed a similar experiment with similar conclusions, but results actually showed that the test subjects (beagles) were sometimes able to distinguish their own bedding from that of a strange litter of the same age. Experiments like these are not evidence of kin recognition.
146 Prato-Previde et al. (2003), Topál et al. (2005).
147 Topál et al. (2005).
148 Topál et al. (2005).
149 Frank and Frank (1982a).
150 Topál et al. (2005).
151 Gácsi et al. (2005).
152 Frank and Frank (1982a: 510).
153 Spotte (2006).
154 Lee (1999: 50).
155 Lee (1999: 95).
156 Mech (1999: 1197).
157 Derix et al. (1993), Lentfer and Sanders (1973), Rabb et al. (1967). In contrast, Fatjó et al. (2007) reported that most agonism in the captive pack they studied took place between males.
158 Derix et al. (1993).
159 As reported by Lentfer and Sanders (1973: 626), during mid-February in a captive colony of gray wolves at Barrow, Alaska, "a 4-year-old female, caged with her mate of the previous season and three of their 10-month-old pups, burrowed at considerable effort through hard-packed snow under a gate into an adjoining cage containing a 3-year-old female and her two 10-month-old pups. There the 4-year-old female killed the 3-year-old female."
160 Lentfer and Sanders (1973), Rabb et al. (1967).
161 Rabb et al. (1967).
162 Rabb et al. (1967).
163 Rabb et al. (1967).
164 Woolpy and Ginsburg (1967).
165 Gartlan (1964).
166 Much of the confusion about dominance has been caused by the different results obtained from observations of captive animals of all kinds versus those made in nature. Gartlan (1964: 76) drew attention to this early on and advised "bearing in mind the fact that most work on this problem has been carried out under highly artificial conditions on different species and genera, notable differences occur in the literature concerning the principal characteristics of dominance." He suggested (Gartlan 1964: 77) that such disparities arise out of ignorance about what constitutes normal behavior under natural conditions: "The fact that cage conditions might exacerbate, if not actually initiate, behaviour which is commonly gathered under the heading of 'dominance' has not been a point of interest to the experimentalists."
167 Zimen (1975, 1976). Also see Packard et al. (1985), who monitored two packs of captive wolves in Minnesota. Their report provides much less detail than Zimen's but enough to highlight the incest and carnage.

168 Zimen (1975).

169 Zimen (1975: 336).

170 Zimen (1975: 337). A later report stated that unrelated pups from different geographic locations were introduced and accepted by the pack, at least initially (Zimen 1976).

171 Rabb *et al.* (1967), Derix *et al.* (1993). Van Hooff and Wensing (1987) found a single linear hierarchy, but their captive wolves knew each other (parents and two successive litters).

172 Scott and Fredericson (1951) were uncertain on this point. These authors wrote before Zimen's publication and were thinking in terms of males competing for females in heat. What Zimen highlighted instead was the dominant female preventing her subordinates from mating.

173 Mech (1999: 1198). Although "peck order" has been discredited when applied to the social structure of wolves it has long been used (Mech 1970: 68–69), and some continue to use it (e.g. Boitani and Ciucci 1995).

174 Derix *et al.* (1993), in contrast, never witnessed a dominant female attempting to suppress mating of a subordinate.

175 This shifting theater is actually predictable on a general scale. Having been defeated, a dominant mouse becomes subordinate not only to its rival but others in the hierarchy (Scott and Fredericson 1951 and references).

176 Zimen (1975: 355) wrote: "When I entered the enclosure he greeted me holding his wagging tail high and stiff. When I approached him he assumed a threatening posture with the hair on his back raised. Other people who came to the enclosure fence were threatened even more, and when he saw strange dogs [through the fence] he turned really wild. The few times I managed to take him out of the enclosure on a leash, he did not threaten me, but he was highly aroused, urinated at every tree and would, if I had not kept him back, have attacked anybody."

177 Scott and Fredericson (1951).

178 Schenkel (1947).

179 Fox (1972a).

180 Drummond (2006: 20).

181 Mech (1988a: 61).

182 Crisler (1958), Mech (1988a), Murie (1944).

183 Crisler (1958: 289).

184 Mech (1999).

185 vonHoldt *et al.* (2008).

186 Olson (1938b).

187 vonHoldt *et al.* (2008). Asa *et al.* (1986) reported captive female Great Lakes wolves denning together and caring for the pups mutually.

188 Murie (1944: 39–40), Peterson *et al.* (2002).

189 Mech (1999).

190 Fritts and Mech (1981), van Ballenberghe (1983a).

191 Fritts and Mech (1981), Harrington and Mech (1979).

192 Mech and Nelson (1990). Ballard *et al.* (1987) reported three cases in which packs produced two litters in the same year but did not state whether more than one male fathered them.

193 Meier *et al.* (1995).

194 Murie (1944).

195 Fritts and Mech (1981), Peterson *et al.* (2002), Stahler *et al.* (2002a), vonHoldt *et al.* (2008).

196 Fritts and Mech (1981). Lone dispersers in BISF usually paired within 8–30 days.

197 Mech and Nelson (1990).

198 Meier *et al.* (1995).

199 Mech (1995a), Peterson *et al.* (2002).

200 Mech and Hertel (1983), Mech *et al.* (1999).

201 Mech (1995a).

202 Mech (1999 and references).

203 vonHoldt *et al.* (2008).

204 Mech (1999).

205 Lentfer and Sanders (1973).

206 Mech (1999).

207 Schenkel (1967).

208 Mech (1999).
209 Mech (1999).
210 According to Mech (1999: 1198), "any parent is dominant to its young offspring, so 'alpha' adds no information. Why not refer to an alpha female as the female parent, the breeding female, the matriarch, or simply the mother? Such a designation emphasizes not the animal's dominant status, which is trivial information, but its role as pack progenitor, which is critical information ... The point here is not so much the terminology but what the terminology falsely implies: a rigid force-based dominance hierarchy." This seems imminently sensible.
211 For example, see Daniels (1983b: 366).
212 Scott (1950).
213 Nesbitt (1975).
214 Berman and Dunbar (1983), Daniels (1983a).
215 Boitani and Ciucci (1995).
216 Boitani and Ciucci (1995 and references).
217 Boitani and Ciucci (1995), Daniels (1983a).
218 Boitani and Ciucci (1995).
219 Boitani and Ciucci (1995).
220 Beck (1973), Daniels (1983a), Daniels and Bekoff (1989b).
221 Daniels (1983a) cited references to document that territoriality is typically associated with scarce resources distributed uniformly. Perhaps this is true in some cases, but the large ungulates hunted by wolves are seldom distributed uniformly and at times can be abundant.
222 Daniels and Bekoff (1989b).
223 Daniels and Bekoff (1989a, 1989b).
224 Ortolani et al. (2009).
225 Daniels (1983a).
226 Macdonald and Carr (1995).
227 Macdonald and Carr (1995); Nesbitt (1975), but see Scott and Causey (1973).
228 Nesbitt (1975).
229 Daniels and Bekoff (1989a), Scott and Causey (1973).
230 Scott and Causey (1973).
231 Scott and Causey (1973).
232 Daniels and Bekoff (1989b).
233 As Scott and Marston (1950: 25) wrote, "the behavior patterns exhibited by dogs toward human beings are essentially the same as those exhibited toward dogs, and ... one sort of social relationship which can be set up between [humans] and dogs is essentially similar to the parent–offspring relationship in either species." Also see Scott (1958: 53).
234 Crisler (1958: 91).
235 Woolpy and Ginsburg (1967).
236 Fox (1970).
237 Palmer and Custance (2008), Prato-Previde et al. (2003), Topál et al. (1998, 2005).
238 Reebs (2000).
239 Ramseyer et al. (2009).
240 Mech (1966: 61–62; 1970: 73).
241 Scott (1950).
242 Mech (1970: 68–76), Peters and Mech (1975).
243 Olson (1938b: 331).
244 Peterson et al. (2002) tried to measure leadership in wolf packs, although with minimal effort to separate dominance behavior. Beauchamp (2000) successfully separated dominance and leadership behaviors in zebra finches (Taenopygia guttata). Camels (Camelus dromedarius) have subtle dominance hierarchies but no leadership (Schulte and Klingel 1991).
245 Mech (1970: 73). Mech, on this same page, deferred to Murie (1944: 28), who described a wolf in the Denali pack he observed as "lord and master" and remarking how "the other wolves approached this one with some diffidence, usually cowering before him." This too describes dominance but not necessarily leadership. In a slightly different version of Mech's definition, and with less emphasis on dominance, Peters and Mech (1975: 630) wrote, "generally the alpha

male is the pack leader, and he takes the initiative in leading attacks on prey and intruders and directs the movements and activities of the pack."

246 Erhart and Overdorff (1999: 927).

247 Not all ungulates are self-organizing. For example, herds of domestic goats with stable matrilineal kinships have identifiable leaders (Escós *et al*. 1993).

248 Krause *et al*. (2000).

249 Tien *et al*. (2004).

250 Conradt and Roper (2005), Stueckle and Zinner (2008).

251 Leca *et al*. (2003).

252 This has also been termed *consistent leadership* (Conradt and Roper 2005; Bonanni *et al*. 2010b), which seems too vague. Any form of leadership can be consistent in the sense of persisting.

253 Seton (1962: 1–21).

254 Stewart and Harcourt (1994).

255 Ramseyer *et al*. (2009).

256 As used here distributed leadership conforms with *variable leadership* (Conradt and Roper 2005; Bonanni *et al*. 2010b).

257 Leca *et al*. (2003).

258 Ramseyer *et al*. (2009).

259 Kummer (1968: 122–148), Stueckle and Zinner (2008).

260 Conradt and Roper (2005).

261 Crisler (1958), Mech (1988a), Murie (1944). Stanwell-Fletcher (1942: 140), whose observations were much less detailed and informed, nonetheless described wolves as "strong, fearless, peace-loving, faithful to each other."

262 Mech (1988a: 64).

263 Mech (1999).

264 Ramseyer *et al*. (2009).

265 Peterson *et al*. (2002).

266 Mech (1970: 73).

267 Mech (1970: 74).

268 Allen (1979: 123).

269 Mech (1970: 75).

270 Mech (1970: 75–76).

271 Peterson *et al*. (2002).

272 Based mainly on Mech (1999, 2000).

273 Caro and Hauser (1992).

274 Seyfarth and Cheney (2003).

275 See, for example, Boitani and Ciucci (1995).

276 Caro and Hauser (1992).

277 Caro and Hauser (1992).

278 Scott (1967).

279 Smith *et al*. (2000). Naïve coyotes chase and kill sheep (Connolly *et al*. 1976); coyotes reared in isolation killed and ate rats at age 30 days (Fox 1969b).

280 Fox *et al*. (1975).

281 Fox *et al*. (1975: 128, example from field notes): "2.50 a.m. Trio sleeping on porch [of abandoned house]. F gets up, gives a yelp bark and goes down steps onto sidewalk with Y. X sleeps on. F returns 5 min later and gives another yelp bark and a tail wag towards X. X gets up and follows her. F face-rubs and tail-wags with X."

282 This sequence is a close paraphrase of a description by Fox *et al*. (1975: 128).

283 Bonanni *et al*. (2010b: 988).

284 Bonanni *et al*. (2010b: 988) considered that "formal dominance" (what I earlier termed paying homage) rather than "agonistic dominance" might be a better predictor of leadership in free-ranging dogs because "the achievement of formal dominance appears to be indistinguishable from the establishment of affiliative relationships with subordinates." This is not a clean separation. Once again, *all* dominance is agonistic if the subordinate animal displays submissive feedback.

285 Bonanni *et al*. (2010b).

286 Murie (1944: 31–34).

287 In observations made by Bonanni *et al.* (2010b) pups never led in this context.

288 Bonanni *et al.* (2010b).

289 Bonanni *et al.* (2010b: 983) measured one form of leadership in free-ranging dogs as "an unsuccessful attempt at leaving."

290 Bonanni *et al.* (2010b: 986) implied a competitive component, writing "dogs that behaved more frequently as leaders were those that were more successful at recruiting followers." However, the measure of such leadership success was simply whether other dogs followed. I realize the term recruitment is sometimes used passively in ecology (e.g. recruitment of planktonic larvae in the sea), but its intended meaning in behavior should be different. Behaviorally, recruitment is an active process requiring directed effort by the recruiter. A dog following another voluntarily is not evidence of leadership, nor does such an observation identify specific qualities that make one dog a leader and the other a follower.

291 Murie (1944: 33).

292 Bonanni *et al.* (2010b).

293 Description based on Bonanni *et al.* (2010a).

294 Bonanni *et al.* (2010a) overstepped the limits of their data by attributing the closeness of "affiliative relationships" to kinship without having first determined kinship ties. Moreover, both formal and agonistic dominant ↔ subordinate relationships are likely based on other factors (e.g. age, sex, degree of familiarity). Groups of dogs split during their study, and others merged, in both cases without evidence of a kinship effect. The report they cited as evidence of a kinship effect (Hepper 1994) is itself flawed by not having controlled for familiarity.

295 Macintosh (1975: 95–95) wrote, "while I have met a number of people who claim and truly believe they have successfully domesticated a nonhybridized dingo, checking out their story and the animal's behavior reveals that they are either self-deluding, or anthropomorphizing which largely amounts to the same thing." Macintosh (1975: 97) continued: "Police dog trainers in Sydney some 20 years ago, even with their great experience, patience, and affection for animals, failed to produce anything resembling obedience."

296 Dayton (2003).

297 Savolainen *et al.* (2004) estimated that dingoes arrived in Australia about 5000 years BP. Evidence of humans at several coastal locations in Australia dates back 21 000 years BP (Macintosh 1975 and references), but the earliest Australians might have arrived 45 000–60 000 years BP (Roberts and Brook 2010), occupying the whole country 15 000 years later (Dayton (2003)).

298 Gollan (1984).

299 Macintosh (1975).

300 The speed at which many behavioral changes occur is astonishing, as shown by long-term experiments at a Siberian fox farm (Trut *et al.* 2009). Wild red foxes do not tail-wag, but fourth-generation foxes selected for tameness wagged their tails when responding to humans. Continuous selection for tameness resulted in more dog-like traits. Offspring of the sixth generation actively sought contact with humans, wagging their tails and whining, whimpering, and licking as pup dogs do. By the 45th generation, a fox had been produced that acted like a socialized dog.

301 Meggitt (1965: 10, footnote 4) wrote, "it may seem remarkable that a people could associate for several millennia with an economically and ritually significant species without domesticating it completely."

302 Meggitt (1965), Nind (1831).

303 Meggitt (1965).

304 Finlayson (1943: 143).

305 Nind (1831).

306 Meggitt (1955: 378).

307 Meggitt (1955: 383) wrote: "Many times, the myriad camp dogs have rushed barking into the bush for no apparent reason, the men have told me this demonstrated the presence of *djanba*. The men naturally would not go out to investigate. Moreover, dogs will attack and hamstring a *djanba* which sneaks up on the camps at night. Either they finish him off by tearing his throat, or they leave him helpless on the ground, to be killed by a medicine man."

308 Kolig (1973).

309 Kolig (1973: 123) stated that in the view of native Australians dingoes "appear as pairs or in packs, but never alone. Without any exception ... they are strongly associated with detrimental features and functions. [Dingoes] are assassins of other mythical beings; they are destroyers ... they never

obey their masters, are vicious and disloyal; they rape and thieve; and they never act as culture heroes as many other mythical beings do."

310 Gould (1969), Meggitt (1965 and references).

311 Nind (1831: 29).

312 Meggitt (1965).

313 Schwartz (1997: 60–92), Young (1944: 175, 193, 185).

314 Troughton (1970: 93) quoted an 1842 publication stating that dingoes were eaten in what is now Papua New Guinea.

315 Krefft (1866: 3).

316 Macintosh (1975: 97).

317 That aborigines in Australia huddled with dingoes (and dogs) on cold nights is often thought to be a myth, but this apparently is not the case (Gould 1970; Macintosh 1975).

318 Nind (1831: 28).

319 Meggitt (1965: 15).

320 Meggitt (1965: 16).

321 Nind (1831: 29).

322 Meggitt (1965).

323 Gould (1969).

324 Nind (1831).

325 Nind (1831).

326 Hayden (1975).

327 Meggitt (1955: 383).

328 Macintosh (1975).

329 Macintosh (1975: 98).

330 Nind (1831).

References

Ackerman, J.M., C.C. Nocera, and J.A. Bargh. (2010). Incidental haptic sensations influence social judgments and decisions. *Science* **328**: 1712–1715.

Adams, D.R. and M.D. Wiekamp. (1984). The canine vomeronasal organ. *Journal of Anatomy* **138**: 771–787.

Adams, J.R., J.A. Leonard, and L.P. Waits. (2003a). Widespread occurrence of a domestic dog mitochondrial DNA haplotype in southeastern US coyotes. *Molecular Ecology* **12**: 541–546.

Adams, J.R., B.T. Kelly, and L.P. Waits. (2003b). Using faecal DNA sampling and GIS to monitor hybridization between red wolves (*Canis rufus*) and coyotes (*Canis latrans*). *Molecular Ecology* **12**: 2175–2186.

Aggarwal, R.K., T. Kivisild, J. Ramadevi, and L. Singh. (2007). Mitochondrial DNA coding region sequences support the phylogenetic distinction of two Indian wolf species. *Journal of Zoological Systematics and Evolutionary Research* **45**: 163–172.

Alexy, K.J., J.W. Gassett, D.A. Osborn, and K.V. Miller. (2003). Bacterial fauna on the tarsal tufts of white-tailed deer (*Odocoileus virginianus*). *American Midland Naturalist* **149**: 237–240.

Allen, B.L. (2010). Skin and bone: observations of dingo scavenging during a chronic food shortage. *Australian Mammalogy* **32**: 207–208.

Allen, D.L. (1979). *Wolves of Minong: Their Vital Role in a Wild Community*. Boston, MA: Houghton Mifflin, xxv + 449 pp.

Allen, G.M. (1920). Dogs of the American aborigines. *Bulletin of the Museum of Comparative Zoölogy* **63**(9): 431–517 + 12 plates.

Anderson, T.M., B.M. vonHoldt, S.I. Candille, M. Musiani, C. Greco, and D.R. Stahler *et al.* (2009). Molecular and evolutionary history of melanism in North American gray wolves. *Science* **323**: 1339–1343.

Andersone, Ž., V. Lucchini, E. Randi, and J. Ozolinš. (2002). Hybridisation between wolves and dogs in Latvia as documented using mitochondrial and microsatellite DNA markers. *Mammalian Biology* **67**: 79–90.

Anonymous. (1999). Wisconsin Wolf Management Plan. Appendix G, Wisconsin Department of Natural Resources, Madison. http://dnr.wi.gov/org/land/er/publications/wolfplan/toc.htm.

Anonymous. (2010a). Tough food makes coyotes better biters. http://news.sciencemag.org/sciencenow/2010/07/tough-food-makes-coyotes-better.-html.

Anonymous. (2010b). Dog depredations by wolves in Wisconsin – 2010. Wisconsin Department of Natural Resources, 27 pp. http://dnr.wi.gov/org/land/er/mammals/wolf/dogdepred.htm.

Anonymous. (2011). Vegetable-eating dog lives to ripe old age of 27. http://dogsinthenews. com/issues/0209/articles/020918a.htm.

Aoki, T. and M. Wada. (1951). Functional activity of the sweat glands in the hairy skin of the dog. *Science* **114**: 123–124.

Arjo, W. M. and D. H. Pletscher. (1999). Behavioral responses of coyotes to wolf recolonization in northwestern Montana. *Canadian Journal of Zoology* **77**: 1919–1927.

Arjo, W. M., D. H. Pletscher, and R. R. Ream. (2002). Dietary overlap between wolves and coyotes in northwestern Montana. *Journal of Mammalogy* **83**: 754–766.

Armitage, K. B. (1987). Social dynamics of mammals: reproductive success, kinship and individual fitness. *Trends in Ecology and Evolution* **2**: 279–284.

Arnason, U., A. Gullberg, A. Janke, and M. Kullberg. (2007). Mitogenomic analyses of caniform relationships. *Molecular Phylogenetics and Evolution* **45**: 863–874.

Arnould, C., C. Malosse, J.-P. Signoret, and C. Descoins. (1998). Which chemical constituents from dog feces are involved in its food repellent effect in sheep? *Journal of Chemical Ecology* **24**: 559–576.

Asa, C. S. (1996). Hormonal and experiential factors in the expression of social and parental behavior in canids. In *Cooperative Breeding in Mammals*, J. A. French and N. G. Solomon (eds.). Cambridge: Cambridge University Press, pp. 129–149.

Asa, C. S. and C. Valdespino. (1998). Canid reproductive biology: an integration of proximate mechanisms and ultimate causes. *American Zoologist* **38**: 251–259.

Asa, C. S., E. K. Peterson, U. S. Seal, and L. D. Mech. (1985a). Deposition of anal-sac secretions by captive wolves (*Canis lupus*). *Journal of Mammalogy* **66**: 89–93.

Asa, C. S., L. D. Mech, and U. S. Seal. (1985b). The use of urine, faeces, and anal-gland secretions in scent marking by a captive wolf (*Canis lupus*) pack. *Animal Behaviour* **33**: 1034–1036.

Asa, C. S., U. S. Seal, E. D. Plotka, M. A. Letellier, and L. D. Mech. (1986). Effect of anosmia on reproduction in male and female wolves (*Canis lupus*). *Behavioral and Neural Biology* **46**: 272–284.

Asa, C. S., U. S. Seal, M. Letellier, E. D. Plotka, and E. K. Peterson. (1987). Pinealectomy or superior cervical ganglionectomy do not alter reproduction in the wolf (*Canis lupus*). *Biology of Reproduction* **37**: 14–21.

Asa, C. S., L. D. Mech, U. S. Seal, and E. D. Plotka. (1990). The influence of social and endocrine factors on urine-marking by captive wolves (*Canis lupus*). *Hormones and Behavior* **24**: 497–509.

Asa, C. S., J. E. Bauman, T. J. Coonan, and M. M. Gray. (2007). Evidence for induced estrus or ovulation in a canid, the island fox (*Urocyon littoralis*). *Journal of Mammalogy* **88**: 436–440.

Aspi, J., E. Roininen, M. Ruokonen, I. Kojola, and C. Vilà. (2006). Genetic diversity, population structure, effective population size and demographic history of the Finnish wolf population. *Molecular Ecology* **15**: 1561–1576.

Atkins, D. L. and L. S. Dillon. (1971). Evolution of the cerebellum in the genus *Canis*. *Journal of Mammalogy* **52**: 96–107.

Atoji, Y., Y. Suzuki, and M. Sugimura. (1988). Lectin histochemistry of the interdigital gland in the Japanese serow (*Capricornis crispus*) in winter. *Journal of Anatomy* **161**: 159–170.

Atwood, T. C. (2006). Behavioral interactions between coyotes, *Canis latrans*, and wolves, *Canis lupus*, at ungulate carcasses in southwestern Montana. *Western North American Naturalist* **66**: 390–394.

Atwood, T. C. and E. M. Gese. (2010). Importance of resource selection and social behavior to partitioning of hostile space by sympatric canids. *Journal of Mammalogy* **91**: 490–499.

August, P. V. and J. G. T. Anderson. (1987). Mammal sounds and motivation–structural rules: a test of the hypothesis. *Journal of Mammalogy* **68**: 1–9.

Ausband, D. E., J. Holyan, and C. Mack. (2009). Longevity and adaptability of a reintroduced gray wolf. *Northwestern Naturalist* **90**: 44–47.

Ausband, D. E., M. S. Mitchell, K. Doherty, P. Zager, C. M. Mack, and J. Holyan. (2010). Surveying predicted rendezvous sites to monitor gray wolf populations. *Journal of Wildlife Management* **74**: 1043–1049.

Ballard, W. B. (1982). Gray wolf–brown bear relationships in the Nelchina Basin of south-central Alaska. In *Wolves of the World: Perspectives of Behavior, Ecology, and Conservation*, F. H. Harrington and P. C. Paquet (eds.). Park Ridge, NJ: Noyes Publications, pp. 71–80.

Ballard, W. B., R. Farnell, and R. O. Stephenson. (1983). Long distance movement by gray wolves, *Canis lupus. Canadian Field-Naturalist* **97**: 333.

Ballard, W. B., J. W. Whitman, and C. L. Gardner. (1987). Ecology of an exploited wolf population in south-central Alaska. *Wildlife Monographs* (**98**): 54 pp.

Ballard, W. B., L. A. Ayres, C. L. Gardner, and J. W. Foster. (1991). Den site activity patterns of gray wolves, *Canis lupus*, in southcentral Alaska. *Canadian Field-Naturalist* **105**: 497–504.

Ballard, W. B., L. A. Ayres, P. R. Krausman, D. J. Reed, and S. G. Fancy. (1997). Ecology of wolves in relation to a migratory caribou herd in northwest Alaska. *Wildlife Monographs* (**135**): 47 pp.

Ballard, W. B., M. Edwards, S. G. Fancy, S. Boe, and P. R. Krausman. (1998). Comparison of VHF and satellite telemetry for estimating sizes of wolf territories in northwest Alaska. *Wildlife Society Bulletin* **26**: 823–829.

Bandyopadhyay, M. and J. Chattopadhyay. (2005). Ratio-dependent predator–prey model: effect of environmental fluctuation and stability. *Nonlinearity* **18**: 913–936.

Banfield, A. W. F. (1954). The role of ice in the distribution of mammals. *Journal of Mammalogy* **35**: 104–107.

Barja, I. (2009). Prey and prey-age preference by the Iberian wolf *Canis lupus signatus* in a multiple-prey ecosystem. *Wildlife Biology* **15**: 147–154.

Barja, I., F. Javier de Miguel, and F. Bárcena. (2004). The importance of crossroads in faecal marking behaviour of wolves (*Canis lupus*). *Naturwissenschaften* **91**: 489–492.

Barja, I., F. J. de Miguel, and F. Bárcena. (2005). Faecal marking behaviour of Iberian wolf [*sic*] in different zones of their territory. *Folia Zoologica* **54**: 21–29.

Barja, I., G. Silván, and J. C. Illera. (2008). Relationships between sex and stress hormone levels in feces and marking behavior in a wild population of Iberian wolves (*Canis lupus signatus*). *Journal of Chemical Ecology* **34**: 697–701.

Barja Nuñez, I. and F. Javier de Miguel. (2004). Variation in stimulus, seasonal context, and response to urine marks by captive Iberian wolves (*Canis lupus signatus*). *Acta Ethologica* **7**: 51–57.

Barnard, C. (1991). Kinship and social behaviour: the trouble with relatives. *Trends in Ecology and Evolution* **6**: 310–312.

Barrette, C. and F. Messier. (1980). Scent-marking in free-ranging coyotes. *Canis latrans. Animal Behaviour* **28**: 814–819.

Barton, N. H. and G. M. Hewitt. (1989). Adaptation, speciation and hybrid zones. *Nature* **341**: 497–503.

Batchelor, A., E. T. Bell, and D. W. Christie. (1972). Urinary oestrogen excretion in the beagle bitch. *British Veterinary Journal* **128**: 560–566.

Bate, D. M. A. (1942). The fossil mammals of Shukbah. *Proceedings of the Prehistoric Society* **8**: 15–20.

Baverstock, P. and B. Green. (1977). Water recycling in lactation. *Science* **187**: 657–658.

Beach, F. A. (1970). Coital behaviour in dogs. VIII. Social affinity, dominance and sexual preference in the bitch. *Behaviour* **36**: 131–147.

Beach, F. A. (1974). Effects of gonadal hormones on urinary behavior in dogs. *Physiology and Behavior* **12**: 1005–1013.

Beach, F. A. and R. W. Gilmore. (1949). Response of male dogs to urine from females in heat. *Journal of Mammalogy* **30**: 391–392.

Beach, F. A. and B. J. LeBoeuf [*sic*]. (1967). Coital behaviour in dogs. I. Preferential mating in the bitch. *Animal Behaviour* **15**: 546–558.

Beach, F. A. and A. Merari. (1968). Coital behavior in dogs, IV. Effects of progesterone in the bitch. *Proceedings of the National Academy of Sciences* **61**: 442–446.

Beauchamp, G. (2000). Individual differences in activity and exploration influence leadership in pairs of foraging zebra finches. *Behaviour* **137**: 301–314.

Beaver, B. V., M. Fischer, and C. E. Atkinson. (1992). Determination of favorite components of garbage by dogs. *Applied Animal Behaviour Science* **34**: 129–136.

Beck, A. M. (1971). The life and times of Shag, a feral dog in Baltimore. *Natural History Magazine* **80**: 58–65.

Beck, A. M. (1973). *The Ecology of Stray Dogs: A Study of Free-ranging Urban Animals.* Baltimore, MD: York Press, xiv + 98 pp.

Beck, A. M. (1975). The ecology of "feral" and free-roving dogs in Baltimore. In *The Wild Canids: Their Systematics, Behavioral Ecology and Evolution*, M. W. Fox (ed.). New York, NY: Van Nostrand Reinhold, pp. 380–390.

Bekoff, M. (1972). The development of social interaction, play, and metacommunication in mammals: an ethological perspective. *Quarterly Review of Biology* **47**: 412–434.

Bekoff, M. (1974). Social play in coyotes, wolves, and dogs. *Bioscience* **24**: 225–230.

Bekoff, M. (1979a). Scent-marking by free-ranging domestic dogs: olfactory and visual components. *Biology of Behavior* **4**: 123–139.

Bekoff, M. (1979b). Ground scratching by male domestic dogs: a composite signal. *Journal of Mammalogy* **60**: 847–848.

Bekoff, M. and M. C. Wells. (1981). Behavioural budgeting by wild coyotes: the influence of food resources and social organization. *Animal Behaviour* **29**: 794–801.

Bekoff, M. and M. C. Wells. (1986). Social ecology and behavior of coyotes. *Advances in the Study of Behavior* **16**: 251–338.

Belyaev, D. K., I. Z. Plyusnina, and L. N. Trut. (1985). Domestication in the silver fox (*Vulpes fulvus* Desm): changes in physiological boundaries of the sensitive period of primary socialization. *Applied Animal Behaviour Science* **13**: 359–370.

Benecke, N. (1987). Studies on early dog remains from northern Europe. *Journal of Archaeological Science* **14**: 31–49.

Benhamou, S. (1989). An olfactory orientation model for mammals' movements in their home ranges. *Journal of Theoretical Biology* **139**: 379–388.

Berg, I. A. (1944). Development of behavior: the micturition pattern in the dog. *Journal of Experimental Psychology* **34**: 343–368.

Berg, W. E. and D. W. Kuehn. (1982). Ecology of wolves in north-central Minnesota. In *Wolves of the World: Perspectives of Behavior, Ecology, and Conservation*, F. H. Harrington and P. C. Paquet (eds.). Park Ridge, NJ: Noyes Publications, pp. 4–11.

Berger, K. M. and E. M. Gese. (2007). Does interference competition with wolves limit the distribution and abundance of coyotes? *Journal of Animal Ecology* **76**: 1075–1085.

Bergerud, A. T. and J. P. Elliott. (1998). Wolf predation in a multiple-ungulate system in northern British Columbia. *Canadian Journal of Zoology* **76**: 1551–1569.

Berman, M. and I. Dunbar. (1983). The social behaviour of free-ranging suburban dogs. *Applied Animal Ethology* **10**: 5–17.

Bertorelle, G. and L. Excoffier. (1998). Inferring admixture proportions from molecular data. *Molecular Biology and Evolution* **15**: 1298–1311.

Bibikov, D. I. (1982). Wolf ecology and management in the USSR. In *Wolves of the World: Perspectives of Behavior, Ecology, and Conservation*, F. H. Harrington, and P. C. Paquet (eds.). Park Ridge, NJ: Noyes Publications, pp. 120–133.

Bino, R. (1996). Notes on behaviour of New Guinea singing dogs (*Canis lupus dingo*). *Science in New Guinea* **22**: 43–47.

Bjärvall, A. and E. Nilsson. (1976). Surplus-killing of reindeer by wolves. *Journal of Mammalogy* **57**: 585.

Bjärvall, A. and E. Isakson. (1982). Winter ecology of a pack of three wolves in northern Sweden. In *Wolves of the World: Perspectives of Behavior, Ecology, and Conservation*, F. H. Harrington and P. C. Paquet (eds.). Park Ridge, NJ: Noyes Publications, pp. 146–157.

Black, J. D. (1936). Mammals of northwestern Arkansas. *Journal of Mammalogy* **17**: 29–35.

Blanco, J. C., S. Reig, and L. de la Cuesta. (1992). Distribution, status and conservation problems of the wolf *Canis lupus* in Spain. *Biological Conservation* **60**: 73–80.

Bleicher, N. (1963). Physical and behavioral analysis of dog vocalizations. *American Journal of Veterinary Research* **24**: 415–427.

Boehm, T. and F. Zufall. (2006). MHC peptides and the sensory evaluation of genotype. *Trends in Neurosciences* **29**: 100–107.

Boehrer, B. (1999). Shylock and the rise of the household pet: thinking social exclusion in *The Merchant of Venice*. *Shakespeare Quarterly* **50**: 152–170.

Boggess, E. K., R. D. Andrews, and R. A. Bishop. (1978). Domestic animal losses to coyotes and dogs in Iowa. *Journal of Wildlife Management* **42**: 362–372.

Boisjoly, D., J.-P. Ouellet, and R. Courtois. (2010). Coyote habitat selection and management implications for the Gaspésie caribou. *Journal of Wildlife Management* **74**: 3–11.

Boitani, L. (1982). Wolf management in intensively used areas of Italy. In *Wolves of the World: Perspectives of Behavior, Ecology, and Conservation*, F. H. Harrington and P. C. Paquet (eds.). Park Ridge, NJ: Noyes Publications, pp. 158–172.

Boitani, L. (1992). Wolf research and conservation in Italy. *Biological Conservation* **61**: 125–132.

Boitani, L. and P. Ciucci. (1995). Comparative social ecology of feral dogs and wolves. *Ethology Ecology and Evolution* **7**: 49–72.

Boland, C. R. J., R. Heinsohn, and A. Cockburn. (1997). Deception by helpers in cooperatively breeding white-winged choughs and its experimental manipulation. *Behavioral Ecology and Sociobiology* **41**: 251–256.

Bonanni, R., P. Valsecchi, and E. Natoli. (2010a.) Pattern of individual participation and cheating in conflicts between groups of free-ranging dogs. *Animal Behaviour* **79**: 957–968.

Bonanni, R., S. Cafazzo, P. Valsecchi, and E. Natoli. (2010b). Effect of affiliative and agonistic relationships on leadership behaviour in free-ranging dogs. *Animal Behaviour* **79**: 981–991.

Bond, R. M. (1939). Coyote food habits on the Lava Beds National Monument. *Journal of Wildlife Management* **3**: 180–198.

Bourke, J., S. Wroe, K. Moreno, C. McHenry, and P. Clausen. (2008). Effects of gape and tooth position on bite force and skull stress in the dingo (*Canis lupus dingo*) using a 3-dimensional finite element approach. *PLoS One* **3**: e2200.

Bowen, W. D. (1981). Variation in coyote social organization: the influence of prey size. *Canadian Journal of Zoology* **59**: 639–652.

Boyd, D. K. and M. D. Jimenez. (1994). Successful rearing of young by wild wolves without mates. *Journal of Mammalogy* **75**: 14–17.

Boyd, D. K. and D. H. Pletscher. (1999). Characteristics of dispersal in a colonizing wolf population in the central Rocky Mountains. *Journal of Wildlife Management* **63**: 1094–1108.

Boyko, A. R., R. H. Boyko, C. M. Boyko, H. G. Parker, M. Castelhano, and L. Corey *et al.* (2009). Complex population structure in African village dogs and its implications for inferring dog domestication history. *Proceedings of the National Academy of Sciences* **106**: 13 903–13 908.

Boyko, A. R., P. Quignon, L. Li, J. J. Schoenebeck, J. D. Degenhardt, and K. E. Lohmueller *et al.* (2010). A simple genetic architecture underlies morphological variation in dogs. *PLoS Biology* **8**: e1000451.

Brand Miller, J. C. B. and S. Colagiuri. (1994). The carnivore connection: dietary carbohydrate in the evolution of NIDDM. *Diabetologia* **37**: 1280–1286.

Brewster, W. G. and S. H. Fritts. 1995. Taxonomy and genetics of the gray wolf in western North America: a review. In *Ecology and Conservation of Wolves in a Changing World*, Occasional Publication No. 35, L. N. Carbyn, S. H. Fritts, and D. R. Seip (eds.). Edmonton, AB: Canadian Circumpolar Institute, pp. 353–373.

Brisbin, I. L. Jr. and S. N. Austad. (1991). Testing the individual odour theory of canine olfaction. *Animal Behaviour* **42**: 63–69.

Briscoe, B. K., M. A. Lewis, and S. E. Parrish. (2002). Home range formation in wolves due to scent marking. *Bulletin of Mathematical Biology* **64**: 261–284.

Broad, K. D., J. P. Curley, and E. B. Keverne. (2006). Mother–infant bonding and the evolution of mammalian social relationships. *Philosophical Transactions of the Royal Society* **361B**: 2199–2214.

Brodbeck, A. J. (1954). An exploratory study on the acquisition of dependency behavior in puppies. *Bulletin of the Ecological Society of America* **35**: 73. [Abstract]

Broom, M., A. Koenig, and C. Borries. (2009). Variation in dominance hierarchies among group-living animals: modeling stability and the likelihood of coalitions. *Behavioral Ecology* **20**: 844–855.

Brouette-Lahlou, I., F. Godinot, and E. Vernet-Maury. (1999). The mother rat's vomeronasal organ is involved in detection of dodecyl proprinate, the pup's preputial gland pheromone. *Physiology and Behavior* **66**: 427–436.

Brown, C. E. (1936). Rearing wild animals in captivity, and gestation periods. *Journal of Mammalogy* **17**: 10–13.

Brown, N. R. and R. G. Lanning. (1954). The mammals of Renfrew County, Ontario. *Canadian Field-Naturalist* **68**: 171–180.

Brownlee, R.G., R.M. Silverstein, D. Müller-Schwarze, and A.G. Singer. (1969). Isolation, identification and function of the chief component of the male tarsal scent in black-tailed deer. *Nature* **221**: 284–285.

Brownlow, C.A. (1996). Molecular taxonomy and the conservation of the red wolf and other endangered carnivores. *Conservation Biology* **10**: 390–396.

Brummett, P. (1995). Dogs, women, cholera, and other menaces in the streets: cartoon satire in the Ottoman revolutionary press, 1908–11. *International Journal of Middle East Studies* **27**: 433–460.

Brundin, A. and G. Andersson. (1979). Seasonal variation of three ketones in the interdigital gland secretion of reindeer (*Rangifer tarandus* L.). *Journal of Chemical Ecology* **5**: 881–889.

Brundin, A., G. Andersson, K. Andersson, T. Mossing, and L. Källquist. (1978). Short-chain aliphatic acids in the interdigital gland secretion of reindeer (*Rangifer tarandus* L.), and their discrimination by reindeer. *Journal of Chemical Ecology* **4**: 613–622.

Buck, L.B. (2000). The molecular architecture of odor and pheromone sensing in mammals. *Cell* **100**: 611–618.

Buck, L.B. (2004). Olfactory receptors and odor coding in mammals. *Nutrition Reviews* **62**: S184-S188.

Buck, L.B. and R. Axel. (1991). A novel multigene family may encode odorant receptors: a molecular basis for odor recognition. *Cell* **65**: 175–187.

Burghardt, G.M. (2005). *The Genesis of Animal Play: Testing the Limits*. Cambridge, MA: MIT Press, xvi + 501 pp.

Burkholder, B.L. (1959). Movements and behavior of a wolf pack in Alaska. *Journal of Wildlife Management* **23**: 1–11.

Burt, W.H. (1943). Territoriality and home range concepts as applied to mammals. *Journal of Mammalogy* **24**: 346–352.

Butler, D. (1994). Bid to protect wolves from genetic pollution. *Nature* **370**: 497.

Butler, J.R.A., J.T. du Toit, and J. Bingham. (2004). Free-ranging domestic dogs (*Canis familiaris*) as predators and prey in rural Zimbabwe: threats of competition and disease to large wild carnivores. *Biological Conservation* **115**: 369–378.

Cadieu, E., M.W. Neff, P. Quignon, K. Walsh, K. Chase, and H.G. Parker *et al.* (2009). Coat variation in the domestic dog is governed by variants in three genes. *Science* **326**: 150–153.

Campos, C.B., C.F. Esteves, K.M.P.M.B. Ferraz, P.G. Crawshaw Jr., and L.M. Verdade. (2007). Diet of free-ranging cats and dogs in a suburban and rural environment, south-eastern Brazil. *Journal of Zoology (London)* **273**: 14–20.

Capello, L., D. Roppolo, V.P. Jungo, P. Feinstein, and I. Rodriguez. (2009). A common gene exclusion mechanism used by two chemosensory systems. *European Journal of Neuroscience* **29**: 671–678.

Carazo, P. and E. Font. (2010). Putting information back into biological communication. *Journal of Evolutionary Biology* **23**: 661–669.

Carbone, C., G.M. Mace, S.C. Roberts, and D.W. Macdonald. (1999). Energetic constraints on the diet of terrestrial carnivores. *Nature* **402**: 286–288.

Carbyn, L.N. (1982). Coyote population fluctuations and spatial distribution in relation to wolf territories in Riding Mountain National Park, Manitoba. *Canadian Field-Naturalist* **96**: 176–183.

Carbyn, L.N. (1983). Wolf predation on elk in Riding Mountain National Park, Manitoba. *Journal of Wildlife Management* **47**: 963–976.

Careau, V., J. Morand-Ferron, and D. Thomas. (2007). Basal metabolic rate of Canidae from hot deserts to cold arctic climates. *Journal of Mammalogy* **88**: 394–400.

Carmichael, L. E., J. A. Nagy, N. C. Larter, and C. Strobeck. (2001). Prey specialization may influence patterns of gene flow in wolves of the Canadian Northwest. *Molecular Ecology* **10**: 2787–2798.

Caro, T. M. and M. D. Hauser. (1992). Is there teaching in nonhuman animals? *Quarterly Review of Biology* **67**: 151–174.

Carrera, R., W. Ballard, P. Gipson, B. T. Kelly, P. R. Krausman, and M. C. Wallace *et al.* (2008). Comparison of Mexican wolf and coyote diets in Arizona and New Mexico. *Journal of Wildlife Management* **72**: 376–381.

Carroll, J. F. (2001). Interdigital gland substances of white-tailed deer and the response of host-seeking ticks (Acari: Ixodidae). *Journal of Medical Entomology* **38**: 114–117.

Catling, P. C., L. K. Corbett, and A. E. Newsome. (1992). Reproduction in captive and wild dingoes (*Canis familiaris dingo*) in temperate and arid environments of Australia. *Wildlife Research* **19**: 195–209.

Causey, M. K. and C. A. Cude. (1980). Feral dog and white-tailed deer interactions in Alabama. *Journal of Wildlife Management* **44**: 481–484.

Ceacero, F., T. Landete-Castillejos, A. J. García, J. A. Estévez, and L. Gallego. (2007). Kinship discrimination and effects on social rank and aggressiveness levels in Iberian red deer hinds. *Ethology* **113**: 1133–1140.

Chabot, D., P. Gagnon, and E. A. Dixon. (1996). Effect of predator odors on heart rate and metabolic rate of wapiti (*Cervus elaphus canadensis*). *Journal of Chemical Ecology* **22**: 839–868.

Chambers, R. E. (1992). Reproduction of coyotes in their northeastern range. In *Ecology and Management of the Eastern Coyote*, A. H. Boer (ed.). Fredericton, NB: Wildlife Research Unit, University of New Brunswick, pp. 39–52.

Chapais, B., C. Gauthier, J. Prud'homme, and P. Vasey. (1997). Relatedness threshold for nepotism in Japanese macaques. *Animal Behaviour* **53**: 1089–1101.

Chapais, B., L. Savard, and C. Gauthier. (2001). Kin selection and the distribution of altruism in relation to degree of kinship in Japanese macaques (*Macaca fuscata*). *Behavioral Ecology and Sociobiology* **49**: 493–502.

Chapman, D. M. (1985). Histology of moose (*Alces alces andersoni*) interdigital glands and associated green hairs. *Canadian Journal of Zoology* **63**: 899–911.

Cheney, D. and R. Seyfarth. (1990). Attending to behaviour versus attending to knowledge: examining monkeys' attribution of mental states. *Animal Behaviour* **40**: 742–753.

Cheney, D. L., R. M. Seyfarth, and R. Palombit. (1996). The function and mechanisms underlying baboon "contact" barks. *Animal Behaviour* **52**: 507–518.

Choudhuri, D. K., B. Ghosh, and B. Pal. (1984). Studies on the territoriality and home range size of some urban and rural stray dogs. *Burdwan University Journal of Science* **1**: 57–61.

Christie, D. W. and E. T. Bell. (1971). Some observations of the seasonal incidence and frequency of oestrus in breeding bitches in Britain. *Journal of Small Animal Practice* **12**: 159–167.

Ciucci, P., W. Reggioni, L. Maiorano, and L. Boitani. (2009). Long-distance dispersal of a rescued wolf from the northern Apennines to the western Alps. *Journal of Wildlife Management* **73**: 1300–1306.

Claridge, A. W., D. J. Mills, R. Hunt, D. J. Jenkins, and J. Bean. (2009). Satellite tracking of wild dogs in south-eastern mainland Australian forests: implications for management of a problematic top-order carnivore. *Forest Ecology and Management* **258**: 814–822.

Clutton-Brock, J. (1995). Origins of the dog: domestication and early history. In *The Domestic Dog: Its Evolution, Behaviour and Interactions with People*, J. Serpell (ed.). Cambridge: Cambridge University Press, pp. 7–20.

Clutton-Brock, T.H., D. Gaynor, R. Kansky, A.D.C. MacColl, G. Mclrath, and P. Chadwick *et al.* (1998). Costs of cooperative behaviour in suricates (*Suricata suricatta*). *Proceedings of the Royal Society of London* **265B**: 185–190.

Clutton-Brock, T.H., P.N.M. Brotherton, M.J. O'Riain, A.S. Griffin, D. Gaynor, and L. Sharpe *et al.* (2000). Individual contributions to babysitting in a cooperative mongoose, *Suricata suricatta*. *Proceedings of the Royal Society of London* **267B**: 301–305.

Clutton-Brock, T.H., P.N.M. Brotherton, M.J. O'Riain, A.S. Griffin, D. Gaynor, and R. Kansky *et al.* (2001). Contribution to cooperative rearing in meerkats. *Animal Behaviour* **61**: 705–710.

Cohen, J.A. and M.W. Fox. (1976). Vocalizations in wild canids and possible effects of domestication. *Behavioural Processes* **1**: 77–92.

Concannon, P. (1980). Effects of hypophysectomy and of LH administration on luteal phase plasma progesterone levels in the beagle bitch. *Journal of Reproduction and Fertility* **58**: 407–410.

Concannon, P., W. Hansel, and K. McEntee. (1977a). Changes in LH, progesterone and sexual behavior associated with preovulatory luteinization in the bitch. *Biology of Reproduction* **17**: 604–613.

Concannon, P., M.E. Powers, W. Holder, and W. Hansel. (1977b). Pregnancy and parturition in the bitch. *Biology of Reproduction* **16**: 517–526.

Concannon, P., R. Cowan, and W. Hansel. (1979a). LH release in ovariectomized dogs in response to estrogen withdrawal and its facilitation by progesterone. *Biology of Reproduction* **20**: 523–531.

Concannon, P.W. (1993). Biology of gonadotropin secretion in adult and prepubertal female dogs. *Journal of Reproduction and Fertility* (Suppl.) **47**: 3–27.

Concannon, P.W. (2009). Endocrinologic control of normal canine ovarian function. *Reproduction in Domestic Animals* **44** (Suppl. 2): 3–15.

Concannon, P.W. and V.D. Castracane. (1985). Serum androstenedione and testosterone concentrations during pregnancy and nonpregnant cycles in dogs. *Biology of Reproduction* **33**: 1078–1083.

Concannon, P.W., W. Hansel, and W.J. Visek. (1975). The ovarian cycle of the bitch: plasma estrogen, LH and progesterone. *Biology of Reproduction* **13**: 112–121.

Concannon, P.W., W.R. Butler, W. Hansel, P.J. Knight, and J.M. Hamilton. (1978). Parturition and lactation in the bitch: serum progesterone, cortisol and prolactin. *Biology of Reproduction* **19**: 1113–1118.

Concannon, P.W., N. Weigand, S. Wilson, and W. Hansel. (1979b). Sexual behavior in ovariectomized bitches in response to estrogen and progesterone treatment. *Biology of Reproduction* **20**: 799–809.

Concannon, P.W., J.P. McCann, and M. Temple. (1989). Biology and endocrinology of ovulation, pregnancy and parturition in the dog. *Journal of Reproduction and Fertility* (Suppl.) **38**: 3–25.

Concannon, P.W., M. Temple, A. Montanez, and D. Frank. (1993). Synchronous delayed oestrus in beagle bitches given infusions of gonadotrophin-releasing hormone super-agonist following withdrawal of progesterone implants. *Journal of Reproduction and Fertility* (Suppl.) **47**: 522–523.

Connolly, G. E. and W. M. Longhurst. (1975). The effects of control on coyote populations: a simulation model. Bulletin No. 1872, Division of Agricultural Sciences. Berkeley, CA: University of California, 37 pp.

Connolly, G. E., R. M. Timm, W. E. Howard, and W. M. Longhurst. (1976). Sheep killing behavior of captive coyotes. *Journal of Wildlife Management* **40**: 400–407.

Conradt, L. and T. J. Roper. (2005). Consensus decision making in animals. *Trends in Ecology and Evolution* **20**: 449–456.

Cook, R. [R. C.] (1952). The coy-dog: hybrid with a future? *Journal of Heredity* **43**: 71–73.

Coon, C. S. (1951). *Cave Explorations in Iran 1949, Museum Monographs, The University Museum*. Philadelphia, PA: University of Pennsylvania, 125 pp.

Coppinger, R. and R. Schneider. (1995). Evolution of working dogs. In *The Domestic Dog: Its Evolution, Behaviour, and Interactions with People*, J. Serpell (ed.). Cambridge: Cambridge University Press, pp. 21–47.

Coppinger, R. and L. Coppinger. (2001). *Dogs: A Startling New Understanding of Canine Origin, Behavior, and Evolution*. New York, NY: Scribner, 352 pp.

Corbett, L. and A. Newsome. (1975). Dingo society and its maintenance: a preliminary analysis. In *The Wild Canids: Their Systematics, Behavioral Ecology and Evolution*, M. W. Fox (ed.). New York, NY: Van Nostrand Reinhold, pp. 369–379.

Corbett, L. K. (1985). Morphological comparisons of Australian and Thai dingoes: a reappraisal of dingo status, distribution and ancestry. *Proceedings of the Ecological Society of Australia* **13**: 277–291.

Corbett, L. K. (1988). Social dynamics of a captive dingo pack: population regulation by dominant female infanticide. *Ethology* **78**: 177–198.

Corbett, L. K. (1989). Assessing the diet of dingoes from feces: a comparison of 3 methods. *Journal of Wildlife Management* **53**: 343–346.

Corbett, L. K. (1995). *The Dingo in Australia and Asia*. Ithaca, NY: Comstock/Cornell University Press, viii + 200 pp.

Corbett, L. K. and A. E. Newsome. (1987). The feeding ecology of the dingo. III. Dietary relationships with widely fluctuating prey populations in arid Australia: an hypothesis of alternation of predation. *Oecologia* **74**: 215–227.

Cordero-Fernando, G. (1977). The Philippine aso: life and hard times of an underdog. *Filipino Heritage* **2**: 414–420.

Cordy-Collins, A. (1994). An unshaggy dog story. *Natural History Magazine* **103**(2): 34–40.

Coscia, E. M., D. P. Phillips, and J. C. Fentress. (1991). Spectral analysis of neonatal wolf *Canis lupus* vocalizations. *Bioacoustics* **3**: 275–293.

Courchamp, F., F. Clutton-Brock, and B. Grenfell. (1999). Inverse density dependence and the Allee effect. *Trends in Ecology and Evolution* **14**: 405–410.

Cowan, I. M. (1947). The timber wolf in the Rocky Mountain national parks of Canada. *Canadian Journal of Research* **25**: 139–174.

Crabtree, R. L. and J. W. Sheldon. (1999). The ecological role of coyotes on Yellowstone's northern range. *Yellowstone Science* **7**(2): 15–23.

Crandall, L. S. (1964). *The Management of Wild Mammals in Captivity*. Chicago, IL: University of Chicago Press, xv + 769 pp.

Creel, S. (1997). Cooperative hunting and group size: assumptions and currencies. *Animal Behaviour* **54**: 1319–1324.

Creel, S. (2005). Dominance, aggression, and glucocorticoid levels in social carnivores. *Journal of Mammalogy* **86**: 255–264.

Creel, S., N. M. Creel, and S. L. Monfort. (1996). Social stress and dominance. *Nature* **379**: 212.

Crisler, L. (1956). Observations of wolves hunting caribou. *Journal of Mammalogy* **37**: 337–346.

Crisler, L. (1958). *Arctic Wild*. New York, NY: Harper Perennial, xviii + 301 pp. [1973 paperback edition. New York, NY: Harper and Row.]

Critchell-Bullock, J. C. (1930). An expedition to sub-arctic Canada, 1924–1925. *Canadian Field-Naturalist* **44**: 156–157, 207–213.

Csibra, G. (2008). Goal attribution to inanimate agents by 6.5-month-old infants. *Cognition* **107**: 705–717.

Dale, B. W., L. G. Adams, and R. T. Bowyer. (1994). Functional response of wolves preying on barren-ground caribou in a multiple-prey ecosystem. *Journal of Animal Ecology* **63**: 644–652.

Dale, B. W., L. G. Adams, and R. T. Bowyer. (1995). Winter wolf predation in a multiple ungulate prey system, Gates of the Arctic National Park, Alaska. In *Ecology and Conservation of Wolves in a Changing World*, Occasional Publication No. 35, L. N. Carbyn, S. H. Fritts, and D. R. Seip (eds.). Edmonton, AB: Canadian Circumpolar Institute, pp. 223–230.

Daniels, M. J. and L. Corbett. (2003). Redefining introgressed protected mammals: when is a wildcat a wild cat and a dingo a wild dog? *Wildlife Research* **30**: 213–218.

Daniels, T. J. (1983a). The social organization of free-ranging urban dogs. I. Non-estrous social behavior. *Applied Animal Ethology* **10**: 341–363.

Daniels, T. J. (1983b). The social organization of free-ranging urban dogs. II. Estrous groups and the mating system. *Applied Animal Ethology* **10**: 365–373.

Daniels, T. J. (1987). Conspecific scavenging by a young domestic dog. *Journal of Mammalogy* **68**: 416–418.

Daniels, T. J. and M. Bekoff. (1989a.) Spatial and temporal resource use by feral and abandoned dogs. *Ethology* **81**: 300–312.

Daniels, T. J. and M. Bekoff. (1989b.) Population and social biology of free-ranging dogs, *Canis familiaris. Journal of Mammalogy* **70**: 754–762.

Daniels, T. J. and M. Bekoff. (1989c). Ferilization: the making of wild domestic animals. *Behavioural Processes* **19**: 79–94.

Darimont, C. T., P. C. Paquet, and T. E. Reimchen. (2008). Spawning salmon disrupt trophic coupling between wolves and ungulate prey in coastal British Columbia. *BMC Ecology* **8**: 14.

Darwin, C. (1897). *The Variation of Animals and Plants Under Domestication*, Vol. 1, 2nd edn. New York, NY: D. Appleton, xiv + 473 pp.

Darwin, C. (1998). *The Expression of the Emotions in Man and Animals*, 3rd edn. New York, NY: Oxford University Press, xxxvi + 473 pp. [1st and 2nd editions published in 1872 and 1889 by John Murray, London.]

Davis, S. J. M. and F. R. Valla. (1978). Evidence for domestication of the dog 12,000 years ago in the Natufian of Israel. *Nature* **276**: 608–610.

Dawes, P. R., M. Elander, and M. Ericson. (1986). The wolf (*Canis lupus*) in Greenland: a historical review and present status. *Arctic* **39**: 119–132.

Dayan, T. (1994). Early domesticated dogs of the Near East. *Journal of Archaeological Science* **21**: 633–640.

Dayton, L. (2003). On the trail of the first dingo. *Science* **302**: 555–556.

de Gier, J., H. S. Kooistra, S. C. Djajadiningrat-Laanen, S. J. Dieleman, and A. C. Okkens. (2006). Temporal relations between plasma concentrations of luteinizing hormone, follicle-stimulating hormone, estradiol-17β, progesterone, prolactin, and β-melanocyte-stimulating hormone during the follicular, ovulatory, and early luteal phase in the bitch. *Theriogenology* **65**: 1346–1359.

de Vos, A. (1949). Timber wolves (*Canis lupus lycaon*) killed by cars on Ontario highways. *Journal of Mammalogy* **30**: 197.

de Vos, A. (1950). Timber wolf movements on Sibley Peninsula, Ontario. *Journal of Mammalogy* **31**: 169–175.

de Waal, F. B. M. (1989). Dominance 'style' and primate social organization. In *Comparative Socioecology: The Behavioural Ecology of Humans and Other Mammals*, V. Staden and R. A. Foley (eds.). Oxford: Blackwell Scientific, pp. 243–263.

Deeb, B. J. and N. S. Wolf. (1994). Studying longevity and morbidity in giant and small breeds of dogs. *Veterinary Medicine* **89** (Suppl.): 702–713.

Degerbøl, M. (1961). On a find of a preboreal domestic dog (*Canis familiaris* L.) from Star Carr, Yorkshire, with remarks on other Mesolithic dogs. *Proceedings of the Prehistoric Society* **3**: 35–55.

DeMatteo, K. E., I. J. Porton, D. G. Kleiman, and C. S. Asa. (2006). The effect of the male bush dog (*Speothos venaticus*) on the female reproductive cycle. *Journal of Mammalogy* **87**: 723–732.

Dennis, J. C., J. G. Allgier, L. S. Desouza, W. C. Edward, and E. E. Morrison. (2003). Immunohistochemistry of the canine vomeronasal organ. *Journal of Anatomy* **203**: 329–338.

Denny, R. N. (1974). The impact of uncontrolled dogs on wildlife and livestock. *Transactions of the North American Natural Resources Conference* **39**: 257–291.

Derix, R., J. van Hooff, H. de Vries, and J. Wensing. (1993). Male and female mating competition in wolves: female suppression vs. male intervention. *Behaviour* **127**: 141–174.

Detry, C. and J. L. Cardosa. (2010). On some remains of dog (*Canis familiaris*) from the Mesolithic shell-middens of Muge, Portugal. *Journal of Archaeological Science* **37**: 2762–2774.

Dice, L. R. (1942). A family of dog–coyote hybrids. *Journal of Mammalogy* **23**: 186–192.

Doak, R. L., A. Hall, and H. E. Dale. (1967). Longevity of spermatozoa in the reproductive tract of the bitch. *Journal of Reproduction and Fertility* **13**: 51–58.

Doty, R. L. 2010. *The Great Pheromone Myth*. Baltimore, MD: Johns Hopkins University Press, xi + 278 pp.

Doty, R. L. and I. Dunbar. (1974). Attraction of beagles to conspecific urine, vaginal and anal sac secretion odors. *Physiology and Behavior* **12**: 825–833.

Dragoo, J. W. and R. L. Honeycutt. (1997). Systematics of mustelid-like carnivores. *Journal of Mammalogy* **78**: 426–443.

Drews, D. R. (1973). Group formation in captive *Galago crassicaudatus*: notes on the dominance concept. *Zeitschrift für Tierpsychologie* **32**: 425–435.

Driscoll, C. A. and D. W. Macdonald. (2010). Top dogs: wolf domestication and wealth. *Journal of Biology* **9**: 10.

Drummond, H. (2006). Dominance in vertebrate broods and litters. *Quarterly Review of Biology* **81**: 3–32.

Dugatkin, L. A., M. Perlin, and R. Atlas. (2003). The evolution of group-beneficial traits in the absence of between-group selection. *Journal of Theoretical Biology* **220**: 67–74.

Dulac, C. and R. Axel. (1995). A novel family of genes encoding putative pheromone receptors in mammals. *Cell* **83**: 195–206.

Dunbar, I. and M. Buehler. (1980). A masking effect of urine from male dogs. *Applied Animal Ethology* **6**: 297–301.

Dunbar, I., E. Ransom, and M. Buehler. (1981). Pup retrieval and maternal attraction to canine amniotic fluids. *Behavioural Processes* **6**: 249–260.

Dunbar, I. F. (1977). Olfactory preferences in dogs: the response of male and female beagles to conspecific odors. *Behavioral Biology* **20**: 471–481.

Dunne, A. L. (1939). Report on wolves followed during February and March, 1939. *Canadian Field-Naturalist* **53**: 117–118.

Durbin, L. S. (1998). Individuality in the whistle call of the Asiatic wild dog *Cuon alpinus*. *Bioacoustics* **9**: 197–206.

Eide, S. H. and W. B. Ballard. (1982). Apparent case of surplus killing of caribou by gray wolves. *Canadian Field-Naturalist* **96**: 87–88.

Ekman, J., A. Brodin, A. Bylin, and B. Sklepkovych. (1996). Selfish long-term benefits of hoarding in the Siberian jay. *Behavioral Ecology* **7**: 140–144.

Elgin, C. Z. (1983). *With Reference to Reference*. Indianapolis, IN: Hackett Publishing, viii + 200 pp.

Elledge, A. E., L. R. Allen, B-L. Carlsson, A. N. Wilton, and L. K-P. Leung. (2008). An evaluation of genetic analyses, skull morphology and visual appearance for assessing dingo purity: implications for dingo conservation. *Wildlife Research* **35**: 812–820.

Ellegren, H. (1999). Inbreeding and relatedness in Scandinavian grey wolves *Canis lupus*. *Hereditas* **130**: 239–244.

Ellegren, H., P. Savolainen, and B. Rosén. (1996). The genetical history of an isolated population of the endangered grey wolf *Canis lupus*: a study of nuclear and mitochondrial polymorphisms. *Philosophical Transactions of the Royal Society of London* **351B**: 1661–1669.

Elliot, O. and J. A. King. (1960). Effect of early food deprivation upon later consummatory behavior in puppies. *Psychological Reports* **6**: 391–400.

Engle, E. T. (1946). No seasonal breeding cycle in dogs. *Journal of Mammalogy* **27**: 79–81.

Erhart, E. M. and D. J. Overdorff. (1999). Female coordination of group travel in wild *Propithecus* and *Eulemur*. *International Journal of Primatology* **20**: 927–940.

Escós, J., C. L. Alados, and J. Boza. (1993). Leadership in a domestic goat herd. *Applied Animal Behaviour Science* **38**: 41–47.

Estes, R. D. and J. Goddard. (1967). Prey selection and hunting behavior of the African wild dog. *Journal of Wildlife Management* **31**: 52–70.

Evans, E. I. (1933). The transport of spermatozoa in the dog. *American Journal of Physiology* **105**: 287–293.

Evans, H. M. and H. H. Cole. (1931). An introduction to the study of the oestrous cycle in the dog. *Memoirs of the University of California* **9**(2): viii + 65–118.

Fain, S. R., D. J. Straughan, and B. F. Taylor. (2010). Genetic outcomes of wolf recovery in the western Great Lakes. *Conservation Genetics* **11**: 1747–1765.

Fanshawe, J. H. and C. D. FitzGibbon. (1993). Factors influencing the hunting success of an African wild dog pack. *Animal Behaviour* **45**: 479–490.

Faragó, T., P. Pongrácz, F. Range, Z. Virányi, and Á. Miklósi. (2010). 'The Bone is mine': affective and referential aspects of dog growls. *Animal Behaviour* **79**: 917–925.

Fatjó, J., D. Feddersen-Petersen, J. L. Ruiz de la Tore, M. Amat, M. Mets, and B. Braus *et al.* (2007). Ambivalent signals during agonistic interactions in a captive wolf pack. *Applied Animal Behaviour Science* **105**: 274–283.

Feddersen-Petersen, D. U. (2000). Vocalization of European wolves (*Canis lupus lupus* L.) and various dog breeds (*Canis lupus* f. fam.). *Archiv für Tierzucht* **43**: 387–397.

Fener, H. M., J. R. Ginsberg, E. W. Sanderson, and M. E. Gompper. (2005). Chronology of range expansion of the coyote, *Canis latrans*, in New York. *Canadian Field-Naturalist* **119**: 1–5.

Fentress, J. C. (1967). Observations on the behavioral development of a hand-reared male timber wolf. *American Zoologist* **7**: 339–351.

Fentress, J. C. and J. Ryon. (1982). A long-term study of distributed pup feeding in captive wolves. In *Wolves of the World: Perspectives of Behavior, Ecology, and Conservation*, F. H. Harrington and P. C. Paquet (eds.). Park Ridge, NJ: Noyes Publications, pp. 238–261.

Fernandes, P. A., R. A. Bowen, A. C. Kostas, H. R. Sawyer, T. M. Nett, and P. N. Olson. (1987). Luteal function in the bitch: changes during diestrus in pituitary concentration of and the number of luteal receptors for luteinizing hormone and prolactin. *Biology of Reproduction* **37**: 804–811.

Ferrero, D. M. and S. D. Liberles. (2010). The secret codes of mammalian scents. *Wiley Interdisciplinary Reviews: Systems Biology and Medicine* **2**: 23–33.

Finlayson, H. H. (1943). *The Red Centre: Man and Beast in the Heart of Australia*, 5th edn. Sydney: Angus and Robertson, 153 pp. + foldout map.

Fiorello, C., A. J. Noss, and S. L. Deem. (2006). Demography, hunting ecology, and pathogen exposure of domestic dogs in the Isoso of Bolivia. *Conservation Biology* **20**: 762–771.

Flagstad, Ø., C. W. Walker, C. Vilà, A.-K. Sundqvist, B. Fernholm, and A. K. Hufthammer *et al.* (2003). Two centuries of the Scandinavian wolf population: patterns of genetic variability and migration during an era of dramatic decline. *Molecular Ecology* **12**: 869–880.

Font, E. (1987). Spacing and social organization: urban stray dogs revisited. *Applied Animal Behaviour Science* **17**: 319–328.

Font, E. and P. Carazo. (2010). Animals in translation: why there is meaning (but probably no message) in animal communication. *Animal Behaviour* **80**(2): e1–e6.

Forbes, G. J. and J. B. Theberge. (1995). Influences of a migratory deer herd on wolf movements and mortality in and near Algonquin Park, Ontario. In *Ecology and Conservation of Wolves in a Changing World*, Occasional Publication No. 35, L. N. Carbyn, S. H. Fritts, and D. R. Seip (eds.). Edmonton, AB: Canadian Circumpolar Institute, pp. 303–313.

Forbes, L. S. (1989). Prey defences and predator handling behaviour: the dangerous prey hypothesis. *Oikos* **55**: 155–158.

Fox, J. L. and R. S. Chundawat. (1995). Wolves in the transhimalayan region of India: the continued survival of a low-density population. In *Ecology and Conservation of Wolves in a Changing World*, Occasional Publication No. 35, L. N. Carbyn, S. H. Fritts, and D. R. Seip (eds.). Edmonton, AB: Canadian Circumpolar Institute, pp. 95–103.

Fox, M. W. (1969a.) The anatomy of aggression and its ritualization in Canidae: a developmental and comparative study. *Behaviour* **35**: 242–258.

Fox, M. W. (1969b). Ontogeny of prey-killing behavior in Canidae. *Behaviour* **35**: 259–272.

Fox, M. W. (1969c). Behavioral effects of rearing dogs with cats during the 'critical period of socialization.' *Behaviour* **35**: 273–280.

Fox, M. W. (1970). A comparative study of the development of facial expressions in canids; wolf, coyote and foxes. *Behaviour* **36**: 49–73.

Fox, M. W. (1971a). Socio-infantile and socio-sexual signals in canids: a comparative and ontogenetic study. *Zeitschrift für Tierpsychologie* **28**: 185–210.

Fox, M. W. (1971b). *Behaviour of Wolves, Dogs and Related Canids*. New York, NY: Harper and Row, 220 pp.

Fox, M. W. (1972a). Socio-ecological implications of individual differences in wolf litters: a developmental and evolutionary perspective. *Behaviour* **41**: 298–313.

Fox, M. W. (1972b.) The social significance of genital licking in the wolf, *Canis lupus*. *Journal of Mammalogy* **53**: 637–640.

Fox, M. W. (1973). Social dynamics of three captive wolf packs. *Behaviour* **47**: 290–301.

Fox, M. W. (1975). Evolution of social behavior in canids. In *The Wild Canids: Their Systematics, Behavioral Ecology and Evolution*, M. W. Fox (ed.). New York, NY: Van Nostrand Reinhold, pp. 429–460.

Fox, M. W. (1984). *The Whistling Hunters: Field Studies of the Asiatic Wild Dog (Cuon alpinus)*. Albany, NY: State University of New York Press, viii + 150 pp.

Fox, M. W. and J. A. Cohen (1977). Canid communication. In *How Animals Communicate*, T. A. Sebeok (ed.). Bloomington, IN: Indiana University Press, pp. 728–748.

Fox, M. W., A. M. Beck, and E. Blackman. (1975). Behavior and ecology of a small group of urban dogs (*Canis familiaris*). *Applied Animal Ethology* **1**: 119–137.

Frame, L. H., J. R. Malcolm, G. W. Frame, and H. van Lawick. (1979). Social organization of the African wild dogs (*Lycaon pictus*) on the Serengeti plains, Tanzania 1967–1978. *Zeitschrift für Tierpsychologie* **50**: 225–249.

Frank, D., G. Beauchamp, and C. Palestrini. (2010). Systematic review of the use of pheromones for treatment of undesirable behavior in cats and dogs. *Journal of the American Veterinary Medical Association* **236**: 1308–1316.

Frank, H. and M. G. Frank. (1982a). On the effects of domestication on canine social development and behavior. *Applied Animal Ethology* **8**: 507–525.

Frank, H. and M. G. Frank. (1982b). Comparison of problem-solving performance in six-week-old wolves and dogs. *Animal Behaviour* **30**: 95–98.

Frank, M. C. and H. Frank. (1988). Food reinforcement versus social reinforcement in timber wolf pups. *Bulletin of the Psychonomic Society* **26**: 467–468.

Fredrickson, R. J. and P. W. Hedrick. (2006). Dynamics of hybridization and introgression in red wolves and coyotes. *Conservation Biology* **20**: 1272–1283.

Freedman, D. G., J. A. King, and O. Elliot. (1961). Critical period in the social development of dogs. *Science* **133**: 1016–1017.

Frijlink, J. H. (1977). Patterns of wolf pack movements prior to kills as read from tracks in Algonquin Provincial Park, Ont., Canada. *Bijdragen Tot De Dirkunde* **47**: 131–137.

Fritts, S. H. (1983). Record dispersal by a wolf from Minnesota. *Journal of Mammalogy* **64**: 166–167.

Fritts, S. H. and L. D. Mech. (1981). Dynamics, movements, and feeding ecology of a newly protected wolf population in northwestern Minnesota. *Wildlife Monographs* **80**, 79 pp.

Fritts, S. H. and W. J. Paul. (1989). Interactions of wolves and dogs in Minnesota. *Wildlife Society Bulletin* **17**: 121–123.

Frommolt, K. H., M. I. Kaal, N. M. Paschina, and A. A. Nikolskii. (1988). Sound development of the wolf (*Canis lupus* L. Canidae L.) during postnatal ontogeny. *Zoologische Jahrbücher. Abteilung für allgemeine Zoologie und Physiologie der Tiere* **92**: 105–115.

Fryxell, J. M., J. Greever, and A. R. E. Sinclair. (1988). Why are migratory ungulates so abundant? *American Naturalist* **131**: 781–798.

Fuller, J. L. (1956). Photoperiodic control of estrus in the basenji. *Journal of Heredity* **47**: 179–180.

Fuller, T. K. (1989a). Population dynamics of wolves in north-central Minnesota. *Wildlife Monographs* (**105**): 41 pp.

Fuller, T. K. (1989b). Denning behavior of wolves in north-central Minnesota. *American Midland Naturalist* **121**: 184–188.

Fuller, T. K. and L. B. Keith. (1980). Wolf population dynamics and prey relationships in northeastern Alberta. *Journal of Wildlife Management* **44**: 583–602.

Fuller, T. K. and L. B. Keith. (1981). Non-overlapping ranges of coyotes and wolves in northeastern Alberta. *Journal of Mammalogy* **62**: 403–405.

Gácsi, M , J. Topál, Á. Miklósi, A. Dóka, and V. Csányi. (2001). Attachment behavior of adult dogs (*Canis familiaris*) living at rescue centers: forming new bonds. *Journal of Comparative Psychology* **115**: 423–431.

Gácsi, M., B. Győri, Á. Miklósi, Z. Virányi, and E. Kubinyi. (2005). Species-specific differences and similarities in the behavior of hand-raised dog and wolf pups in social situations with humans. *Developmental Psychobiology* **47**: 111–22.

Garcia, M. A. (2005). Ichnologie générale de la grotte Chauvet. *Bulletin de la Société préhistorique française* **102**: 103–108.

García-Moreno, J., M. D. Matocq, M. S. Roy, E. Geffen, and R. K. Wayne. (1996). Relationships and genetic purity of the endangered Mexican wolf based on analysis of microsatellite loci. *Conservation Biology* **10**: 376–389.

Gardner, A. and S. A. West. (2006). Demography, altruism, and the benefits of budding. *Journal of Evolutionary Biology* **19**: 1707–1716.

Garrott, R. A., J. E. Bruggeman, M. S. Becker, S. T. Kalinowski, and P. J. White. (2007). Evaluating prey switching in wolf–ungulate systems. *Ecological Applications* **17**: 1588–1597.

Gartlan, J. S. (1964). Dominance in east African monkeys. *Proceedings of the East African Academy* **2**: 75–79.

Gassett, J. W., D. P. Wiesler, A. G. Baker, D. A. Osborn, K. V. Miller, and R. L. Marchinton *et al.* (1996). Volatile compounds from interdigital gland [*sic*] of male white-tailed deer (*Odocoileus virginianus*). *Journal of Chemical Ecology* **22**: 1689–1696.

Gaston, A. J. (1978). The evolution of group territorial behavior and cooperative breeding. *American Naturalist* **112**: 1091–1100.

Gazit, I. and J. Terkel. (2003). Explosives detection by sniffer dogs following strenuous physical activity. *Applied Animal Behaviour Science* **81**: 149–161.

Gazzano, A., C. Mariti, L. Notari, C. Sighieri, and E. A. McBride. (2008). Effects of early gentling and early environment on emotional development of puppies. *Applied Animal Behaviour Science* **110**: 294–304.

Geffen, E., M. J. Anderson, and R. K. Wayne. (2004). Climate and habitat barriers to dispersal in the highly mobile grey wolf. *Molecular Ecology* **13**: 2481–2490.

Gehrt, S. D., C. Anchor, and L. A. White. (2009). Home range and landscape use of coyotes in a metropolitan landscape: conflict or coexistence? *Journal of Mammalogy* **90**: 1045–1057.

Gerads, J. R., J. A. Jenks, and B. K. Watters. (2001). Food habits of coyotes inhabiting the Black Hills and surrounding prairies in western South Dakota. *Proceedings of the South Dakota Academy of Science* **80**: 95–108.

Germonpré, M., M. V. Sablin, R. E. Stevens, R. E. M. Hedges, M. Hofreiter, and M. Stiller *et al.* (2009). Fossil dogs and wolves from Palaeolithic sites in Belgium, the Ukraine and Russia: osteometry, ancient DNA and stable isotopes. *Journal of Archaeological Science* **36**: 473–490.

Gese, E. M. and L. D. Mech. (1991). Dispersal of wolves (*Canis lupus*) in northeastern Minnesota, 1969–1989. *Canadian Journal of Zoology* **69**: 2946–2955.

Gese, E. M. and R. L. Ruff. (1997). Scent-marking by coyotes, *Canis latrans*: the influence of social and ecological factors. *Animal Behaviour* **54**: 1155–1166.

Ghiselin, M. T. (1974). *The Economy of Nature and the Evolution of Sex*. Berkeley, CA: University of California Press, xii + 346 pp.

Ghiselin, M. T. (1997). *Metaphysics and the Origin of Species*. Albany, NY: State University of New York Press, xi + 377 pp.

Ghosh, B., D. K. Choudhuri, and B. Pal. (1984). Some aspects of the sexual behaviour of stray dogs, *Canis familiaris*. *Applied Animal Behaviour Science* **13**: 113–127.

Gier, H. T. (1957). *Coyotes in Kansas, Contribution No. 258*. Manhattan, KS: Department of Zoology, Kansas Agricultural Experiment Station, 95 pp.

Gier, H. T. (1975). Ecology and behavior of the coyote (*Canis latrans*). In *The Wild Canids: Their Systematics, Behavioral Ecology and Evolution*, M. W. Fox (ed.). New York, NY: Van Nostrand Reinhold, pp. 247–262.

Gilad, Y., V. Wiebe, M. Przeworski, D. Lancet, and S. Pääbo. (2004). Loss of olfactory receptor genes coincides with the acquisition of full trichromatic vision in primates. *PLoS Biology* **2**(1): 0120–0125.

Gipson, P. S. (1983). Evaluation and control implications of behavior of feral dogs in interior Alaska. In *Vertebrate Pest Control and Management Materials: Fourth Symposium*, D. E. Kaukeinen (ed.). Philadelphia, PA: American Society for Testing and Materials, pp. 285–295.

Gipson, P. S. and J. A. Sealander. (1976). Changing food habits of wild *Canis* in Arkansas with emphasis on coyote hybrids and feral dogs. *American Midland Naturalist* **95**: 249–253.

Gipson, P. S. and W. B. Ballard. (1998). Accounts of famous North American wolves, *Canis lupus*. *Canadian Field-Naturalist* **112**: 724–739.

Gipson, P. S., J. A. Sealander, and J. E. Dunn. (1974). The taxonomic status of wild *Canis* in Arkansas. *Systematic Zoology* **23**: 1–11.

Giraldeau, L-A. and T. Caraco. (1993). Genetic relatedness and group size in an aggregation economy. *Evolutionary Ecology* **7**: 429–438.

Gittleman, J. L. (1985). Carnivore body size: ecological and taxonomic correlates. *Oecologia* **67**: 540–554.

Gittleman, J. L. (1991). Carnivore olfactory bulb size: allometry, phylogeny and ecology. *Journal of Zoology* (London) **225**: 253–272.

Gittleman, J. L. and B. Van Valkenburgh. (1997). Sexual dimorphism in the canines and skulls of carnivores: effects of size, phylogeny, and behavioural ecology. *Journal of Zoology (London)* **242**: 97–117.

Glen, A. S., C. R. Dickman, M. E. Soulé, and B. G. Mackey. (2007). Evaluating the role of the dingo as a trophic regulator in Australian ecosystems. *Austral Ecology* **32**: 492–501.

Gobello, C., P. W. Concannon, and J. Verstegen III. (2001). Canine pseudopregnancy: a review. In *Recent Advances in Small Animal Reproduction*, Document No. A1215.0801, P. W. Concannon, G. England, and J. Verstegen III (eds.). Ithaca, NY: International Veterinary Information Service, 11 pp.

Goebel, T., M. R. Waters, and D. H. O'Rourke. (2008). The late Pleistocene dispersal of modern humans in the Americas. *Science* **319**: 1497–1502.

Gogoleva, S. S., J. A. Volodin, E. V. Volodina, and L. N. Trut. (2008). To bark or not to bark: vocalizations by red foxes selected for tameness or aggressiveness toward humans. *Bioacoustics* **18**: 99–132.

Golani, I. and G. Moran. (1983). A motility–immobility gradient in the behavior of the "inferior" wolf during "ritualized fighting." In *Advances in the Study of Mammalian behavior*, Special Publication No. 7, J. F. Eisenberg and D. G. Kleiman (eds.). Shippens-burg, PA: American Society of Mammalogists, pp. 65–94.

Goldman, E. A. (1937). The wolves of North America. *Journal of Mammalogy* **18**: 37–45.

Goldman, E. A. (1944). *The Wolves of North America, Part II. Classification of Wolves*. New York, NY: Dover Publications, xi + pp. 389–636. [1964 edition with corrections.]

Gollan, K. (1984). The Australian dingo: in the shadow of man. In *Vertebrate Zoogeography and Evolution in Australasia: Animals in Space and Time*, M. Archer and G. Clayton (eds.). Carlisle, Western Australia: Hesperian Press, pp. 921–927.

Gomerčič, T., M. Sindičič, A. Galov, H. Arbanasić, J. Kusak, and I. Kocijan *et al.* (2010). High genetic variability of the grey wolf (*Canis lupus* L.) population from Croatia as revealed by mitochondrial DNA control region sequences. *Zoological Studies* **49**: 816–823.

Gompper, M. E. (2002). Top carnivores in the suburbs? Ecological and conservation issues raised by colonization of northeastern North America by coyotes. *Bioscience* **52**: 185–190.

Goodwin, D., J. W. S. Bradshaw, and S. M. Wickens. (1997). Paedomorphosis affects agonistic visual signals of domestic dogs. *Animal Behaviour* **53**: 297–304.

Goodwin, M., K. M. Gooding, and F. Regnier. (1979). Sex pheromone in the dog. *Science* **203**: 559–561.

Gottelli, D., C. Sillero-Zubiri, G. D. Applebaum, M. S. Roy, D. J. Girman, and J. García-Moreno *et al.* (1994). Molecular genetics of the most endangered canid: the Ethiopian wolf *Canis simensis. Molecular Ecology* **3**: 301–312.

Gould, R. A. (1969). Subsistence behaviour among the western desert aborigines of Australia. *Oceania* **39**: 253–274.

Gould, R. A. (1970). Journey to Pulykara. *Natural History Magazine* **74**(10): 56–67.

Grafen, A. (1990). Do animals really recognize kin? *Animal Behaviour* **39**: 42–54.

Gray, D. R. (1970). The killing of a bull muskox by a single wolf. *Arctic* **23**: 197–199.

Gray, M. M. and R. K. Wayne. (2010). Response to Klütsch and Crapon de Caprona. *BMC Biology* **8**: 120.

Gray, M. M., J. M. Granka, C. D. Bustamante, N. B. Sutter, A. R. Boyko, and L. Zhu *et al.* (2009). Linkage disequilibrium and demographic history of wild and domestic canids. *Genetics* **181**: 1493–1505.

Gray, M. M., N. B. Sutter, E. A. Ostrander, and R. K. Wayne. (2010a). The *IGF1* small dog haplotype is derived from Middle Eastern grey wolves. *BMC Biology* **8**: 16.

Gray, M. M., N. B. Sutter, E. A. Ostrander, and R. K. Wayne. (2010b). The *IGF1* small dog haplotype is derived from Middle Eastern gray wolves. *BMC Biology* **8**: 118.

Green, B. and P. Catling. (1977). The biology of the dingo. In *Australian Animals and Their Environments*, H. Messel and S. T. Butler (eds.). Sydney: Shakespeare Head Press, pp. 51–60.

Greer, K. A., S. C. Canterberry, and K. E. Murphy. (2007). Statistical analysis regarding the effects of height and weight on life span of the domestic dog. *Research in Veterinary Science* **82**: 208–214.

Grewal, S. K., P. J. Wilson, T. K. Kung, K. Shami, M. T. Theberge, and J. B. Theberge *et al.* (2004). A genetic assessment of the eastern wolf (*Canis lycaon*) in Algonquin Provincial Park. *Journal of Mammalogy* **85**: 625–632.

Griffin, A. S. and S. A. West. (2002). Kin selection: fact and fiction. *Trends in Ecology and Evolution* **17**: 15–21.

Grosberg, R. K. and J. F. Quinn. (1986). The genetic control and consequences of kin recognition by the larvae of a colonial marine invertebrate. *Nature* **322**: 456–459.

Grus, W. E. and J. Zhang. (2008). Distinct evolutionary patterns between chemoreceptors of 2 vertebrate olfactory systems and the differential tuning hypothesis. *Molecular Biology and Evolution* **25**: 1593–1601.

Grus, W. E., P. Shi, Y-P. Zhang, and J. Zhang. (2005). Dramatic variation of the vomeronasal pheromone receptor gene repertoire among five orders of placental and marsupial mammals. *Proceedings of the National Academy of Sciences* **102**: 5767–5772.

Gula, R. (2008). Wolf depredation on domestic animals in the Polish Carpathian Mountains. *Journal of Wildlife Management* **72**: 283–289.

Hailer, F. and J. A. Leonard. (2008). Hybridization among three native North American *Canis* species in a region of natural sympatry. *PLoS One* **3**(10): e3333.

Halpern, M. and A. Martínez-Marcos. (2003). Structure and function of the vomeronasal system: an update. *Progress in Neurobiology* **70**: 245–318.

Hamilton, W. D. (1963). The evolution of altruistic behavior. *American Naturalist* **97**: 354–356.

Hamilton, W. D. (1964). The genetical evolution of social behaviour. I. *Journal of Theoretical Biology* **7**: 1–16.

Hamilton, W. D. and R. M. May. (1977). Dispersal in stable habitats. *Nature* **269**: 578–581.

Harden, R. H. (1985). The ecology of the dingo in north-eastern New South Wales. I. Movements and home range. *Australian Wildlife Research* **12**: 25–37.

Hare, J. F. and J. O. Murie. (1996). Ground squirrel sociality and the quest for the "holy grail": does kinship influence behavioral discrimination by juvenile Columbian ground squirrels? *Behavioral Ecology* **7**: 76–81.

Harper, F. (1955). *The Barren Ground Caribou of Keewatin, Miscellaneous Publications No. 6.* Lawrence, KS: University of Kansas Museum of Natural History, 163 pp.

Harriman, A. E. and R. H. Berger. (1986). Olfactory acuity in the common raven (*Corvus corax*). *Physiology and Behavior* **36**: 257–262.

Harrington, F. H. (1978). Ravens attracted to wolf howling. *Condor* **80**: 236–237.

Harrington, F. H. (1981). Urine-marking and caching behavior in the wolf. *Behaviour* **76**: 280–288.

Harrington, F. H. (1987). Aggressive howling in wolves. *Animal Behaviour* **35**: 7–12.

Harrington, F. H. (1989). Chorus howling by wolves: acoustic structure, pack size and the Beau Geste effect. *Bioacoustics* **2**: 117–136.

Harrington, F. H. and C. S. Asa. (2003). Wolf communication. In *Wolves: Behavior, Ecology, and Conservation*, L. D. Mech and L. Boitani (eds.). Chicago, IL: University of Chicago Press, pp. 66–103.

Harrington, F. H. and L. D. Mech. (1979). Wolf howling and its role in territory maintenance. *Behaviour* **68**: 207–249.

Harrington, F. H. and L. D. Mech. (1982). Patterns of homesite attendance in two Minnesota wolf packs. In *Wolves of the World: Perspectives of Behavior, Ecology, and Conservation*, F. H. Harrington and P. C. Paquet (eds.). Park Ridge, NJ: Noyes Publications, pp. 81–105.

Harrington, F. H. and L. D. Mech. (1983). Wolf pack spacing: howling as a territory-independent spacing mechanism in a territorial population. *Behavioral Ecology and Sociobiology* **12**: 161–168.

Harrington, F. H., L. D. Mech, and S. H. Fritts. (1983). Pack size and wolf pup survival: their relationship under varying ecological conditions. *Behavioral Ecology and Sociobiology* **13**: 19–26.

Harrison, D. J. (1992). Social ecology of coyotes in northeastern North America: relationships to dispersal, food resources, and human exploitation. In *Ecology and Management of the Eastern Coyote*, A. H. Boer (ed.). Fredericton, NB: Wildlife Research Unit, University of New Brunswick, pp. 53–72.

Hart, B. L. and C. M. Haugen. (1971). Scent marking and sexual behavior maintained in anosmic male dogs. *Communications in Behavioral Biology* **6**: 131–135.

Hatt, R. T. (1959). *The Mammals of Iraq, Miscellaneous Publication No. 16.* Ann Arbor, MI: Museum of Zoology, University of Michigan, 128 pp. 34–37.

Hayden, B. (1975). Dingoes: pets or producers? *Mankind* **10**: 11–15.

Hayes, R. D. and A. Baer. (1992). Brown bear, *Ursus arctos*, preying upon gray wolf, *Canis lupus*, pups at a wolf den. *Canadian Field-Naturalist* **106**: 381–382.

Hayes, R. D. and A. S. Harestad. (2000a). Demography of a recovering wolf population in the Yukon. *Canadian Journal of Zoology* **78**: 36–48.

Hayes, R. D. and A. S. Harestad. (2000b). Wolf functional response and regulation of moose in the Yukon. *Canadian Journal of Zoology* **78**: 60–66.

Hayes, R. D., A. M. Baer, U. Wotschikowsky, and A. S. Harestad. (2000). Kill rate by wolves on moose in the Yukon. *Canadian Journal of Zoology* **78**: 49–59.

Heard, D. C. and T. M. Williams. (1992). Distribution of wolf dens on migratory caribou ranges in the Northwest Territories, Canada. *Canadian Journal of Zoology* **70**: 1504–1510.

Hedrick, P. W. and R. J. Fredrickson. (2008). Captive breeding and the reintroduction of Mexican and red wolves. *Molecular Ecology* **17**: 344–350.

Hedrick, P. W., P. S. Miller, E. Geffen, and R. Wayne. (1997). Genetic evaluation of the three captive Mexican wolf lineages. *Zoo Biology* **16**: 47–69.

Hedrick, P. W., R. N. Lee, and D. Garrigan. (2002). Major histocompatibility complex variation in red wolves: evidence for common ancestry with coyotes and balancing selection. *Molecular Ecology* **11**: 1905–1913.

Heinsohn, R. and S. Legge. (1999). The cost of helping. *Trends in Ecology and Evolution* **14**: 53–57.

Henshaw, R. E. and R. O. Stephenson. (1974). Homing in a gray wolf (*Canis lupus*). *Journal of Mammalogy* **55**: 234–237.

Hepper, P. G. (1994). Long-term retention of kinship recognition established during infancy in the domestic dog. *Behavioural Processes* **33**: 3–14.

Hepper, P. G. and D. L. Wells. (2005). How many footsteps do dogs need to determine the direction of an odour trail? *Chemical Senses* **30**: 291–298.

Herrada, G. and C. Dulac. (1997). A novel family of putative pheromone receptors in mammals with a topographically organized and sexually dimorphic distribution. *Cell* **90**: 763–773.

Higashi, M. and N. Yamamura. (1993). What determines animal group size? Insider–outsider conflict and its resolution. *American Naturalist* **142**: 553–563.

Higham, C. F. W., A. Kijngam, and B. F. J. Manly. (1980). An analysis of prehistoric canid remains from Thailand. *Journal of Archaeological Science* **7**: 149–165.

Hinde, R. A. (1985). Was 'The Expression of Emotions' a misleading phrase? *Animal Behaviour* **33**: 985–992.

Hirsch, E. (1986). *Wild Gratitude*. New York, NY: Alfred A. Knopf, 78 pp.

Ho, S. Y. W., M. J. Phillips, A. Cooper, and A. J. Drummond. (2005). Time dependency of molecular rate estimates and systematic overestimation of recent divergence times. *Molecular Biology and Evolution* **22**: 1561–1568.

Holst, P. A. and R. D. Phemister. (1971). The prenatal development of the dog: preimplantation events. *Biology of Reproduction* **5**: 194–206.

Holst, P. A. and R. D. Phemister. (1974). Onset of diestrus in the beagle bitch: definition and significance. *American Journal of Veterinary Research* **35**: 401–406.

Holst, P. A. and R. D. Phemister. (1975). Temporal sequence of events in the estrous cycle of the bitch. *American Journal of Veterinary Research* **36**: 705–706.

Hoogland, J. L. (1985). Infanticide in prairie dogs: lactating females kill offspring of close kin. *Science* **230**: 1037–1040.

Hoon, M. A., E. Adler, J. Lindemeier, J. F. Battey, N. J. P. Ryba, and C. S. Zuker. (1999). Putative mammalian taste receptors: a class of taste-specific GPCRs with distinct topographic selectivity. *Cell* **96**: 541–551.

Hope, J. (1994). Wolves and wolf hybrids as pets are big business – but a bad idea. *Smithsonian Magazine* **25**(3): 34–45.

Hopkins, K. (2010). *Traffic takes unusual toll on city's wolves*. http://www/adn.com/2010/05/09/1270587/traffic-takes-unusual-toll-on.html.

Hopkins, S. G., T. A. Schubret, and B. L. Hart. (1976). Castration of adult male dogs: effects on roaming, aggression, urine marking, and mounting. *Journal of the American Veterinary Medical Association* **168**: 1108–1110.

Howe, P. E., H. A. Mattel, and P. B. Hawk. (1912). Fasting studies. VI. Distribution of nitrogen during a fast of one hundred and seventeen days. *Journal of Biological Chemistry* **11**: 103–127.

Hradecký, P. (1985). Possible pheromonal regulation of reproduction in wild carnivores. *Journal of Chemical Ecology* **11**: 241–250.

Hutt, N. (2003). Wolves return to Wrangel Island. *International Wolf* **3**(1): 19.

Iljin, N. A. (1941). Wolf-dog genetics. *Journal of Genetics* **42**: 359–414 + plates 19–25.

Illius, A. E., N. B. Haynes, G. E. Lamming, C. M. Howles, N. Fairall, and R. P. Millar. (1983). Evaluation of LH–RH stimulation of testosterone as an index of reproductive status in rams and its application in wild antelope. *Journal of Reproduction and Fertility* **68**: 105–112.

Irion, D. N., A. L. Schaffer, T. R. Famula, M. L. Eggleston, S. S. Hughes, and N. C. Pedersen. (2003). Analysis of genetic variation in 28 dog breed populations with 100 microsatellite markers. *Journal of Heredity* **94**: 81–87.

Ivanter, E. V. and N. A. Sedova. (2008). Ecological monitoring of urban groups of stray dogs: an example of the city of Petrozavodsk. *Russian Journal of Ecology* **39**: 105–110.

Jackson, C. F. (1922). Notes on New Hampshire mammals. *Journal of Mammalogy* **3**: 13–15.

Jamieson, I. G. and J. L. Craig. (1987). Critique of helping behaviour in birds: a departure from functional explanations. In *Perspectives in Ethology*, Vol. 7, P. Bateson and P. Klopfer (eds.). New York, NY: Cambridge University Press, pp. 79–98.

Janicki, Z., A. Hraste, A. Slavica, D. Konjević, Z. Marinović, and Đ. Stubičan. (2003). Morphohistological characteristics of the interdigital gland in the roebuck (*Capreolus capreolus* L.). *Veterinarski Arhiv* **73**: 27–37.

Jankovic, I., B. M. vonHoldt, and N. A. Rosenberg. (2010). Heterozygosity of the Yellowstone wolves. *Molecular Ecology* **19**: 3246–3249.

Jensen, C. and H. E. Ederstrom. (1955). Development of temperature regulation in the dog. *American Journal of Physiology* **183**: 340–344.

Jhala, Y. V. (1993). Predation on blackbuck [*sic*] by wolves in Velavadar National Park, Gujarat, India. *Conservation Biology* **7**: 874–881.

Jöchle, W. and A. C. Andersen. (1977). The estrous cycle in the dog: a review. *Theriogenology* **7**: 113–140.

Johnson, C. E. (1921). A note of the habits of the timber wolf. *Journal of Mammalogy* **2**: 11–15.

Johnson, C. N., J. L. Isaac, and D. O. Fisher. (2007). Rarity of a top predator triggers continent-wide collapse of mammal prey: dingoes and marsupials in Australia. *Proceedings of the Royal Society of London* **274B**: 341–346.

Johnson, M. L. and M. S. Gaines. (1990). Evolution of dispersal: theoretical models and empirical tests using birds and mammals. *Annual Review of Ecology and Systematics* **21**: 449–480.

Jolicoeur, P. (1959). Multivariate geographical variation in the wolf. *Canis lupus* L. *Evolution* **13**: 283–299.

Jones, E. (1990). Physical characteristics and taxonomic status of wild canids, *Canis familiaris*, from the eastern highlands of Victoria. *Australian Wildlife Research* **17**: 69–81.

Jones, E. (2009). Hybridisation between the dingo, *Canis lupus dingo*, and the domestic dog, *Canis lupus familiaris*, in Victoria: a critical review. *Australian Mammalogy* **31**: 1–7.

Jones, E. and P. L. Stevens. (1988). Reproduction in wild canids, *Canis familiaris* from the eastern highlands of Victoria. *Australian Wildlife Research* **15**: 385–394.

Jordan, P. A., P. C. Shelton, and D. L. Allen. (1967). Numbers, turnover, and social structure of the Isle Royale wolf population. *American Zoologist* **7**: 233–252.

Jorgenson, J. W., M. Novotny, M. Carmack, G. B. Copland, S. R. Wilson, and S. Katona et al. (1978). Chemical scent constituents in the urine of the red fox (*Vulpes vulpes* L.) during the winter season. *Science* **199**: 796–798.

Joslin, P. (1982). Status, growth and other facets of the Iranian wolf. In *Wolves of the World: Perspectives of Behavior, Ecology, and Conservation*, F. H. Harrington and P. C. Paquet (eds.). Park Ridge, NJ: Noyes Publications, pp. 196–203.

Joslin, P. W. B. (1967). Movements and home sites of timber wolves in Algonquin Park. *American Zoologist* **7**: 279–288.

Jost, C., G. Devulder, J. A. Vucetich, R. O. Peterson, and R. Arditi. (2005). The wolves of Isle Royale display scale-invariant satiation and ratio-dependent predation on moose. *Journal of Animal Ecology* **74**: 809–816.

Kaartinen, S., M. Luoto, and I. Kojola. (2010). Selection of den sites by wolves in boreal forests in Finland. *Journal of Zoology (London)* **281**: 99–104.

Kalinowski, S. T., P. W. Hedrick, and P. S. Miller. (1999). No inbreeding depression observed in Mexican and red wolf captive breeding programs. *Conservation Biology* **13**: 1371–1377.

Kambere, M. B. and R. P. Lane. (2007). Co-regulation of a large and rapidly evolving repertoire of odorant receptor genes. *BMC Neuroscience* **8** (Suppl. 3): S2.

Kamler, J. F., K. Keeler, G. Wiens, C. Richardson, and P. S. Gipson. (2003). Feral dogs, *Canis familiaris*, kill coyote, *Canis latrans*. *Canadian Field-Naturalist* **117**: 123–124.

Karlson, P. and M. Lüscher. (1959). 'Pheromones': a new term for a class of biologically active substances. *Nature* **183**: 55–56.

Kay, C. E. (1995). An alternative interpretation of the historical evidence relating to the abundance of wolves in the Yellowstone ecosystem. In *Ecology and Conservation of Wolves in a Changing World*, Occasional Publication No. 35, L. N. Carbyn, S. H. Fritts, and D. R. Seip (eds.). Edmonton, AB: Canadian Circumpolar Institute, pp. 77–84.

Kays, R., A. Curtis, and J. J. Kirchman. (2010). Rapid adaptive evolution of northeastern coyotes via hybridization with wolves. *Biology Letters* **6**: 89–93.

Kays, R. W., M. E. Gompper, and J. C. Ray. (2008). Landscape ecology of eastern coyotes based on large-scale estimates of abundance. *Ecological Applications* **18**: 1014–1027.

Keane, B., S. R. Creel, and P. M. Waser. (1996). No evidence of inbreeding avoidance or inbreeding depression in a social carnivore. *Behavioral Ecology* **7**: 480–489.

Kennelly, J. J. and B. E. Johns. (1976). The estrous cycle of coyotes. *Journal of Wildlife Management* **40**: 272–277.

Kerns, J. A., M. Olivier, G. Lust, and G. S. Barsh. (2003). Exclusion of *melanocortin-1 receptor* (*Mc1r*) and *Agouti* as candidates for dominant black in dogs. *Journal of Heredity* **94**: 75–79.

Kerr, B., P. Godfrey-Smith, and M. W. Feldman. (2004). What is altruism? *Trends in Ecology and Evolution* **19**: 135–140.

Keverne, E. B. (1999). The vomeronasal organ. *Science* **286**: 716–720.

King, J. A. (1954). Closed social groups among domestic dogs. *Proceedings of the American Philosophical Society* **98**: 327–336.

Kleiman, D. (1966). Scent marking in the Canidae. *Symposium of the Zoological Society of London* **18**: 167–177.

Kleiman, D. G. (1968). Reproduction in the Canidae. *International Zoo Yearbook* **8**: 3–8.

Klütsch, C. F. C. and M. D. Crapon de Caprona. (2010). The IGF1 small dog haplotype is derived from Middle Eastern grey wolves: a closer look at statistics, sampling, and the alleged Middle Eastern origin of small dogs. *BMC Biology* **8**: 119.

Knell, R. J. (2009). Population density and the evolution of male aggression. *Journal of Zoology (London)* **278**: 83–90.

Koblmüller, S., M. Nord, R. K. Wayne, and J. A. Leonard. (2009). Origin and status of the Great Lakes wolf. *Molecular Ecology* **18**: 2313–2326.

Kojola, I., J. Aspi, A. Hakala, S. Heikkinen, C. Ilmoni, and S. Ronkainen. (2006). Dispersal in an expanding wolf population in Finland. *Journal of Mammalogy* **87**: 281–286.

Kokko, H. and J. Ekman. (2002). Delayed dispersal as a route to breeding: territorial inheritance, safe havens, and ecological constraints. *American Naturalist* **160**: 468–484.

Kokko, H. and P. Lundberg. (2001). Dispersal, migration, and offspring retention in saturated habitats. *American Naturalist* **157**: 188–202.

Kokko, H., R. A. Johnstone, and T. H. Clutton-Brock. (2001). The evolution of cooperative breeding through group augmentation. *Proceedings of the Royal Society of London* **268B**: 187–196.

Kolenosky, G. B. (1971). Hybridization between wolf and coyote. *Journal of Mammalogy* **52**: 446–449.

Kolenosky, G. B. (1972). Wolf predation on wintering deer in east-central Ontario. *Journal of Wildlife Management* **36**: 357–369.

Kolenosky, G. B. and D. H. Johnston. (1967). Radio-tracking timber wolves in Ontario. *American Zoologist* **7**: 289–303.

Kolenosky, G. B. and R. O. Standfield. (1975). Morphological and ecological variation among gray wolves (*Canis lupus*) of Ontario, Canada. In *The Wild Canids: Their Systematics, Behavioral Ecology and Evolution*, M. W. Fox (ed.). New York, NY: Van Nostrand Reinhold, 62–72.

Koler-Matznick, J. (2002). The origin of the dog revisited. *Anthrozoös* **15**: 98–118.

Kolig, E. (1973). Aboriginal man's best foe? *Mankind* **9**: 122–123.

Kooistra, H. S. and A. C. Okkens. (2002). Secretion of growth hormone and prolactin during progression of the luteal phase in healthy dogs: a review. *Molecular and Cellular Endocrinology* **197**: 167–172.

Kooistra, H. S., A. C. Okkens, M. M. Bevers, C. Popp-Snijders, B. van Haaften, and S. J. Dieleman *et al.* (1999). Concurrent pulsatile secretion of luteinizing hormone and follicle-stimulating hormone during different phases of the estrous cycle and anestrus in beagle bitches. *Biology of Reproduction* **60**: 65–71.

Koskinen, M. T. (2003). Individual assignment using microsatellite DNA reveals unambiguous breed identification in the domestic dog. *Animal Genetics* **34**: 297–301.

Kovács, Á. M., E. Téglás, and A. D. Endress. (2010). The social sense: susceptibility to others' beliefs in human infants and adults. *Science* **330**: 1830–1834.

Krause, J., D. J. Hoare, D. Croft, J. Lawrence, A. Ward, and G. D. Ruxton *et al.* (2000). Fish shoal composition: mechanisms and constraints. *Proceedings of the Royal Society of London* **267B**: 2011–2017.

Kreeger, T. J., U. S. Seal, Y. Cohen, E. D. Plotka, and C. S. Asa. (1991). Characterization of prolactin secretion in gray wolves (*Canis lupus*). *Canadian Journal of Zoology* **69**: 1366–1374.

Kreeger, T. J., G. D. DelGiudice, and L. D. Mech. (1997). Effects of fasting and refeeding [*sic*] on body composition of captive gray wolves (*Canis lupus*). *Canadian Journal of Zoology* **75**: 1549–1552.

Krefft, G. (1866). On the vertebrated animals of the Lower Murray and Darling, their habits, economy, and geographical distribution. *Transactions of the Philosophical Society of New South Wales 1862–1865*: 1–33.

Kruse, S. M. and W. E. Howard. (1983). Canid sex attractant studies. *Journal of Chemical Ecology* **9**: 1503–1510.

Kruuk, H. and H. Snell. (1981). Prey selection by feral dogs from a population of marine iguanas (*Amblyrhynchus cristatus*). *Journal of Applied Ecology* **18**: 197–204.

Kuang, Y. and E. Beretta. (1998). Global qualitative analysis of a ratio-dependent predator–prey system. *Journal of Mathematical Biology* **36**: 389–406.

Kummer, H. (1968). *Social Organization of Hamadryas Baboons: A Field Study*. Chicago, IL: University of Chicago Press, vi + 139 pp.

Kunkel, K. E., D. H. Pletscher, D. K. Boyd, R. R. Ream, and M. W. Fairchild. (2004). Factors correlated with foraging behavior of wolves in and near Glacier National Park, Montana. *Journal of Wildlife Management* **68**: 157–178.

Kuyt, E. (1962). Movements of young wolves in the Northwest Territories of Canada. *Journal of Mammalogy* **43**: 270–271.

Kyle, C. J., A. R. Johnson, B. R. Patterson, P. J. Wilson, K. Shami, and S. K. Grewal *et al.* (2006). Genetic nature of eastern wolves: past, present and future. *Conservation Genetics* **7**: 273–287.

Laikre, L. and N. Ryman. (1991). Inbreeding depression in a captive wolf (*Canis lupus*) population. *Conservation Biology* **5**: 33–40.

Larivière, S. and M. Crête. (1993). The size of eastern coyotes (*Canis latrans*): a comment. *Journal of Mammalogy* **74**: 1072–1074.

Lavigne, G. R. (1992). Sex/age composition and physical condition of deer killed by coyotes during winter in Maine. In *Ecology and Management of the Eastern Coyote*, A. H. Boer (ed.). Fredericton, NB: Wildlife Research Unit, University of New Brunswick, pp. 141–159.

Lawrence, B. (1967). Early domestic dogs. *Zeitschrift für Säugetierkunde* **32**: 44–59.

Lawrence, B. and W. H. Bossert. (1967). Multiple character analysis of *Canis lupus, latrans,* and *familiaris,* with a discussion of the relationships of *Canis niger. American Zoologist* **7**: 223–232.

Lawrence, B. and W. H. Bossert. (1969). The cranial evidence for hybridization in New England *Canis. Breviora* (**330**): 1–13.

Lawrence, B. and W. H. Bossert. (1975). Relationships of North American *Canis* shown by a multiple character analysis of selected populations. In *The Wild Canids: Their Systematics, Behavioral Ecology and Evolution*, M. W. Fox (ed.). New York, NY: Van Nostrand Reinhold, 73–86.

Lawson, R. E., R. J. Putman, and A. H. Fielding. (2000). Individual signatures in scent gland secretions of Eurasian deer. *Journal of Zoology (London)* **251**: 399–410.

Le Boeuf, B. J. (1967). Interindividual [*sic*] associations in dogs. *Behaviour* **29**: 268–295.

Leaver, S. D. A. and T. E. Reimchen. (2008). Behavioural responses of *Canis familiaris* to different tail lengths of a remotely-controlled life-size dog replica. *Behaviour* **145**: 377–390.

Leca, J-B., N. Gunst, B. Thierry, and O. Petit. (2003). Distributed leadership in semifree-ranging white-faced capuchin monkeys. *Animal Behaviour* **66**: 1045–1052.

Lee, K. (1999). *The Natural and the Artefactual: The Implications of Deep Science and Deep Technology for Environmental Philosophy*. Lanham, MD: Lexington Books, ix + 285 pp.

Legge, S. (1996). Cooperative lions escape the prisoner's dilemma. *Trends in Ecology and Evolution* **11**: 2–3.

Lehman, N. and R. K. Wayne. (1991). Analysis of coyote mitochondrial DNA genotype frequencies: estimation of the effective number of alleles. *Genetics* **128**: 405–416.

Lehman, N., A. Eisenhawer, K. Hansen, L. D. Mech, R. O. Peterson, and P. J. P. Gogan. (1991). Introgression of coyote mitochondrial DNA into sympatric North American gray wolf populations. *Evolution* **45**: 104–119.

Lehman, N., P. Clarkson, L. D. Mech, T. J. Meier, and R. K. Wayne. (1992). A study of the genetic relationships within and among wolf packs using DNA fingerprinting and mitochondrial DNA. *Behavioral Ecology and Sociobiology* **30**: 83–94.

Lehner, P. N. (1978). Coyote vocalizations: a lexicon and comparisons with other canids. *Animal Behaviour* **26**: 712–722.

Lentfer, J. W. and D. K. Sanders. (1973). Notes on the captive wolf (*Canis lupus*) colony, Barrow, Alaska. *Canadian Journal of Zoology* **51**: 623–627.

Leonard, J. A. and R. K. Wayne. (2008). Native Great Lakes wolves were not restored. *Biology Letters* **4**: 95–98.

Leonard, J. A., R. K. Wayne, J. Wheeler, R. Valadez, S. Guillén, and C. Vilà. (2002). Ancient DNA evidence for Old World origin of New World dogs. *Science* **298**: 1613–1616.

Leonard, J. A., C. Vilà, and R. K. Wayne. (2005). From wild wolf to domestic dog. In *The Dog and Its Genome*, E. A. Ostrander, U. Giger, and K. Lindblad-Toh (eds.). Cold Spring Harbor, NY: Cold Spring Harbor Press, pp. 95–117.

Leonard, J. A., C. Vilà, K. Fox-Dobbs, P. L. Koch, R. K. Wayne, and B. van Valkenburgh. (2007). Megafaunal extinctions and the disappearance of a specialized wolf ecomorph. *Current Biology* **17**: 1146–1150.

Lepais, O., R. J. Petit, E. Guichoux, J. E. Lavabre, F. Alberto, and A. Kremer *et al.* (2009). Species relative abundance and direction of introgression in oaks. *Molecular Ecology* **18**: 2228–2242.

Lesniak, A., M. Walczak, T. Jezierski, M. Sacharczuk, M. Gawkowski, and K. Jaszczak. (2008). Canine olfactory receptor gene polymorphism and its relation to odor detection performance by sniffer dogs. *Journal of Heredity* **99**: 518–527.

Letnic, M. and F. Koch. (2010). Are dingoes a trophic regulator in arid Australia? A comparison of mammal communities on either side of the dingo fence. *Austral Ecology* **35**: 167–175.

Letnic, M., F. Koch, C. Gordon, M. S. Crowther, and C. R. Dickman. (2009). Keystone effects of an alien top-predator stem extinctions of native mammals. *Proceedings of the Royal Society of London* **276B**: 3249–3256.

Levitis, D. A., W. Z. Lidicker Jr., and G. Freund. (2009). Behavioural biologists do not agree on what constitutes behaviour. *Animal Behaviour* **78**: 103–111.

Levy, S. (2009). The dingo dilemma. *Bioscience* **59**: 465–469.

Lewis, M. A. and J. D. Murray. (1993). Modelling territoriality and wolf-deer interactions. *Nature* **336**: 738–740.

Lewis, M. A., K. A. J. White, and J. D. Murray. (1997). Analysis of a model for wolf territories. *Journal of Mathematical Biology* **35**: 749–774.

Li, Q., Z. Liu, X. Li, X. Zhao, L. Dong, and Z. Pan *et al.* (2008). Origin and phylogenetic analysis of the Tibetan mastiff based on the mitochondrial DNA sequence. *Journal of Genetics and Genomics* **35**: 335–340.

Li, Y., B. Deeb, W. Pendergrass, and N. Wolf. (1996). Cellular proliferation capacity and life span in small and large dogs. *Journal of Gerontology* **51A**: B403–B408.

Liberg, O., H. Andrén, H-C. Pedersen, H. Sand, D. Sejberg, and P. Wabakken *et al.* (2005). Severe inbreeding depression in a wild wolf *Canis lupus* population. *Biology Letters* **1**: 17–20.

Liberles, S. D. and L. B. Buck. (2006). A second class of chemosensory receptors in the olfactory epithelium. *Nature* **442**: 645–650.

Lickliter, R. and J. W. Ness. (1990). Domestication and comparative psychology: status and strategy. *Journal of Comparative Psychology* **104**: 211–218.

Lindblad-Toh, K., C. M. Wade, T. S. Mikkelsen, E. K. Karlsson, D. B. Jaffe, and M. Kamal *et al.* (2005). Genome sequence, comparative analysis and haplotype structure of the domestic dog. *Nature* **438**: 803–810.

Linnell, J. D. C., H. Brøseth, E. J. Solberg, and S. M. Brainerd. (2005). The origins of the southern Scandinavian wolf *Canis lupus* population: potential for natural immigration in relation to dispersal distances, geography and Baltic ice. *Wildlife Biology* **11**: 383–391.

Lockwood, R. (1979). Dominance in wolves: useful construct or bad habit? In *The Behavior and Ecology of Wolves*, E. Klinghammer (ed.). New York, NY: Garland STPM Press, pp. 225–244.

Loew, F. M. and A. F. Fraser. (1977). The anti-social behaviour of urban dogs. *Applied Animal Ethology* **3**: 101–104.

Lord, K., M. Feinstein, and R. Coppinger. (2009). Barking and mobbing. *Behavioural Processes* **81**: 358–368.

Lorenz, K. (1953). *Man Meets Dog*. New York, NY: Kodansha International, pp. xviii and 211 [1994 English language edition.]

Lorenz, K. (1995). Foreword. In *The Wild Canids: Their Systematics, Behavioral Ecology and Evolution*, M. W. Fox (ed.). New York, NY: Van Nostrand Reinhold, pp. vii–xii.

Losee, R. M. (1997). A discipline independent definition of information. *Journal of the American Society for Information Science and Technology* **48**: 254–269.

Lundberg, P. and J. M. Fryxell. (1995). Expected population density versus productivity in ratio-dependent and prey-dependent models. *American Naturalist* **146**: 153–161.

Lydell, K. and R. L. Doty. (1972). Male rat odor preferences for female urine as a function of sexual experience, urine age, and urine source. *Hormones and Behavior* **3**: 205–212.

Lyons, C. A., P. M. Ghezzi, and C. D. Cheney. (1982). Reinforcement of cooperative behavior in captive wolves. In *Wolves of the World: Perspectives of Behavior, Ecology, and Conservation*, F. H. Harrington and P. C. Paquet (eds.). Park Ridge, NJ: Noyes Publications, pp. 262–271.

MacCracken, J. G. (1982). Coyote foods in a southern California suburb. *Wildlife Society Bulletin* **10**: 280–281.

Macdonald, D. W. and G. M. Carr. (1995). Variation in dog society: between resource dispersion and social flux. In *The Domestic Dog: Its Evolution, Behaviour and Interactions with People*, J. Serpell (ed.). Cambridge: Cambridge University Press, pp. 199–216.

MacDonald, J. B. and B. E. Ginsburg. (1981). Induction of normal prepubertal behavior in wolves with restricted rearing. *Behavioral and Neural Biology* **33**: 133–162.

MacFarlane, R. R. (1905). Notes on mammals collected and observed in the northern Mackenzie River district, Northwest Territories of Canada. *Proceedings of the United States National Museum* **28**: 673–764. [pp. 692–694.]

Macintosh, N. W. G. (1964). A 3000 year old dingo from Shelter 6 (Fromm's Landing, South Australia). *Proceedings of the Royal Society of Victoria* **7**: 498–507.

Macintosh, N. W. G. (1975). The origin of the dingo: an enigma. In *The Wild Canids: Their Systematics, Behavioral Ecology and Evolution*, M. W. Fox (ed.). New York, NY: Van Nostrand Reinhold, pp. 87–106.

Magrath, R. D. and S. M. Yezerinac. (1997). Facultative helping does not influence reproductive success or survival in cooperatively breeding white-browed scrubwrens. *Journal of Animal Ecology* **66**: 658–670.

Maher, C. R. and D. F. Lott. (1995). Definitions of territoriality used in the study of variation in vertebrate spacing systems. *Animal Behaviour* **49**: 1581–1597.

Maher, L. A., J. T. Stock, S. Finney, J. J. N. Heywood, P. T. Miracle, and E. B. Banning. (2011). A unique human–fox burial from a pre-Natufian cemetery in the Levant (Jordan). *PLoS One* **6**: e15815.

Mahrenke, P. III. (1971). An observation of four wolves killing another wolf. *Journal of Mammalogy* **52**: 630–631.

Malcolm, J. R. and K. Marten. (1982). Natural selection and the communal rearing of pups in African wild dogs (*Lycaon pictus*). *Behavioral Ecology and Sociobiology* **10**: 1–13.

Malm, K. (1995). Regurgitation in relation to weaning in the domestic dog: a questionnaire study. *Applied Animal Behaviour Science* **43**: 111–122.

Marlowe, F. W. (2004). What explains Hadza food sharing? *Research in Economic Anthropology* 23: 69–88.

Maros, K., P. Pongrácz, G. Bárdos, C. Molnár, T. Faragó, and Á. Miklósi. (2008). Dogs can discriminate barks from different situations. *Applied Animal Behaviour Science* 114: 159–167.

Marsack, P. and G. Campbell. (1990). Feeding behaviour and diet of dingoes in the Nullarbor Region, Western Australia. *Wildlife Research* 17: 349–357.

Martin, P. and T. M. Caro. (1985). On the functions of play and its role in behavioral development. *Advances in the Study of Behavior* 15: 59–103.

Martins, T. and J. R. Valle. (1948). Hormonal regulation of the micturition behavior of dogs. *Journal of Comparative and Physiological Psychology* 41: 301–311.

Matsunami, H. and L. B. Buck. (1997). A multigene family encoding a diverse array of putative pheromone receptors in mammals. *Cell* 90: 775–784.

Matthew, W. D. (1930). The phylogeny of dogs. *Journal of Mammalogy* 11: 117–138.

Maximilian, A. P. (1906). Travels in the interior of North America, 1832–1834. In *Early Western Travels 1748–1846*, Volume 22, Part 1, R. G. Thwaites (ed.). Cleveland, OH: Arthur H. Clark, 393 pp.

Maynard Smith, J. (1974). The theory of games and the evolution of animal conflicts. *Journal of Theoretical Biology* 47: 209–221.

Maynard Smith, J. (1979). Game theory and the evolution of behaviour. *Proceedings of the Royal Society of London* 205B: 475–488.

McCarley, H. (1962). The taxonomic status of wild *Canis* (Canidae) in the south central United States. *Southwestern Naturalist* 7: 227–235.

McCarley, H. (1975). Long-distance vocalizations of coyotes (*Canis latrans*). *Journal of Mammalogy* 56: 847–856.

McCarley, H. (1978). Vocalizations of red wolves (*Canis rufus*). *Journal of Mammalogy* 58: 27–35.

McLeod, P. J. (1990). Infanticide by female wolves. *Canadian Journal of Zoology* 68: 402–404.

McLeod, P. J. (1996). Developmental changes in associations among timber wolf (*Canis lupus*) postures. *Behavioural Processes* 38: 105–118.

McLeod, P. J. and J. C. Fentress. (1997). Developmental changes in the sequential behavior of interacting timber wolf pups. *Behavioural Processes* 39: 127–136.

McLoughlin, P. D., L. R. Walton, H. D. Cluff, P. C. Paquet, and M. A. Ramsay. (2004). Hierarchical habitat selection by tundra wolves. *Journal of Mammalogy* 85: 576–580.

McNamara, J. M., A. I. Houston, and J. R. Krebs. (1990). Why hoard? The economics of food storing in tits, *Parus* spp. *Behavioral Ecology* 1: 12–23.

McNay, M. E. (2002). Wolf–human interactions in Alaska and Canada: a review of the case history. *Wildlife Society Bulletin* 30: 831–843.

Mech, L. D. (1966). *The Wolves of Isle Royale, Fauna of the National Parks of the United States, Fauna Series 7*. Washington, DC: US Government Printing Office, xiv + 210 pp.

Mech, L. D. (1970). *The Wolf: The Ecology and Behavior of an Endangered Species*. Garden City, NY: Natural History Press, xx + 384 pp.

Mech, L. D. (1974). *Canis lupus, Mammalian Species No. 37*. Lawrence, KS: American Society of Mammalogists, 6 pp.

Mech, L. D. (1977). Productivity, mortality, and population trend of wolves in northeastern Minnesota. *Journal of Mammalogy* 58: 559–574.

Mech, L. D. (1987). Age, season, distance, direction, and social aspects of wolf dispersal from a Minnesota pack. In *Mammalian Dispersal Patterns: The Effects of Social Structure on Population Genetics*, B. D. Chepko-Sade and Z. T. Halpin (eds.). Chicago, IL: University of Chicago Press, pp. 55–74.

Mech, L. D. (1988a). *The Arctic Wolf: Living with the Pack*. Stillwater, MN: Voyageur Press, 128 pp.

Mech, L. D. (1988b). Longevity in wild wolves. *Journal of Mammalogy* **69**: 197–198.

Mech, L. D. (1991). *The Way of the Wolf*. Stillwater, MN: Voyageur Press, 120 pp.

Mech, L. D. (1992). Daytime activity of wolves during winter in northeastern Minnesota. *Journal of Mammalogy* **73**: 570–571.

Mech, L. D. (1993a). Details of a confrontation between two wild wolves. *Canadian Journal of Zoology* **71**: 1900–1903.

Mech, L. D. (1993b). Resistance of young wolf pups to inclement weather. *Journal of Mammalogy* **74**: 485–486.

Mech, L. D. (1994a). Buffer zones of territories of gray wolves as regions of intraspecific strife. *Journal of Mammalogy* **75**: 199–202.

Mech, L. D. (1994b). Regular and homeward travel speeds of arctic wolves. *Journal of Mammalogy* **75**: 741–742.

Mech, L. D. (1995a). A ten-year history of the demography and productivity of an arctic wolf pack. *Arctic* **48**: 329–332.

Mech, L. D. (1995b). Summer movements and behavior of an arctic wolf, *Canis lupus*, pack without pups. *Canadian Field-Naturalist* **109**: 473–475.

Mech, L. D. (1999). Alpha status, dominance, and division of labor in wolf packs. *Canadian Journal of Zoology* **77**: 1196–1203.

Mech, L. D. (2000). Leadership in wolf, *Canis lupus*, packs. *Canadian Field-Naturalist* **114**: 259–263.

Mech, L. D. (2010). What is the taxonomic identity of Minnesota wolves? *Canadian Journal of Zoology* **88**: 129–138.

Mech, L. D. and L. D. Frenzel Jr. (1969). Continuing timber wolf studies. *Naturalist* **20**: 30–35.

Mech, L. D. and S. T. Knick. (1978). Sleeping distance in wolf pairs in relation to the breeding season. *Behavioral Biology* **23**: 521–525.

Mech, L. D. and H. H. Hertel. (1983). An eight-year demography of a Minnesota wolf pack. *Acta Zoologica Fennica* **174**: 249–250.

Mech, L. D. and U. S. Seal. (1987). Premature reproductive activity in wild wolves. *Journal of Mammalogy* **68**: 871–873.

Mech, L. D. and M. E. Nelson. (1989). Polygyny in a wild wolf pack. *Journal of Mammalogy* **70**: 675–676.

Mech, L. D. and M. E. Nelson. (1990). Non-family wolf, *Canis lupus*, packs. *Canadian Field-Naturalist* **104**: 482–483.

Mech, L. D. and S. M. Goyal. (1995). Effects of canine parvovirus on gray wolves in Minnesota. *Journal of Wildlife Management* **59**: 565–570.

Mech, L. D. and N. E. Federoff. (2002). α_1-antitrypsin polymorphism and systematics of eastern North American wolves. *Canadian Journal of Zoology* **80**: 961–963.

Mech, L. D. and L. Boitani. (2003). Wolf social ecology. In *Wolves: Behavior, Ecology, and Conservation*, L. D. Mech and L. Boitani (eds.). Chicago, IL: University of Chicago Press, pp. 1–34.

Mech, L. D. and W. J. Paul. (2008). Wolf body mass cline across Minnesota related to taxonomy? *Canadian Journal of Zoology* **86**: 933–936.

Mech, L. D., U. S. Seal, and S. M. Arthur. (1984). Recuperation of a severely debilitated wolf. *Journal of Wildlife Diseases* **20**: 166–168.

Mech, L. D., L. G. Adams, T. J. Meier, J. W. Burch, and B. W. Dale. (1998). *The Wolves of Denali*. Minneapolis, MN: University of Minnesota Press, x + 225 pp.

Mech, L. D., P. C. Wolf, and J. M. Packard. (1999). Regurgitative food transfer among wild wolves. *Canadian Journal of Zoology* **77**: 1192–1195.

Medjo, D. C. and L. D. Mech. (1976). Reproductive activity in nine- and ten-month-old wolves. *Journal of Mammalogy* **57**: 406–408.

Meggitt, M. (1955). Djanba among the Walbiri, Central Australia. *Anthropos* **50**: 375–403.

Meggitt, M. J. (1965). The association between Australian Aborigines and dingoes. In *Man, Culture, and Animals: The Role of Animals in Human Ecological Adjustments*, Publication No. 78, A. Leeds and A. P. Vayda (eds.). Washington, DC: American Association for the Advancement of Science, pp. 7–26.

Meier, T. J., T. W. Burch, L. D. Mech, and L. G. Adams. (1995). Pack structure and genetic relatedness among wolf packs in a naturally-regulated population. In *Ecology and Conservation of Wolves in a Changing World*, Occasional Publication No. 35, L. N. Carbyn, S. H. Fritts, and D. R. Seip (eds.). Edmonton, AB: Canadian Circumpolar Institute, pp. 293–302.

Mekosh-Rosenbaum, V., W. J. Carr, J. L. Goodwin, P. L. Thomas, A. D'Ver, and C. J. Wysock. (1994). Age-dependent responses to chemosensory cues mediating kin recognition in dogs (*Canis familiaris*). *Physiology and Behavior* **55**: 495–499.

Mendelssohn, H. (1982). Wolves in Israel. In *Wolves of the World: Perspectives of Behavior, Ecology, and Conservation*, F. H. Harrington and P. C. Paquet (eds.). Park Ridge, NJ: Noyes Publications, pp. 173–195.

Mengel, R. M. (1971). A study of the dog–coyote hybrids and implications concerning hybridization In *Canis*. *Journal of Mammalogy* **52**: 316–336.

Meredith, M. (2001). Human vomeronasal organ function: a critical review of best and worst cases. *Chemical Senses* **26**: 433–445.

Merrill, S. B. and L. D. Mech. (2000). Details of extensive movements by Minnesota wolves (*Canis lupus*). *American Midland Naturalist* **144**: 428–433.

Messier, F. (1985a). Solitary living and extraterritorial movements of wolves in relation to social status and prey abundance. *Canadian Journal of Zoology* **63**: 239–245.

Messier, F. (1985b). Social organization, spatial distribution, and population density of wolves in relation to moose density. *Canadian Journal of Zoology* **63**: 1068–1077.

Messier, F. (1991). The significance of limiting and regulating factors on the demography of moose and white-tailed deer. *Journal of Animal Ecology* **60**: 377–393.

Messier, F. (1994). Ungulate population models with predation: a case study with the North American moose. *Ecology* **75**: 478–488.

Messier, F. and C. Barrette. (1982). The social system of the coyote (*Canis latrans*) in a forested habitat. *Canadian Journal of Zoology* **60**: 1743–1753.

Messier, F. and M. Crête. (1984). Body condition and population regulation by food resources in moose. *Oecologia* **65**: 44–50.

Messier, F. and M. Crête. (1985). Moose–wolf dynamics and the natural regulation of moose populations. *Oecologia* **65**: 503–512.

Milakovic, B. and K. L. Parker. (2011). Using stable isotopes to define diets of wolves in northern British Columbia, Canada. *Journal of Mammalogy* **92**: 295–304.

Milham, P. and P. Thompson. (1976). Relative antiquity of human occupation and extinct fauna at Madura Cave, south-eastern Western Australia. *Mankind* **10**: 175–180.

Miller, D. B. (1977). Social displays of mallard ducks (*Anas platyrhynchos*): effects of domestication. *Journal of Comparative and Physiological Psychology* **91**: 221–232.

Miller, F. L., A. Gunn, and E. Broughton. (1985). Surplus killing as exemplified by wolf predation on newborn caribou. *Canadian Journal of Zoology* **63**: 295–300.

Miller, G. S. (1920). Remarks on some South American Canidae. *Journal of Mammalogy* **1**: 149–150.

Miller, G. S. Jr. (1912). The names of the large wolves of northern and western North America. *Smithsonian Miscellaneous Collections* **59**(15): 5 pp.

Miller, K. V., B. Jemiolo, J. W. Gassett, I. Jelinek, D. Wiesler, and M. Novotny. (1998). Putative chemical signals from white-tailed deer (*Odocoileus virginianus*): social and seasonal effects on urinary volatile excretion in males. *Journal of Chemical Ecology* **24**: 673–684.

Mills, K. J., B. R. Patterson, and D. L. Murray. (2008). Direct estimation of early survival and movements in eastern wolf pups. *Journal of Wildlife Management* **72**: 949–954.

Mitchell, B. D. and P. B. Banks. (2005). Do wild dogs exclude foxes? Evidence for competition from dietary and spatial overlaps. *Austral Ecology* **30**: 581–591.

Molnár, C., P. Pongrácz, T. Faragó, A. Dóka, and Á. Miklósi. (2009). Dogs discriminate between barks: the effect of context and identity of the caller. *Behavioural Processes* **82**: 198–201.

Mombaerts, P. (2004). Genes and ligands for odorant, vomeronasal and taste receptors. *Nature Reviews in Neuroscience* **5**: 263–278.

Moore, G. C. and J. S. Millar. (1986). Food habits and average weights of a fall–winter sample of eastern coyotes, *Canis latrans*. *Canadian Field-Naturalist* **100**: 105–106.

Morey, D. F. (1986). Studies on Amerindian dogs: taxonomic analysis of canid crania from the northern Plains. *Journal of Archaeological Science* **13**: 119–145.

Morey, D. F. (1994). The early evolution of the domestic dog. *American Scientist* **82**: 336–347.

Morey, P. S., E. M. Gese, and S. Gehrt. (2007). Spatial and temporal variation in the diet of coyotes in the Chicago metropolitan area. *American Midland Naturalist* **158**: 147–161.

Morton, E. S. (1977). On the occurrence and significance of motivation–structural rules in some bird and mammal sounds. *American Naturalist* **111**: 855–869.

Moss, G. L. and D. B. Croft. (1999). Body condition of the red kangaroo (*Macropus rufus*) in arid Australia: the effect of environmental condition, sex and reproduction. *Australian Journal of Ecology* **24**: 97–109.

Müller-Schwarze, D., R. Altieri, and N. Porter. (1984). Alert odor from skin gland in deer. *Journal of Chemical Ecology* **10**: 1707–1729.

Muñoz-Fuentes, V., C. T. Darimont, R. K. Wayne, P. C. Paquet, and J. A. Leonard. (2009). Ecological factors drive differentiation in wolves from British Columbia. *Journal of Biogeography* **36**: 1516–1531.

Murie, A. (1940). *Ecology of the Coyote in the Yellowstone, Fauna of the National Parks of the United States, Fauna Series 4*. Washington, DC: US Government Printing Office, x + 206 pp.

Murie, A. (1944). *The Wolves of Mount McKinley, Fauna of the National Parks of the United States, Fauna Series 5*. Washington, DC: US Government Printing Office, xix + 238 pp.

Musiani, M., J. A. Leonard, H. D. Cluff, C. C. Gates, S. Mariani, and P. C. Paquet *et al.* (2007). Differentiation of tundra/taiga and boreal coniferous forest wolves: genetics, coat colour and association with migratory caribou. *Molecular Ecology* **16**: 4149–4170.

Mykytowycz, R. (1972). The behavioural role of the mammalian skin glands. *Naturwissenschaften* **59**: 133–139.

Nagel, T. (1974). What is it like to be a bat? *Philosophical Review* **83**: 435–450.

Natynczuk, S., J. W. S. Bradshaw, and D. W. Macdonald. (1989). Chemical constituents of the anal sacs of domestic dogs. *Biochemical Systematics and Ecology* **17**: 83–87.

Neff, M. W., K. R. Robertson, A. K. Wong, N. Safra, K. W. Broman, and M. Slatkin *et al.* (2004). Breed distribution and history of canine *mdr1–1Δ*, a pharmacogenetic mutation that marks the emergence of breeds from the collie lineage. *Proceedings of the National Academy of Sciences* **101**: 11725–11730.

Nesbitt, W. H. (1975). Ecology of a feral dog pack on a wildlife refuge. In *The Wild Canids: Their Systematics, Behavioral Ecology and Evolution*, M. W. Fox (ed.). New York, NY: Van Nostrand Reinhold, pp. 391–396.

Newsome, A. E. and L. Corbett. (1982). The identity of the dingo. II. Hybridization with domestic dogs in captivity and in the wild. *Australian Journal of Zoology* **30**: 365–374.

Newsome, A. E. and L. K. Corbett. (1985). The identity of the dingo III. The incidence of dingoes, dogs and hybrids and their coat colours in remote and settled regions of Australia. *Australian Journal of Zoology* **33**: 363–375.

Newsome, A. E., L. K. Corbett, and S. M. Carpenter. (1980). The identity of the dingo I. Morphological discriminants of dingo and dog skulls. *Australian Journal of Zoology* **28**: 615–625.

Newsome, A. E., L. K. Corbett, and R. J. Burt. (1983a). The feeding ecology of the dingo. I. Stomach contents from trapping in south-eastern Australia, and the non-target wildlife also caught in dingo traps. *Australian Wildlife Research* **10**: 477–486.

Newsome, A. E., P. C. Catling, and L. K. Corbett. (1983b). The feeding ecology of the dingo. II. Dietary and numerical relationships with fluctuating prey populations in south-eastern Australia. *Australian Journal of Ecology* **8**: 345–366.

Newton-Fisher, N., S. Harris, P. White, and G. Jones. (1993). Structure and function of red fox *Vulpes vulpes* vocalisations. *Bioacoustics* **5**: 1–31.

Nind, S. (1831). Description of the natives of King George's Sound (Swan River Colony) and adjoining country. *Journal of the Royal Geographical Society of London* **1**: 21–51.

Nolte, D. L., J. R. Mason, G. Epple, E. Arnov, and D. E. Campbell. (1994). Why are predator urines aversive to prey? *Journal of Chemical Ecology* **20**: 1501–1516.

Nöth, W. (1990). *Handbook of Semiotics*. Bloomington, IN: Indiana University Press, xii + 576 pp.

Nowak, R. M. (1979). *North American Quaternary Canis*. Lawrence, KS: Monograph No. 6, University of Kansas Museum of Natural History, 154 pp.

Nowak, R. M. (1983). A perspective on the taxonomy of wolves in North America. In *Wolves in Canada and Alaska: Their Status, Biology, and Management*, Canadian Wildlife Service Report Series No. 45, L. N. Carbyn (ed.). Edmonton, AB: Canadian Wildlife Service, pp. 10–19.

Nowak, R. M. (1992). The red wolf is not a hybrid. *Conservation Biology* **6**: 593–595.

Nowak, R. M. (1995). Another look at wolf taxonomy. In *Ecology and Conservation of Wolves in a Changing World*, Occasional Publication No. 35, L. N. Carbyn, S. H. Fritts, and D. R. Seip (eds.). Edmonton, AB: Canadian Circumpolar Institute, pp. 375–397.

Nowak, R. M. (2002). The original status of wolves in eastern North America. *Southeastern Naturalist* **1**: 95–130.

Nowak, R. M. and N. E. Federoff. (1998). Validity of the red wolf: response to Roy *et al.* *Conservation Biology* **12**: 722–725.

Ognev, S. I. (1931). [Mammals of Eastern Europe and Northern Asia, Vol. II, Carnivora (Fissipedia)]. Moscow and Leningrad: Glavnauka-Gosudarstvennoe Izdatel'stvo, 590 pp. + indices. [1962 translation by Israel Program for Scientific Translations, Jerusalem.]

Ohl, F. (1996). Ontogeny of vocalizations in domestic dogs, breed standard-poodle (*Canis lupus* f. *familiaris*). *Zoologische Beiträge* **37**: 199–215.

Okkens, A. C. and H. S. Kooistra. (2006). Anoestrus in the dog: a fascinating story. *Reproduction in Domestic Animals* **41**: 291–296.

Okkens, A. C., S. J. Dieleman, H. S. Kooistra, and M. M. Bevers. (1997). Plasma concentrations of prolactin in overtly pseudopregnant Afghan hounds and the effect of metergoline. *Journal of Reproduction and Fertility* (Suppl.) **51**: 295–301.

Okumura, N., N. Ishiguro, M. Nakano, A. Matsui, and M. Sahara. (1996). Intra- and interbreed genetic variations of mitochondrial DNA major non-coding regions in Japanese native dog breeds (*Canis familiaris*). *Animal Genetics* **27**: 397–405.

Olender, T., T. Fuchs, C. Linhart, R. Shamir, M. Adams, and F. Kalush *et al.* (2004). The canine olfactory subgenome. *Genomics* **83**: 361–372.

Olsen, S. J. (1974). Early domestic dogs in North America and their origins. *Journal of Field Archaeology* **1**: 343–345.

Olsen, S. J. and J. W. Olsen. (1977). The Chinese wolf, ancestor of New World dogs. *Science* **197**: 533–535.

Olson, P. N., R. A. Bowen, M. D. Behrendt, J. D. Olson, and T. M. Nett. (1984a). Concentrations of testosterone in canine serum during late anestrus, proestrus, estrus, and early diestrus. *American Journal of Veterinary Research* **45**: 145–148.

Olson, P. N., R. A. Bowen, M. D. Behrendt, J. D. Olson, and T. M. Nett. (1984b). Concentrations of progesterone and luteinizing hormone in the serum of diestrous bitches before and after hysterectomy. *American Journal of Veterinary Research* **45**: 149–153.

Olson, P. N., T. M. Nett, R. A Bowen, H. R. Sawyer, and G. D. Niswender. (1989). Endocrine regulation of the corpus luteum of the bitch as a potential target for altering fertility. *Journal of Reproduction and Fertility* (Suppl.) **39**: 27–40.

Olson, S. F. (1938a). Organization and range of the pack. *Ecology* **19**: 168–170.

Olson, S. F. (1938b). A study in predatory relationship with particular reference to the wolf. *Scientific Monthly* **46**: 323–336.

Onclin, K., B. Murphy, and J. P. Verstegen. (2002). Comparisons of estradiol, LH and FSH patterns in pregnant and nonpregnant beagle bitches. *Theriogenology* **57**: 1957–1972.

Oosenbrug, S. M. and L. N. Carbyn. (1982). Winter predation on bison and activity patterns of a wolf pack in Wood Buffalo National Park. In *Wolves of the World: Perspectives of Behavior, Ecology, and Conservation*, F. H. Harrington and P. C. Paquet (eds.). Park Ridge, NJ: Noyes Publications, pp. 43–70.

Oppenheimer, E. and J. R. Oppenheimer. (1975). Certain behavioral features in the pariah dog (*Canis familiaris*) in West Bengal. *Applied Animal Ethology* **2**: 81–92.

Ortolani, A., H. Vernooij, and R. Coppinger. (2009). Ethiopian village dogs: behavioural responses to a stranger's approach. *Applied Animal Behaviour Science* **119**: 210–218.

Ostrander, E. A. (2007). Genetics and the shape of dogs. *American Scientist* **95**: 406–413.

Packard, J. M. (2003). Wolf behavior: reproductive, social, and intelligent. In *Wolves: Behavior, Ecology, and Conservation*, L. D. Mech and L. Boitani (eds.). Chicago, IL: University of Chicago Press, pp. 35–65.

Packard, J. M., L. D. Mech, and U. S. Seal. (1983). Social influences on reproduction in wolves. In *Wolves in Canada and Alaska: Their Status, Biology, and Management*, Canadian Wildlife Service Report Series No. 45, L. N. Carbyn (ed.). Edmonton, AB: Canadian Wildlife Service, pp. 78–85.

Packard, J. M., U. S. Seal, L. D. Mech, and E. D. Plotka. (1985). Causes of reproductive failure in two family groups of wolves (*Canis lupus*). *Zeitschrift für Tierpsychologie* **68**: 24–40.

Packard, J. M., L. D. Mech, and R. R. Ream. (1992). Weaning in an arctic wolf pack: behavioral mechanisms. *Canadian Journal of Zoology* **70**: 1269–1275.

Packer, C. and L. Ruttan. (1988). The evolution of cooperative hunting. *American Naturalist* **132**: 159–198.

Packer, C., D. Scheel, and A. E. Pusey. (1990). Why lions form groups: food is not enough. *American Naturalist* **136**: 1–19.

Pal, S. K. (2003). Reproductive behaviour of free-ranging rural dogs in West Bengal, India. *Acta Theriologica* **48**: 271–281.

Pal, S. K. (2005). Parental care in free-ranging dogs, *Canis familiaris*. *Applied Animal Behaviour Science* **90**: 31–47.

Pal, S. K. (2010). Play behaviour during early ontogeny in free-ranging dogs (*Canis familiaris*). *Applied Animal Behaviour Science* **126**: 140–153.

Pal, S. K., B. Ghosh, and S. Roy. (1998). Agonistic behaviour of free-ranging dogs (*Canis familiaris*) in relation to season, sex and age. *Applied Animal Behaviour Science* **59**: 331–348.

Palacios, V., E. Font, and R. Márquez. (2007). Iberian wolf howls: acoustic structure, individual variation, and comparison with North American populations. *Journal of Mammalogy* **88**: 606–613.

Palmer, R. and D. Custance. (2008). A counterbalanced version of Ainsworth's Strange Situation procedure reveals secure-base effects in dog–human relationships. *Applied Animal Behaviour Science* **109**: 306–319.

Pang, J-F., C. Kluetsch, X-J. Zou, A-b. Zhang, L-Y. Luo, and H. Angleby *et al.* (2009). mtDNA data indicate a single origin for dogs south of Yangtze River, less than 16,300 years ago, from numerous wolves. *Molecular Biology and Evolution* **26**: 2849–2864.

Paquet, P. C. (1992). Prey use strategies of sympatric wolves and coyotes in Riding Mountain National Park, Manitoba. *Journal of Mammalogy* **73**: 337–343.

Paquet, P. C., S. Bragdon, and S. McCusker. (1982). Cooperative rearing of simultaneous litters in captive wolves. In *Wolves of the World: Perspectives of Behavior, Ecology, and Conservation*, F. H. Harrington and P. C. Paquet (eds.). Park Ridge, NJ: Noyes Publications, pp. 223–237.

Paradiso, J. L. (1968). Canids recently collected in east Texas, with comments on the taxonomy of the red wolf. *American Midland Naturalist* **80**: 529–534.

Paradiso, J. L. and R. M. Nowak. (1971). A report on the taxonomic status and distribution of the red wolf, Special Scientific Report – Wildlife 145. Washington, DC: US Fish and Wildlife Service, 36 pp.

Parillo, F. and S. Diverio. (2009). Glycocomposition of the apocrine gland secretions in the fallow deer (*Dama dama*). *Research in Veterinary Science* **86**: 194–199.

Parker, G. (1995). *Eastern Coyote: The Story of Its Success*. Halifax, NS: Nimbus Publishing, x + 254 pp.

Parker, G. R. (1973). Distribution and densities of wolves within barren-ground caribou range in northern mainland Canada. *Journal of Mammalogy* **54**: 341–348.

Parker, H. G., L. V. Kim, N. B. Sutter, S. Carlson, T. D. Lorentzen, and T. B. Malek *et al.* (2004). Genetic structure of the purebred domestic dog. *Science* **304**: 1160–1164.

Parmelee, D. F. (1964). Myth of the wolf. *The Beaver* **295**: 4–9.

Parsons, D. R. (1998). "Green fire" returns to the southwest: reintroduction of the Mexican wolf. *Wildlife Society Bulletin* **26**: 799–807.

Parsons, M. H. and D. T. Blumstein. (2010a). Feeling vulnerable? Indirect risk cues differently influence how two marsupials respond to novel dingo urine. *Ethology* **116**: 972–980.

Parsons, M. H. and D. T. Blumstein. (2010b). Familiarity breeds contempt: kangaroos persistently avoid areas with experimentally deployed dingo scents. *PLoS One* **5**: e10403.

Parsons, M. H., B. B. Lamont, B. R. Kovacs, and S. J. J. F. Davies. (2007). Effects of novel and historic predator urines on semi-wild western grey kangaroos. *Journal of Wildlife Management* **71**: 1225–1228.

Pasitschniak-Arts, M., M. E. Taylor, and L. D. Mech. (1988). Note on skeletal injuries in an adult arctic wolf. *Arctic and Alpine Research* **20**: 360–365.

Patronek, G. J., D. J. Waters, and L. T. Glickman. (1997). Comparative longevity of pet dogs and humans: implications for gerontology research. *Journal of Gerontology* **52A**: B171–B178.

Paulraj, S., N. Sundararajan, A. Manimozhi, and S. Walker. (1992). Reproduction of the Indian wild dog (*Cuon alpinus*) in captivity. *Zoo Biology* **11**: 235–241.

Pavey, C. R., S. R. Eldridge, and M. Heywood. (2008). Population dynamics and prey selection of native and introduced predators during a rodent outbreak in arid Australia. *Journal of Mammalogy* **89**: 674–683.

Payne, R. B. (1977). The ecology of brood parasitism in birds. *Annual Review of Ecology and Systematics* **8**: 1–28.

Peaker, M. (1995). Endocrine signals from the mammary gland. *Journal of Endocrinology* **147**: 189–193.

Pekins, P. J. (1992). Winter diet and bioenergetics of eastern coyotes: a review. In *Ecology and Management of the Eastern Coyote*, A. H. Boer (ed.). Fredericton, NB: Wildlife Research Unit, University of New Brunswick, pp. 87–99.

Penn, D. C. and D. J. Povinelli. (2007). On the lack of evidence that non-human animals possess anything remotely resembling a 'theory of mind'. *Philosophical Transactions of the Royal Society* **362B**: 731–744.

Peters, R. P. and L. D. Mech. (1975). Scent-marking in wolves. *American Scientist* **63**: 628–637.

Peterson, E. K., M. A. Letellier, J. A. Parsons, E. D. Plotka, L. D. Mech, and U. S. Seal. (1981). Olfactory pedunculotomy induced anosmia in the wolf (*Canis lupus*). *Physiology and Behavior* **27**: 543–546.

Peterson, R. O. (1977). *Wolf Ecology and Prey Relationships on Isle Royale*, National Park Service Scientific Monograph Series No. 11. Washington, DC: US Government Printing Office, xx + 210 pp.

Peterson, R. O. (1979). Social rejection following mating of a subordinate wolf. *Journal of Mammalogy* **60**: 219–221.

Peterson, R. O. and R. E. Page. (1988). The rise and fall of Isle Royal wolves, 1975–1986. *Journal of Mammalogy* **69**: 89–99.

Peterson, R. O., J. D. Woolington, and T. N. Bailey. (1984). Wolves of the Kenai Peninsula, Alaska. *Wildlife Monographs* **88**: 52 pp.

Peterson, R. O., N. J. Thomas, J. M. Thurber, J. A. Vucetich, and T. A. Waite. (1998). Population limitation and the wolves of Isle Royale. *Journal of Mammalogy* **79**: 828–841.

Peterson, R. O., A. K. Jacobs, T. D. Drummer, L. D. Mech, and D. W. Smith. (2002). Leadership behavior in relation to dominance and reproductive status in gray wolves, *Canis lupus. Canadian Journal of Zoology* **80**: 1405–1412.

Pferd, W. III. (1987). *Dogs of the American Indians.* Fairfax, VA: Denlinger's Publishers, 192 pp.

Phemister, R. D., P. A. Holst, J. S. Spano, and M. L. Hopwood. (1973). Time of ovulation in the beagle bitch. *Biology of Reproduction* **8**: 74–82.

Phillips, M. K. and V. G. Henry. (1992). Comments on red wolf taxonomy. *Conservation Biology* **6**: 596–599.

Phillips, M. K. V. G. Henry, and B. T. Kelly. (2003). Restoration of the red wolf. In *Wolves: Behavior, Ecology, and Conservation*, L. D. Mech and L. Boitani (eds.). Chicago, IL: University of Chicago Press, pp. 272–288.

Pilgrim, K. L., D. K. Boyd, and S. H. Forbes. (1998). Testing for wolf–coyote hybridization in the Rocky Mountains using mitochondrial DNA. *Journal of Wildlife Management* **62**: 683–689.

Pilot, M., W. Jędrzejewski, W. Branicki, V. E. Sidorovich, B. Jędrzejewski, and K. Stachura *et al.* (2006). Ecological factors influence population genetic structure of European grey wolves. *Molecular Ecology* **15**: 4533–4553.

Pimlott, D. H. (1967). Wolf predation and ungulate populations. *American Zoologist* **7**: 267–278.

Plotnik, R., F. A. King, and L. Roberts. (1968). Effects of competition on the aggressive behavior of squirrel and cebus monkeys. *Behaviour* **32**: 315–332.

Pocock, R. L. (1935). The races of *Canis lupus. Proceedings of the Zoological Society of London*, pp. 647–686.

Pongrácz, P., C. Molnár, and Á. Miklósi. (2010). Barking in family dogs: an ethological approach. *Veterinary Journal* **183**: 141–147.

Potvin, F. (1987). Wolf movements and population dynamics in Papineau-Labelle Reserve, Quebec. *Canadian Journal of Zoology* **66**: 1266–1273.

Potvin, M. J., R. O. Peterson, and J. A. Vucetich. (2004). Wolf homesite attendance patterns. *Canadian Journal of Zoology* **82**: 1512–1518.

Powers, M. A., S. S. Schiffman, D. C. Lawson, T. N. Pappas, and I. L. Taylor. (1990). The effect of taste on gastric and pancreatic responses in dogs. *Physiology and Behavior* **47**: 1295–1297.

Prato-Previde, E., D. M. Custance, C. Spiezio, and F. Sabatini. (2003). Is the dog–human relationship an attachment bond? An observational study using Ainsworth's Strange Situation. *Behaviour* **140**: 225–254.

Preti, G., E. L. Muetterties, J. M. Furman, J. J. Kennelly, and B. E. Johns. (1976). Volatile constituents of dog (*Canis familiaris*) and coyote (*Canis latrans*) anal sacs. *Journal of Chemical Ecology* **2**: 177–186.

Price, E. O. (1984). Behavioral aspects of animal domestication. *Quarterly Review of Biology* **59**: 1–32.

Pringle, L. P. (1960). Notes on coyotes in southern New England. *Journal of Mammalogy* **41**: 278.

Puja, I. K., D. N. Irion, A. L. Schaffer, and N. C. Pedersen. (2005). The Kintamani dog: genetic profile of an emerging breed from Bali, Indonesia. *Journal of Heredity* **96**: 854–859.

Pulliainen, E. (1965). Studies on the wolf (*Canis lupus* L.) in Finland. *Annales Zoologici Fennici* **2**: 215–259.

Pulliainen, E. (1967). A contribution to the study of the social behavior of the wolf. *American Zoologist* **7**: 313–317.

Pulliainen, E. (1982). Behavior and structure of an expanding wolf population in Karelia, Northern Europe. In *Wolves of the World: Perspectives of Behavior, Ecology, and Conservation*, F. H. Harrington and P. C. Paquet (eds.). Park Ridge, NJ: Noyes Publications, pp. 134–145.

Purcell, B. V. (2010). A novel observation of dingoes (*Canis lupus dingo*) attacking a swimming eastern grey kangaroo (*Macropus giganteus*). *Australian Mammalogy* **32**: 201–204.

Pusey, A. E. and C. Packer. (1987). The evolution of sex-biased dispersal in lions. *Behaviour* **101**: 275–310.

Quaranta, A., M. Siniscalchi, and G. Vallortigara. (2007). Asymmetric tail-wagging responses by dogs to different emotive stimuli. *Current Biology* **17**: R199-R201.

Quay, W. B. (1959). Microscopic structure and variation in the cutaneous glands of the deer, *Odocoileus virginianus*. *Journal of Mammalogy* **40**: 114–128.

Queller, D. C. (1994). Genetic relatedness in viscous populations. *Evolutionary Ecology* **8**: 70–73.

Quignon, P, M. Giraud, M. Rambaut, P. Lavigne, S. Teacher, and E. Morin *et al.* (2005). The dog and rat olfactory receptor repertoires. *Genome Biology* **6**: R83.

Qvarnström, A. and E. Forsgren. (1998). Should females prefer dominant males? *Trends in Ecology and Evolution* **13**: 498–501.

Rabb, G. B., J. H. Woolpy, and B. E. Ginsburg. (1967). Social relationships in a group of captive wolves. *American Zoologist* **7**: 305–311.

Räikkönen, J., A. Bignert, P. Mortensen, and B. Fernholm. (2006). Congenital defects in a highly inbred wild wolf population (*Canis lupus*). *Mammalian Biology* **71**: 65–73.

Ralph, E. K. (1955). University of Pennsylvania radiocarbon dates I. *Science* **121**: 149–151.

Ramseyer, A., A. Boissy, B. Dumont, and B. Thierry. (2009). Decision making in group departures of sheep is a continuous process. *Animal Behaviour* **78**: 71–78.

Randi, E. (1993). Effects of fragmentation and isolation on genetic variability of the Italian population of wolf *Canis lupus* and brown bear *Ursus arctos*. *Acta Theriologica* **38** (Suppl. 2): 113–120.

Randi, E. and V. Lucchini. (2002). Detecting rare introgression of domestic dog genes into wild wolf (*Canis lupus*) populations by Bayesian admixture analyses of microsatellite variation. *Conservation Genetics* **3**: 31–45.

Randi, E., V. Lucchini, M. F. Christensen, N. Mucci, S. M. Funk, and G. Dolf *et al.* (2000). Mitochondrial DNA variability in Italian and east European wolves: detecting the consequences of small population size and hybridization. *Conservation Biology* **14**: 464–473.

Ranson, E. and F. A. Beach. (1985). Effects of testosterone on ontogeny of urinary behavior in male and female dogs. *Hormones and Behavior* **19**: 36–51.

Rasmussen, G. S. A., M. Gusset, F. Courchamp, and D. W. Macdonald. (2008). Achilles' Heel of sociality revealed by energetic poverty trap in cursorial hunters. *American Naturalist* **172**: 508–518.

Rausch, R. A. (1967). Some aspects of the population ecology of wolves, Alaska. *American Zoologist* **7**: 253–265.

Raymer, J., D. Wiesler, M. Novotny, C. Asa, U. S. Seal, and L. D. Mech. (1984). Volatile constituents of wolf (*Canis lupus*) urine as related to gender and season. *Experientia* **40**: 707–709.

Raymer, J., D. Wiesler, M. Novotny, C. Asa, U. S. Seal, and L. D. Mech. (1985). Chemical investigations of wolf (*Canis lupus*) anal-sac secretion in relation to breeding season. *Journal of Chemical Ecology* **11**: 593–608.

Raymer, J., D. Wiesler, M. Novotny, C. Asa, U. S. Seal, and L. D. Mech. (1986). Chemical scent constituents in urine of wolf [*sic*] (*Canis lupus*) and their dependence on reproductive hormones. *Journal of Chemical Ecology* **12**: 297–314.

Reddy, M. J. (1979). The conduit metaphor – a case of frame conflict in our language about language. In *Metaphor and Thought*, A. Ortony (ed.). Cambridge: Cambridge University Press, pp. 284–310.

Reebs, S. G. (2000). Can a minority of informed leaders determine the foraging movements of a fish shoal? *Animal Behaviour* **59**: 403–409.

Reed, C. A. (1959). Animal domestication in the prehistoric Near East. *Science* **130**: 1629–1639.

Rehm, S., D. J. Stanislaus, and A. M. Williams. (2007). Estrous cycle-dependent histology and review of sex steroid receptor expression in dog reproductive tissues and mammary gland and associated hormone levels. *Birth Defects Research* **80B**: 233–245.

Reich, D. E., R. K. Wayne, and D. B. Goldstein. (1999). Genetic evidence for a recent origin by hybridization of red wolves. *Molecular Ecology* **8**: 139–144.

Rendall, D., M. J. Owren, and M. J. Ryan. (2009). What do animal signals mean? *Animal Behaviour* **78**: 233–240.

Rhymer, J. M. and D. Simberloff. (1996). Extinction by hybridization and introgression. *Annual Review of Ecology and Systematics* **27**: 83–109.

Richens, V. B. and R. D. Hugie. (1974). Distribution, taxonomic status, and characteristics of coyotes in Maine. *Journal of Wildlife Management* **38**: 447–454.

Riede, T. and T. Fitch. (1999). Vocal tract length and acoustics of vocalization in the domestic dog (*Canis familiaris*). *Journal of Experimental Biology* **202**: 2859–2867.

Riedman, M. L. (1982). The evolution of alloparental care and adoption in mammals and birds. *Quarterly Review of Biology* **57**: 405–435.

Riesenfeld, A. and M. I. Siegel. (1970). The relationship between facial proportions and root length in the dentition of dogs. *American Journal of Physical Anthropology* **33**: 429–432.

Riewe, R. R. (1975). The high arctic wolf in the Jones Sound region of the Canadian high arctic. *Arctic* **28**: 209–212.

Riley, G. A. and R. T. McBride. (1975). A survey of the red wolf (*Canis rufus*). In *The Wild Canids: Their Systematics, Behavioral Ecology and Evolution*, M. W. Fox (ed.). New York, NY: Van Nostrand Reinhold, pp. 263–277.

Roberts, R. G. and B. W. Brook. (2010). And then there were none? *Science* **327**: 420–422.

Robertshaw, J. D. and R. H. Harden. (1985). The ecology of the dingo in north-eastern New South Wales. II. Diet. *Australian Wildlife Research* **12**: 39–50.

Robertshaw, J. D. and R. H. Harden. (1986). The ecology of the dingo in north-eastern New South Wales. IV. Prey selection by dingoes, and its effect on the major prey species, the swamp wallaby, *Wallabia bicolor* (Demarest). *Australian Wildlife Research* **13**: 141–163.

Robley, A., A. Gormley, D. M. Forsyth, A. N. Wilton, and D. Stephens. (2010). Movements and habitat selection by wild dogs in eastern Victoria. *Australian Mammalogy* **32**: 23–32.

Rodman, P. S. (1981). Inclusive fitness and group size with a reconsideration of group sizes in lions and wolves. *American Naturalist* **118**: 275–283.

Rodriguez, I. (2004). Pheromone receptors in mammals. *Hormones and Behavior* **46**: 219–230.

Rodriguez, I. (2005). Remarkable diversity of mammalian pheromone receptor repertoires. *Proceedings of the National Academy of Sciences* **102**: 6639–6640.

Rodríquez-Muñoz, R., A. Bretman, J. Slate, C. A. Walling, and T. Tregenza. (2010). Natural and sexual selection in a wild insect population. *Science* **328**: 1269–1272.

Romsos, D. R., H. J. Palmer, K. L. Muiruri, and M. R. Bennink. (1981). Influence of low carbohydrate diet on performance of pregnant and lactating dogs. *Journal of Nutrition* **111**: 678–689.

Roppolo, D., S. Vollery, Chen-Da Kan, C. Lüscher, M-C. Broillet, and I. Rodriguez. (2007). Gene cluster lock after pheromone receptor gene choice. *EMBO Journal* **26**: 3423–3430.

Rothman, R. J. and L. D. Mech. (1979). Scent-marking in lone wolves and newly formed pairs. *Animal Behaviour* **27**: 750–760.

Rothstein, S. I. (1982). Successes and failures in avian egg and nestling recognition with comments on the utility of optimality reasoning. *American Zoologist* **22**: 547–560.

Rouquier, S. and D. Giorgi. (2007). Olfactory receptor gene repertoires in mammals. *Mutation Research* **616**: 95–102.

Rowell, T. E. (1974). The concept of social dominance. *Behavioral Biology* **11**: 131–154.

Roy, M. S., E. Geffen, D. Smith, E. A. Ostrander, and R. K. Wayne. (1994). Patterns of differentiation and hybridization in North American wolflike canids, revealed by analysis of microsatellite loci. *Molecular Biology and Evolution* **11**: 443–570.

Roy, M. S., E. Geffen, D. Smith, and R. K. Wayne. (1996). Molecular genetics of pre-1940 red wolves. *Conservation Biology* **10**: 1413–1424.

Ruas, J. P., C. Detry, and J. L. Cardosa. (2010). On some remains of dog (*Canis familiaris*) from the Mesolithic shell-middens of Muge, Portugal. *Journal of Archaeological Science* **37**: 2762–2774.

Rubin, H. D. and A. M. Beck. (1982). Ecological behavior of free-ranging urban pet dogs. *Applied Animal Ethology* **8**: 161–168.

Runstadler, J. A., M. M. Angles, and N. C. Pedersen. (2006). Dog leucocyte antigen class II diversity and relationships among indigenous dogs of the island nations of Indonesia (Bali), Australia and New Guinea. *Tissue Antigens* **68**: 418–426.

Rutledge, L. Y., B. R. Patterson, K. J. Mills, K. M. Loveless, D. L. Murray, and B. N. White. (2010a). Protection from harvesting restores the natural social structure of eastern wolf packs. *Biological Conservation* **143**: 322–339.

Rutledge, L. Y., C. J. Garroway, K. M. Loveless, and B. R. Patterson. (2010b). Genetic differentiation of eastern wolves in Algonquin Park despite bridging gene flow between coyotes and grey wolves. *Heredity* **105**: 520–531.

Rutledge, L. Y., K. I. Bos, R. J. Pearce, and B. N. White. (2010c). Genetic and morphometric analysis of sixteenth century *Canis* skull fragments: implications for historic [*sic*] eastern and gray wolf distribution in North America. *Conservation Genetics* **11**: 1273–1281.

Rutter, R. J. and D. H. Pimlott. 1968. *The World of the Wolf*. Philadelphia, PA: J. B. Lippincott, 202 pp.

Ryabov, L. S. (1979). Stray and feral dogs in the Voronezhskaya Oblast. *Bulletin of the Moscow Society of Naturalists* **84**: 18–27. [Russian with English summary.]

Ryba, N. J. P. and R. Tirindelli. (1997). A new multigene family of putative pheromone receptors. *Neuron* **19**: 371–379.

Ryon, C. J. (1977). Den digging and related behavior in a captive timber wolf pack. *Journal of Mammalogy* **58**: 87–89.

Ryon, J., J. C. Fentress, F. H. Harrington, and S. Bragdon. (1986). Scent rubbing in wolves (*Canis lupus*): the effect of novelty. *Canadian Journal of Zoology* **64**: 573–577.

Sablin, M. V. and G. A. Khlopachev. (2002). The earliest Ice Age dogs: evidence from Eliseevichi I. *Current Anthropology* **43**: 795–799.

Saetre, P., J. Lindberg, J. A. Leonard, K. Olsson, U. Pettersson, and H. Ellegren *et al.* (2004). From wild wolf to domestic dog: gene expression changes in the brain. *Molecular Brain Research* **126**: 198–206.

Salazar, I., P. C. Barber, and J. M. Cifuentes. (1992). Anatomical and immunohistological demonstration of the primary neural connections in the vomeronasal organ in the dog. *Anatomical Record* **233**: 309–313.

Sam, M., S. Vora, B. Malnic, W. Ma, M. V. Novotny, and L. B. Buck. (2001). Odorants may arouse instinctive behaviours. *Nature* **412**: 142.

Sands, J. and S. Creel. (2004). Social dominance, aggression and faecal glucocorticoid levels in a wild population of wolves, *Canis lupus*. *Animal Behaviour* **67**: 387–396.

Sands, M. W., R. P. Coppinger, and C. J. Phillips. (1977). Comparisons of thermal sweating and histology of sweat glands of selected canids. *Journal of Mammalogy* **58**: 74–78.

Savile, D. B. O. and D. R. Oliver. (1964). Bird and mammal observations at Hazen Camp, Northern Ellesmere Island, in 1962. *Canadian Field-Naturalist* **78**: 1–7.

Savolainen, P., Ya-ping Zang, J. Luo, J. Lundeberg, and T. Leitner. (2002). Genetic evidence for an east Asian origin of domestic dogs. *Science* **298**: 1610–1613.

Savolainen, P., T. Leitner, A. N. Wilton, E. Matisoo-Smith, and J. Lundeberg. (2004). A detailed picture of the origin of the Australian dingo, obtained from the study of mitochondrial DNA. *Proceedings of the National Academy of Sciences* **101**: 12 387–12 390.

Sawyer, T. G., K. V. Miller, and R. L. Marchinton. (1993). Patterns of urination and rub-urination in female white-tailed deer. *Journal of Mammalogy* **74**: 477–479.

Schassburger, R. M. (1993). *Vocal Communication in the Timber Wolf, Canis lupus,* [sic] *Linnaeus: Structure, Motivation, and Ontogeny, Advances in Ethology No. 30*. Berlin and Hamburg: Paul Parey, 84 pp.

Schenkel, R. (1947). Ausdrucks-Studien an Wölfen: Gefangenschafts-Beobachtungen. [Studies of expressions in wolves: captive observations.] *Behaviour* **1**: 81–129.

Schenkel, R. (1967). Submission: its features and function in the wolf and dog. *American Zoologist* **7**: 319–329.

Schilder, M. B. H. and J. A. M. van der Borg. (2004). Training dogs with help of the shock collar: short and long term behavioural effects. *Applied Animal Behaviour Science* **85**: 319–334.

Schleidt, W. M. (1973). Tonic communication: continual effects of discrete signs in animal communication systems. *Journal of Theoretical Biology* **42**: 359–386.

Schmidt, P. A. and L. D. Mech. (1997). Wolf pack size and food acquisition. *American Naturalist* **150**: 513–517.

Schmitz, O. J. and G. B. Kolenosky. (1985). Wolves and coyotes in Ontario: morphological relationships and origins. *Canadian Journal of Zoology* **63**: 1130–1137.

Schmitz, O. J. and D. M. Lavigne. (1987). Factors affecting body size in sympatric Ontario *Canis*. *Journal of Mammalogy* **68**: 92–99.

Schmutz, S. M., T. G. Berryere, J. L. Barta, K. D. Reddick, and J. K. Schmutz. (2007). Agouti sequence polymorphisms in coyotes, wolves and dogs suggest hybridization. *Journal of Heredity* **98**: 351–355.

Schullery, P. and L. Whittlesey. (1995). Summary of the documentary record of wolves and other wildlife species in the Yellowstone National Park area prior to 1882. In *Ecology and Conservation of Wolves in a Changing World*, Occasional Publication No. 35, L. N. Carbyn, S. H. Fritts, and D. R. Seip (eds.). Edmonton, AB: Canadian Circumpolar Institute, pp. 63–76.

Schulte, N. and H. Klingel. (1991). Herd structure, leadership, dominance and site attachment of the camel, *Camelus dromedarius*. *Behaviour* **118**: 103–114.

Schultz, T. H., S. M. Kruse, and R. A. Flath. (1985). Some volatile constituents of female dog urine. *Journal of Chemical Ecology* **11**: 169–175.

Schultz, T. H., R. A. Flath, R. J. Stern, T. R. Mon, R. Teranishi, and S. M. Kruse *et al.* (1988). Coyote estrous urine volatiles. *Journal of Chemical Ecology* **14**: 701–712.

Schwartz, M. (1997). *A History of Dogs in the Early Americas*. New Haven, CT: Yale University Press, x + 233 pp.

Scott, B. M. V. and D. M. Shackleton. (1982). A preliminary study of the social organization of the Vancouver Island wolf (*Canis lupus crassodon*; [sic] Hall, 1932). In *Wolves of the World: Perspectives of Behavior, Ecology, and Conservation*, F. H. Harrington and P. C. Paquet (eds.). Park Ridge, NJ: Noyes Publications, pp. 12–25.

Scott, J. P. (1950). The social behavior of dogs and wolves: an illustration of sociobiological systematics. *Annals of the New York Academy of Sciences* **51**: 1009–1021.

Scott, J. P. (1958). Critical periods in the development of social behavior in puppies. *Psychosomatic Medicine* **20**: 42–54.

Scott, J. P. (1962). Critical periods in behavioral development. *Science* **138**: 949–958.

Scott, J. P. (1964). Genetics and the development of social behavior in dogs. *American Zoologist* **4**: 161–168.

Scott, J. P. (1967). The evolution of social behavior in dogs and wolves. *American Zoologist* **7**: 373–381.

Scott, J. P. (1968). Evolution and domestication of the dog. *Evolutionary Biology* **2**: 243–275.

Scott, J. P. and M-'V. Marston. (1950). Critical periods affecting the development of normal and mal-adjustive social behavior of puppies. *Journal of Genetics and Psychology* **77**: 25–60.

Scott, J. P. and E. Fredericson. (1951). The causes of fighting in mice and rats. *Physiological Zoölogy* **24**: 273–309.

Scott, J. P. and J. L. Fuller. (1965). *Genetics and the Social Behavior of the Dog*. Chicago, IL: University of Chicago Press, xviii + 468 pp.

Scott, M. D. and K. Causey. (1973). Ecology of feral dogs in Alabama. *Journal of Wildlife Management* **37**: 253–265.

Scott-Phillips, T. C. (2008). Defining biological communication. *Journal of Evolutionary Biology* **21**: 387–395.

Scott-Phillips, T. C. (2010). Animal communication: insights from linguistic pragmatics. *Animal Behaviour* **79**: e1–e4.

Seal, U.S., E.D. Plotka, J.M. Packard, and L.D. Mech. (1979). Endocrine correlates of reproduction in the wolf. I. Serum progesterone, estradiol and LH during the estrous cycle. *Biology of Reproduction* **21**: 1057–1066.

Sears, H.J., J.B. Theberge, M.T. Theberge, I. Thornton, and G.D. Campbell. (2003). Landscape influence on *Canis* morphological and ecological variation in a coyote–wolf *C. lupus* × *latrans* hybrid zone, southeastern Ontario. *Canadian Field-Naturalist* **117**: 589–600.

Seton, E. T. (1962). *Wild Animals I Have Known*. St. Louis, MO: McGraw-Hill, 138 pp.

Severinghaus, C.W. (1974). Notes on the history of wild canids in New York. *New York State Fish and Game Journal* **21**: 117–125.

Seyfarth, R.M. and D.L. Cheney. (2003). Signalers and receivers in animal communication. *Annual Review of Psychology* **54**: 145–173.

Sharma, D.K., J.E. Maldonado, Y.V. Jhala, and R.C. Fleischer. (2004). Ancient wolf lineages in India. *Proceedings of the Royal Society of London* **271B** (Suppl.): S1–S4.

Shelley, E.L. and D.T. Blumstein. (2005). The evolution of vocal alarm communication in rodents. *Behavioral Ecology* **16**: 169–177.

Shepherd, N.C. (1981). Predation of red kangaroos, *Macropus rufus*, by the dingo, *Canis familiaris dingo* (Blumenbach), in north-western New South Wales. *Australian Wildlife Research* **8**: 255–262.

Sherman, P.W. (1980). The meaning of nepotism. *American Naturalist* **116**: 604–606.

Short, J., J.E. Kinnear, and A. Robley. (2002). Surplus killing by introduced predators in Australia – evidence for ineffective anti-predator adaptations in native prey species? *Biological Conservation* **103**: 283–301.

Silk, J.B., J. Altmann, and S.C. Alberts. (2006). Social relationships among adult female baboons (*papio* [*sic*] *cynocephalus*) I. Variation in the strength of social bonds. *Behavioral Ecology and Sociobiology* **61**: 183–195.

Sillero-Zubiri, C.D. Gottelli, and D.W. Macdonald. (1996). Male philopatry, extra-pack copulations and inbreeding avoidance in Ethiopian wolves (*Canis simensis*). *Behavioral Ecology and Sociobiology* **38**: 331–340.

Silver, H. and W.T. Silver. (1969). Growth and behavior of the coyote-like canid of northern New England with observations on canid hybrids. *Wildlife Monographs* **17**: 41 pp.

Slater, G.J., E.R. Dumont, and B. Van Valkenburgh. (2009). Implications of predatory specialization for cranial form and function in canids. *Journal of Zoology (London)* **278**: 181–188.

Slocombe, K.E. and K. Zuberbühler. (2005). Functionally referential communication in a chimpanzee. *Current Biology* **15**: 1779–1784.

Slotnick, B.D. Restrepo, H. Schellinck, G. Archbold, S. Price, and W. Lin. (2010). Accessory olfactory bulb function is modulated by input from the main olfactory system. *European Journal of Neuroscience* **31**: 1108–1116.

Smith, D., T. Meier, E. Geffen, L.D. Mech, J.W. Burch, and L.G. Adams *et al.* (1997). Is incest common in gray wolf packs? *Behavioral Ecology* **8**: 384–391.

Smith, D.W., L.D. Mech, M. Meagher, W.E. Clark, R. Jaffe, and M.K. Phillips *et al.* (2000). Wolf–bison interactions in Yellowstone National Park. *Journal of Mammalogy* **81**: 1128–1135.

Smith, D.W., E.E. Bangs, J.K. Oakleaf, C. Mack, J. Fontaine, and D. Boyd *et al.* (2010). Survival of colonizing wolves in the northern Rocky Mountains of the United States, 1982–2004. *Journal of Wildlife Management* **74**: 620–634.

Smith, W. J. (1997). The behavior of communicating, after twenty years. *Perspectives in Ecology* **12**: 7–53.

Snow, C. J. (1967). Some observations on the behavioral and morphological development of coyote pups. *American Zoologist* **7**: 353–355.

Sobel, N., V. Prabhakaran, J. E. Desmond, G. H. Glover, R. L. Goode, and E. V. Sullivan *et al.* (1998). Sniffing and smelling: separate subsystems in the human olfactory cortex. *Nature* **392**: 282–286.

Sokolov, V. Y., A. S. Severtsov, and A. V. Shubkina. (1990). Modelling of the selective behavior of the predator towards prey: the use of borzois for catching saigas. *Zoologicheskiĭ Zhurnal* **69**: 117–125. [Russian with English summary.]

Sparkman, A. M., J. Adams, A. Beyer, T. D. Steury, L. Waits, and D. L. Murray. (2011). Helper effects on pup lifetime fitness in the cooperatively breeding red wolf (*Canis rufus*). *Proceedings of the Royal Society of London* **278B**: 1381–1389.

Speakman, J. R., A. van Acker, and E. J. Harper. (2003). Age-related changes in the metabolism and body composition of three dog breeds and their relationship to life expectancy. *Aging Cell* **2**: 265–275.

Spehr, M., J. Spehr, K. Ukhanov, K. R. Kelliher, T. Leinders-Zufall, and F. Zufall. (2006a). Parallel processing of social signals by the mammalian main and accessory olfactory systems. *Cellular and Molecular Life Sciences* **63**: 1476–1484.

Spehr, M., K. R. Kelliher, X-H. Li, T. Boehm, T. Leinders-Zufall, and F. Zufall. (2006b). Essential role of the main olfactory system in social recognition of major histocompatibility complex peptide ligands. *Journal of Neuroscience* **26**: 1961–1970.

Spong, G. and S. Creel. (2004). Effects of kinship on territorial conflicts among groups of lions, *Panthera leo*. *Behavioral Ecology and Sociobiology* **55**: 325–331.

Spotte, S. (2006). *Zoos in Postmodernism: Signs and Simulation*. Madison, NJ: Fairleigh Dickinson University Press, 208 pp.

Stahler, D. R., D. W. Smith, and R. Landis. (2002a). The acceptance of a new breeding male into a wild wolf pack. *Canadian Journal of Zoology* **80**: 360–365.

Stahler, D., B. Heinrich, and D. Smith. (2002b). Common ravens, *Corvus corax*, preferentially associate with grey wolves, *Canis lupus*, as a foraging strategy in winter. *Animal Behaviour* **64**: 283–290.

Stanwell-Fletcher, J. (1942). Three years in the wolves' wilderness. *Natural History Magazine* **49**(3): 136–147.

Stebler, A. M. (1944). The status of the wolf in Michigan. *Journal of Mammalogy* **25**: 37–43.

Stephenson, R. O. and D. James. (1982). Wolf movements and food habits in northwest Alaska. In *Wolves of the World: Perspectives of Behavior, Ecology, and Conservation*, F. H. Harrington and P. C. Paquet (eds.). Park Ridge, NJ: Noyes Publications, pp. 26–42.

Sternthal, S. (2010). Moscow's stray dogs. London: *Financial Times* (http://www.ft.com/cms/s/2/628a8500-ff1c-11de-a677-00144feab49a.html).

Stevens, J. R. and D. W. Stephens. (2002). Food sharing: a model of manipulation by harassment. *Behavioral Ecology* **13**: 393–400.

Stewart, K. J. and A. H. Harcourt. (1994). Gorillas' vocalizations during rest periods: signals of impending departure? *Behaviour* **130**: 29–40.

Stiehl, R. B. and S. N. Trautwein. (1991). Variations in diets of nesting common ravens. *Wilson Bulletin* **103**: 83–92.

Street, J. M. (1962). Feral animals in Hispaniola. *Geographical Review* **52**: 400–406.

Stueckle, S. and D. Zinner. (2008). To follow or not to follow: decision making and leadership during the morning departure in chacma baboons. *Animal Behaviour* **75**: 1995–2004.

Switalski, T. A. (2003). Coyote foraging ecology and vigilance in response to gray wolf reintroduction in Yellowstone National Park. *Canadian Journal of Zoology* **81**: 985–993.

Tacher, S., P. Quignon, M. Rimbault, S. Dreano, C. Andre, and F. Galibert. (2005). Olfactory receptor sequence polymorphism within and between breeds of dogs. *Journal of Heredity* **96**: 812–816.

Taha, M. B., D. E. Noakes, and W. E. Allen. (1981). The effect of season of the year on the characteristics and composition of dog semen. *Journal of Small Animal Practice* **22**: 177–184.

Takami, S. (2002). Recent progress in the neurobiology of the vomeronasal organ. *Microscopy Research and Technique* **58**: 228–250.

Takigami, S., Y. Mori, Y. Tanioka, and M. Ichikawa. (2004). Morphological evidence of two types of mammalian vomeronasal system. *Chemical Senses* **29**: 301–310.

Taylor, A. M., D. Reby, and K. McComb. (2009). Context-related variation in the vocal growling behaviour of the domestic dog (*Canis familiaris*). *Ethology* **115**: 905–915.

Taylor, A. M., D. Reby, and K. McComb. (2010). Size communication in domestic dog, *Canis familiaris*, growls. *Animal Behaviour* **79**: 205–210.

Tembrock, G. (1968). Land mammals. In *Animal Communication: Techniques of Study and Results of Research*, T. A. Sebeok (ed.). Bloomington, IN: Indiana University Press, pp. 338–404.

Tembrock, G. (1976). Canid vocalizations. *Behavioural Processes* **1**: 57–75.

Tener, J. S. (1954). A preliminary study of the musk-oxen of Fosheim Peninsula, Ellesmere Island, N. W. T., Wildlife Management Bulletin Series 1, No. 9. Ottawa, ON: Canadian Wildlife Service, 34 pp. + 7 figs.

Theberge, J. H. and J. B. Falls. (1967). Howling as a means of communication in timber wolves. *American Zoologist* **7**: 331–338.

Theuerkauf, J., W. Jędrzejewski, K. Schmidt, H. Okarma, I. Ruczyński, and S. Śnieżko *et al.* (2003). Daily patterns and duration of wolf activity in the Białowieża Forest, Poland. *Journal of Mammalogy* **84**: 243–253.

Thompson, D. Q. (1952). Travel, range, and food habits of timber wolves in Wisconsin. *Journal of Mammalogy* **33**: 429–442.

Thomson, P. C. (1992a). The behavioural ecology of dingoes in north-western Australia. I. The Fortescue River study area and details of captured dingoes. *Wildlife Research* **19**: 509–518.

Thomson, P. C. (1992b). The behavioural ecology of dingoes in north-western Australia. II. Activity patterns, breeding season and pup rearing. *Wildlife Research* **19**: 519–530.

Thomson, P. C. (1992c). The behavioural ecology of dingoes in north-western Australia. III. Hunting and feeding behaviour, and diet. *Wildlife Research* **19**: 531–541.

Thomson, P. C. (1992d). The behavioural ecology of dingoes in north-western Australia. IV. Social and spatial organisation, and movements. *Wildlife Research* **19**: 543–563.

Thomson, P. C., K. Rose, and N. E. Kok. (1992). The behavioural ecology of dingoes in north-western Australia. VI. Temporary extraterritorial movements and dispersal. *Wildlife Research* **19**: 585–595.

Thornhill, R., S. W. Gangestad, R. Miller, G. Scheyd, J. K. McCollough, and M. Franklin. (2003). Major histocompatibility complex genes, symmetry, and body scent attractiveness in men and women. *Behavioral Ecology* **14**: 668–678.

Thurber, J. M. and R. O. Peterson. (1991). Changes in body size associated with range expansion in the coyote (*Canis latrans*). *Journal of Mammalogy* **72**: 750–755.

Thurber, J. M. and R. O. Peterson. (1993). Effects of population density and pack size on the foraging ecology of gray wolves. *Journal of Mammalogy* **74**: 879–889.

Tien, J. H., S. A. Levin, and D. I. Rubenstein. (2004). Dynamics of fish shoals: identifying key decision rules. *Evolutionary Ecology Research* **6**: 555–565.

Tilson, R. L. and J. R. Henschel. (1986). Spatial arrangement of spotted hyaena groups in a desert environment, Namibia. *African Journal of Ecology* **24**: 173–180.

Tinbergen, N. (1963). On aims and methods of ethology. *Zeitschrift für Tierpsychologie* **20**: 410–433.

Tome, P. (1854). *Pioneer Life; or, Thirty Years a Hunter. Scenes and Adventures in the Life of Philip Tome.* Buffalo, NY: Self-published, 238 pp. http://www.archive.org/details/pioneerlifeorthi00tome.

Tooze, Z. J., F. H. Harrington, and J. C. Fentress. (1990). Individually distinct vocalizations in timber wolves, *Canis lupus*. *Animal Behaviour* **40**: 723–730.

Topál, J., Á. Miklósi, V. Csányi, and A. Dóka. (1998). Attachment behavior in dogs (*Canis familiaris*): a new application of Ainsworth's (1969) Strange Situation test. *Journal of Comparative Psychology* **112**: 219–229.

Topál, J., M. Gácsi, Á. Miklósi, Z. Virányi, E. Kubinyi, and V. Csányi. (2005). Attachment to humans: a comparative study on hand-reared wolves and differently socialized dog puppies. *Animal Behaviour* **70**: 1367–1375.

Troughton, E. (1970). The early history and relationships of the New Guinea highland dog (*Canis hallstromi*). *Proceedings of the Linnean Society of New South Wales* **96**: 93–98.

Trut, L. N. (1999). Early canid domestication: the farm-fox experiment. *American Scientist* **87**: 160–169.

Trut, L., I. Oskina, and A. Kharlamova. (2009). Animal evolution during domestication: the domesticated fox as a model. *BioEssays* **31**: 349–360.

Tsutsui, T., N. Kirihara, T. Hori, and P. W. Concannon. (2007). Plasma progesterone and prolactin concentrations in overtly pseudopregnant bitches: a clinical study. *Theriogenology* **67**: 1032–1038.

Turnbull, P. F. and C. A. Reed. (1974). The fauna from the Terminal Pleistocene of Palegawra Cave, a Zarzian occupation site in northeastern Iraq. *Fieldiana Anthropology* **63**(3): 81–146. [pp. 99–106.]

van Ballenberghe, V. (1983a). Extraterritorial movements and dispersal of wolves in south-central Alaska. *Journal of Mammalogy* **64**: 168–171.

van Ballenberghe, V. (1983b). Two litters raised in one year by a wolf pack. *Journal of Mammalogy* **64**: 171–172.

van Ballenberghe, V. and A. W. Erickson. (1973). A wolf pack kills another wolf. *American Midland Naturalist* **90**: 490–493.

van Ballenberghe, V. and L. D. Mech. (1975). Weights, growth, and survival of timber wolf pups in Minnesota. *Journal of Mammalogy* **56**: 44–63.

van Ballenberghe, V., A. W. Erickson, and D. Byman. (1975). Ecology of the timber wolf in northeastern Minnesota. *Wildlife Monographs* **(43)**: 43 pp.

Van Camp, J. and R. Gluckie. (1979). A record long-distance move by a wolf (*Canis lupus*). *Journal of Mammalogy* **60**: 236–237.

van Gelder, R. W. (1977). Mammalian hybrids and generic limits. *American Museum Novitates* **(2635)**: 25 pp.

van Gelder, R. W. (1978). A review of canid classification. *American Museum Novitates* (**2646**): 10 pp.

van Haaften, B., M. M. Bevers, W. E. van den Brom, A. C. Okkens, F. J. van Sluijs, and A. H. Willemse *et al.* (1994). Increasing sensitivity of the pituitary to GnRH from early to late anoestrus in the beagle bitch. *Journal of Reproduction and Fertility* **101**: 221–225.

van Hooff, J. A. R. A. M. and J. A. B. Wensing. (1987). Dominance and its behavioral measures in a captive wolf pack. In *Man and Wolf: Advances, Issues, and Problems in Captive Wolf Research*, H. Frank (ed.). Dordrecht, the Netherlands: Dr W. Junk, pp. 219–252.

van Lawick-Goodall, H. (1971). Wild dogs: nomads of the plains. In *Innocent Killers*, H. van Lawick-Goodall and J. van Lawick Goodall (eds.). Boston, MA: Houghton Mifflin, pp. 48–101.

Van Vuren, D. and S. E. Thomson Jr. (1982). Opportunistic feeding by coyotes. *Northwest Science* **56**: 131–135.

Vaughan, C. (1983). Coyote range expansion in Costa Rica and Panama. *Brenesia* **21**: 27–32.

Verardi, A., V. Lucchini, and E. Randi. (2006). Detecting introgressive hybridization between free-ranging domestic dogs and wild wolves (*Canis lupus*) by admixture linkage disequilibrium analysis. *Molecular Ecology* **15**: 2845–2855.

Verginelli, F., C. Capelli, V. Coia, M. Musiani, M. Falchetti, and L. Ottini, *et al.* (2005). Mitochondrial DNA from prehistoric canids highlights relationships between dogs and south-east European wolves. *Molecular Biology and Evolution* **22**: 2541–2551.

Vernes, K., A. Dennis, and J. Winter. (2001). Mammalian diet and broad hunting strategy of the dingo (*Canis familiaris dingo*) in the wet tropical rain forests of northeastern Australia. *Biotropica* **33**: 339–345.

Verstegen, J., K. Onclin, L. Silva, and P. Concannon. (1997). Termination of obligate anoestrus and induction of fertile ovarian cycles in dogs by administration of purified pig LH. *Journal of Reproduction and Fertility* **111**: 35–40.

Verstegen-Onclin, K. and J. Verstegen. (2008). Endocrinology of pregnancy in the dog: a review. *Theriogenology* **70**: 291–299.

Vézina, A. F. (1985). Empirical relationships between predator and prey size among terrestrial vertebrate predators. *Oecologia* **67**: 555–565.

Vilà, C. and R. K. Wayne. (1999). Hybridization between wolves and dogs. *Conservation Biology* **13**: 195–198.

Vilà, C., V. Urios, and J. Castroviejo. (1994). Use of faeces for scent marking in Iberian wolves (*Canis lupus*). *Canadian Journal of Zoology* **72**: 374–377.

Vilà, C., P. Savolainen, J. E. Maldonado, I. R. Amorim, J. E. Rice, and R. L. Honeycutt *et al.* (1997). Multiple and ancient origins of the domestic dog. *Science* **276**: 1687–1689.

Vilà, C., J. E. Maldonado, and R. K. Wayne. (1999a). Phylogenetic relationships, evolution, and genetic diversity of the domestic dog. *Journal of Heredity* **90**: 71–77.

Vilà, C., R. Amorim, J. A. Leonard, D. Posada, J. Castroviejo, and F. Petrucci-Fonseca *et al.* (1999b). Mitochondrial DNA phylogeography and population history of the grey wolf *Canis lupus*. *Molecular Ecology* **8**: 2089–2103.

Vilà, C., A-K. Sundqvist, Ø. Flagstad, J. Seddon, S. Björnerfeldt, and I. Kojola *et al.* (2003a). Rescue of a severely bottlenecked wolf (*Canis lupus*) population by a single immigrant. *Proceedings of the Royal Society of London* **270B**: 91–97.

Vilà, C., C. Walker, A-K. Sundqvist, Ø. Flagstad, Z. Andersone, and A. Casulli *et al.* (2003b). Combined use of maternal, paternal and bi-parental genetic markers for the identification of wolf–dog hybrids. *Heredity* **90**: 17–24.

Vilà, C., J. Seddon, and H. Ellegren. (2005). Genes of domestic mammals augmented by backcrossing with wild ancestors. *Trends in Genetics* **21**: 214–218.

Voigt, D. R. and W. E. Berg. (1987). Coyote. In *Wild Furbearer Management and Conservation in North America*, M. Novak, J. A. Baker, M. E. Obbard, and B. Malloch (eds.). Peterborough, ON: Ontario Trappers Association, pp. 345–357.

vonHoldt, B. M., D. R. Stahler, D. W. Smith, D. A. Early, J. P. Pollinger, and R. K. Wayne. (2008). The genealogy and genetic viability of reintroduced Yellowstone grey wolves. *Molecular Ecology* **17**: 252–274.

vonHoldt, B. M., J. P. Pollinger, K. E. Lohmueller, E. Han, H. G. Parker, and P. Quignon *et al.* (2010). Genome-wide SNP and haplotype analyses reveal a rich history underlying dog domestication. *Nature* **464**: 898–903.

vonHoldt, B. M., J. P. Pollinger, D. A. Earl, J. C. Knowles, A. R. Boyko, and H. Parker *et al.* (2011). A genome-wide perspective on the evolutionary history of enigmatic wolf-like canids. *Genome Research*: doi.10.1101/gr.116301.110.

von Schreber, J. C. D. (1775). *Die säugthiere in abbildungen nach der Natur mit beschreibungen, Part 3*: 281–590, Suppl. 1: plates 1–165. [p. 353, plate 89.] Heidelberg: Walther. "Name *Canis lycaon* used on plate 8, 1775, reference to "loup noir" of Buffon, Vol. 3, p. 353, 1776, and name again appears in index, p. 585, 1778." [From Goldman 1944: 571.]

Vos, J. (2000). Food habits and livestock depredation of two Iberian wolf packs (*Canis lupus signatus*) in the north of Portugal. *Journal of Zoology (London)* **251**: 457–462.

Vucetich, J. A., R. O. Peterson, and C. L. Schaefer. (2002). The effect of prey and predator densities on wolf predation. *Ecology* **83**: 3003–3013.

Wabakken, P., H. Sand, O. Liberg, and A. Bjärvall. (2001). The recovery, distribution, and population dynamics of wolves on the Scandinavian peninsula, 1978–1998. *Canadian Journal of Zoology* **79**: 710–725.

Wabakken, P., H. Sand, I. Kojola, B. Zimmermann, J. M. Arnemo, and H. C. Pedersen *et al.* (2007). Multistage, long-range natal dispersal by a global positioning system-collared Scandinavian wolf. *Journal of Wildlife Management* **71**: 1631–1634.

Walton, L. R., H. D. Cluff, P. C. Paquet, and M. A. Ramsay. (2001). Movement patterns of barren-ground wolves in the central Canadian arctic. *Journal of Mammalogy* **82**: 867–876.

Wang, X. and R. H. Tedford. (2008). *Dogs: Their Fossil Relatives and Evolutionary History*. New York, NY: Columbia University Press, pp. viii and 219.

Wang, X., R. H. Tedford, B. van Valkenburgh, and R. K. Wayne. (2004). Phylogeny, classification, and evolutionary ecology of the Canidae. In *Canids: Foxes, Wolves, Jackals and Dogs*, C. Sillero-Zubiri, M. Hoffmann, and D. W. Macdonald (eds.). Gland and Cambridge: IUCN, pp. 8–20.

Watts, D. E., L. G. Butler, B. W. Dale, and R. D. Cox. (2010). The Ilnik wolf *Canis lupus* pack: use of marine mammals and offshore sea ice. *Wildlife Biology* **16**: 144–149.

Way, J. G., D-L. M. Szumylo, and E. G. Strauss. (2006). An ethogram developed on captive eastern coyotes *Canis latrans*. *Canadian Field-Naturalist* **120**: 263–288.

Way, J. G., L. Rutledge, T. Wheeldon, and B. N. White. (2010). Genetic characterization of eastern "coyotes" in eastern Massachusetts. *Northeastern Naturalist* **17**: 189–204.

Wayne, R. K. (1992). On the use of morphologic and molecular genetic characters to investigate species status. *Conservation Biology* **6**: 590–592.

Wayne, R. K. (1993). Molecular evolution of the dog family. *Trends in Genetics* **9**: 218–224.

Wayne, R. K. and S. M. Jenks. (1991). Mitochondrial DNA analysis implying extensive hybridization of the endangered red wolf *Canis rufus*. *Nature* **351**: 565–568.

Wayne, R. K. and E. A. Ostrander. (1999). Origin, genetic diversity, and genome structure of the domestic dog. *BioEssays* **21**: 247–257.

Wayne, R. K., N. Lehman, M. W. Allard, and R. L. Honeycutt. (1992). Mitochondrial DNA variability of the gray wolf: genetic consequences of population decline and habitat fragmentation. *Conservation Biology* **6**: 559–569.

Wayne, R. K., N. Lehman, and T. K. Fuller. (1995). Conservation genetics of the gray wolf. In *Ecology and Conservation of Wolves in a Changing World*, Occasional Publication No. 35, L. N. Carbyn, S. H. Fritts, and D. R. Seip (eds.). Edmonton, AB: Canadian Circumpolar Institute, pp. 399–407.

Wayne, R. K., M. S. Roy, and J. L. Gittleman. (1998). Origin of the red wolf: response to Nowak and Federoff and Gardner. *Conservation Biology* **12**: 726–729.

Wayne, R. K., J. A. Leonard, and C. Vilà. (2006). Genetic analysis of dog domestication. In *Documenting Domestication: New Genetic and Archaeological Paradigms*, M. A. Zeder, D. Decker-Walters, D. Bradley, and B. D. Smith (eds.). Berkeley, CA: University of California Press, pp. 279–293.

Weaver, J. L., C. Arvidson, and P. Wood. (1992). Two wolves, *Canis lupus*, killed by a moose, *Alces alces*, in Jasper National Park, Alberta. *Canadian Field-Naturalist* **106**: 126–127.

Weiler, E., R. Apfelbach, and A. I. Farbman. (1999). The vomeronasal organ of the male ferret. *Chemical Senses* **24**: 127–136.

Wells, D. L. and P. G. Hepper. (2006). Prenatal olfactory learning in the domestic dog. *Animal Behaviour* **72**: 681–686.

Wells, H., E. G. Strauss, M. A. Rutter, and P. H. Wells. (1998). Mate location, population growth and species extinction. *Biological Conservation* **86**: 317–324.

West, S. A., I. Pen, and A. S. Griffin. (2002). Cooperation and competition between relatives. *Science* **296**: 72–76.

West, S. A., M. G. Murray, C. A. Machado, A. S. Griffin, and E. A. Herre. (2001). Testing Hamilton's rule with competition between relatives. *Nature* **409**: 510–513.

Wheeldon, T. and B. N. White. (2009). Genetic analysis of historic western Great Lakes region wolf samples reveals early *Canis lupus/lycaon* hybridization. *Biology Letters* **5**: 101–104.

Wheeldon, T. J., B. R. Patterson, and B. N. White. (2010). Sympatric wolf and coyote populations of the western Great Lakes region are reproductively isolated. *Molecular Ecology* **19**: 4428–4440.

White, K. A. J., M. A. Lewis, and J. D. Murray. (1996). A model for wolf-pack territory formation and maintenance. *Journal of Theoretical Biology* **178**: 29–43.

Whitehouse, S. J. O. (1977). The diet of the dingo in Western Australia. *Australian Wildlife Research* **4**: 145–150.

Whitney, L. F. (1971). *How to Breed Dogs*, rev. edn. New York, NY: Howell Book House, 384 pp.

Whitten, W. K., M. C. Wilson, S. R. Wilson, J. W. Jorgenson, M. Novotny, and M. Carmack. (1980). Induction of marking behavior in wild red foxes (*Vulpes vulpes* L.) by synthetic urinary constituents. *Journal of Chemical Ecology* **6**: 49–55.

Widdig, A., P. Nürnberg, M. Krawczak, W. J. Streich, and F. Bercovitch. (2002). Affiliation and aggression among adult female rhesus macaques: a genetic analysis of paternal cohorts. *Behaviour* **139**: 371–391.

Wildt, D. E., P. K. Chakraborty, W. B. Panko, and S. W. J. Seager. (1978). Relationship of reproductive behavior, serum luteinizing hormone and time of ovulation in the bitch. *Biology of Reproduction* **18**: 561–570.

Wildt, D. E., W. B. Panko, P. K. Chakraborty, and S. W. J. Seager. (1979). Relationship of serum estrone, estradiol-17β and progesterone to LH, sexual behavior and time of ovulation in the bitch. *Biology of Reproduction* **20**: 648–658.

Wildt, D. E., E. J. Baas, P. K. Chakraborty, T. L. Wolfle, and A. P. Stewart. (1982). Influence of inbreeding on reproductive performance, ejaculate quality and testicular volume in the dog. *Theriogenology* **17**: 445–452.

Wiley, R. H. and D. G. Richards. (1978). Physical constraints on acoustic communication in the atmosphere: implications for the evolution of animal vocalizations. *Behavioral Ecology and Sociobiology* **3**: 69–94.

Wiley, R. H. and K. N. Rabenold. (1984). The evolution of cooperative breeding by delayed reciprocity and queuing for favorable social positions. *Evolution* **38**: 609–621.

Wilkinson, G. S. (1985). The social organization of the common vampire bat. I. Pattern and cause of association. *Behavioral Ecology and Sociobiology* **17**: 111–121.

Wilmers, C. C., R. L. Crabtree, D. W. Smith, K. M. Murphy, and W. M. Getz. (2003). Trophic facilitation by introduced top predators: grey wolf subsidies to scavengers in Yellowstone National Park. *Journal of Animal Ecology* **72**: 909–916.

Wilson, H. C. (1963). An inquiry into the nature of Plains Indian cultural development. *American Anthropologist* **65**: 355–369.

Wilson, P. J., S. Grewal, I. D. Lawford, J. N. M. Heal, A. G. Granacki, and D. Pennock et al. (2000). DNA profiles of the eastern Canadian wolf and the red wolf provide evidence for a common evolution independent of the gray wolf. *Canadian Journal of Zoology* **78**: 2156–2166.

Wilson, P. J., S. Grewal, T. McFadden, R. C. Chambers, and B. N. White. (2003). Mitochondrial DNA extracted from eastern North American wolves killed in the 1800s is not of gray wolf origin. *Canadian Journal of Zoology* **81**: 936–940.

Wilson, P. J., S. K. Grewal, F. F. Mallory, and B. N. White. (2009). Genetic characterization of hybrid wolves across Ontario. *Journal of Heredity* **100**: S80-S89.

Wilton, A. N., D. J. Steward, and K. Zafiris. (1999). Microsatellite variation in the Australian dingo. *Journal of Heredity* **90**: 108–111.

Wolff, J. O. (1993). Why are female small mammals territorial? *Oikos* **68**: 364–370.

Wolff, J. O. (1997). Population regulation in mammals: an evolutionary perspective. *Journal of Animal Ecology* **66**: 1–13.

Wood, W. F., T. B. Shaffer, and A. Kubo. (1995). Volatile ketones from interdigital glands of black-tailed deer, *Odocoileus hemionus columbianus*. *Journal of Chemical Ecology* **21**: 1401–1408.

Wood, W. F., A. Kubo, and T. B. Shaffer. (2010). Antimicrobial activity of long-chain (*E*)-3-alken-2-ones. *Bioorganic and Medicinal Chemistry Letters* **20**: 1819–1820.

Woodall, P. F., P. Pavlov, and K. L. Twyford. (1996). Dingoes in Queensland, Australia: skull dimensions and identity of wild canids. *Wildlife Research* **23**: 581–587.

Wood Jones, F. (1921). The status of the dingo. *Transactions of the Royal Society of South Australia* **45**: 254–263.

Woodley, S. K. and M. J. Baum. (2004). Differential activation of glomeruli in the ferret's main olfactory bulb by anal scent gland odours from males and females: an early step in mate identification. *European Journal of Neuroscience* **20**: 1025–1032.

Woolhouse, A. D. and D. R. Morgan. (1995). An evaluation of repellents to suppress browsing by possums. *Journal of Chemical Ecology* **21**: 1571–1583.

Woolpy, J. H. (1968). The social organization of wolves. *Natural History Magazine* **77**(5): 46–55.

Woolpy, J. H. and B. E. Ginsburg. (1967). Wolf socialization: a study of temperament in a wild social species. *American Zoologist* **7**: 357–363.

Wright, B. S. (1960). Predation on big game in east Africa. *Journal of Wildlife Management* **24**: 1–15.

Wright, G. J., R. O. Peterson, D. W. Smith, and T. O. Lemke. (2006). Selection of northern Yellowstone elk by gray wolves and hunters. *Journal of Wildlife Management* **70**: 1070–1078.

Wronski, T. and W. Macasero. (2008). Evidence for the persistence of Arabian wolf [*sic*] (*Canis lupus pallipes*) in the Ibex Reserve, Saudi Arabia and its preferred prey species. *Zoology in the Middle East* **45**: 11–18.

Wydeven, A. P., R. N. Schultz, and R. P. Thiel. (1995). Monitoring a recovering gray wolf population in Wisconsin, 1979–1991. In *Ecology and Conservation of Wolves in a Changing World*, Occasional Publication No. 35, L. N. Carbyn, S. H. Fritts, and D. R. Seip (eds.). Edmonton, AB: Canadian Circumpolar Institute, pp. 147–156.

Wydeven, A. P., J. E. Weidenhoeft, B. E. Kohn, R. P. Thiel, R. N. Schultz, and S. R. Boales. (1999). Progress report of wolf population monitoring in Wisconsin for the period April–September 1999. Park Falls, WI: Wisconsin Department of Natural Resources, unpaginated. http://www.timberwolfinformation.org/updates/oct201999/october1999 wolfprogressreport.pdf.

Yin, S. (2002). A new perspective on barking in dogs (*Canis familiaris*). *Journal of Comparative Psychology* **116**: 189–193.

Yin, S. and B. McCowan. (2004). Barking in domestic dogs: context specificity and individual identification. *Animal Behaviour* **68**: 343–355.

Young, J. M. and B. J. Trask. (2007). V2R gene families degenerated in primates, dog and cow, but expanded in opossum. *Trends in Genetics* **23**: 212–215.

Young, J. M., M. Kambere, B. J. Trask, and R. P. Lane. (2005). Divergent V1R repertoires in five species: amplification in rodents, decimation in primates, and a surprisingly small repertoire in dogs. *Genome Research* **15**: 231–240.

Young, S. P. (1944). *The Wolves of North America, Part I. Their History, Life Habits, Economic Status, and Control.* New York, NY: Dover Publications, xvi + pp. 1–385. [1964 edition with corrections.]

Zimen, E. (1975). Social dynamics of the wolf pack. In *The Wild Canids: Their Systematics, Behavioral Ecology and Evolution*, M. W. Fox (ed.). New York, NY: Van Nostrand Reinhold, 336–362.

Zimen, E. (1976). On the regulation of pack size in wolves. *Zeitschrift für Tierpsychologie* **40**: 300–341.

Zimen, E. (1981). *The Wolf: A Species in Danger.* New York, NY: Delacorte, vi + 373 pp.

Zimen, E. (1982). A wolf pack sociogram. In *Wolves of the World: Perspectives of Behavior, Ecology, and Conservation*, F. H. Harrington and P. C. Paquet (eds.). Park Ridge, NJ: Noyes Publications, pp. 282–322.

Index

Note: page numbers in *italics* refer to figures and tables. Page numbers with suffix 'n' refer to Endnotes.

Aboriginal cultures 235–236, 310–311n
  hunting 238
accessory olfactory bulb (AOB) 61
accessory olfactory system (AOS)
      61–62
  size 65–66
admixture 1, 5, 241n
  see also named species
affective state 51, 56–57
  vocalizations 75
African wild dog (*Lycaon pictus*) xii
  dominant 43
  food loss to hyaenas 279n
  hunting 133–134
    technique 281n
  infanticide 105
  pack size 276n, 277n
  pack structure 277n
  stalking 280n
aggression 41
  ambivalent 49
  assault 51
  burden 255n
  captive wolves 222–223
    zoo animals 307n
  captivity 253n
  competitive 41
  conflicted 49
  dogs to strangers 196
  dominance relationship 252n
  free-ranging dogs 111–112, 234
  leadership 234
  littermate 189
  mating
    dingoes 167
    dogs 162, 164
  noncompetitive 41
  reproductive cycle 151
  territorial
    conspecific 95
    intraspecific 95
  threat 51

agonistic behavior 40–42n, 252n
  captive wolves 225
  dogs 55–56
  dominance 41, 52, 309n
  haptic 45
  pups 53
air temperature, activity of wolves 127
Algonquin wolf (*Canis lycaon*) xi, 4–5, 9, 14–15
  synonyms 5
Allee effect 11, 29, 243n
allelomimetic behavior, pups 210
alpha wolf 40n, 227, 252, 308n
  leadership 308n
altricial young 99
altruism 142, 193–204
  apparent 194
  dispersal impact 197
  helper advantages 202
  natural selection 299n
  pay-to-stay 200–201
  relatedness 195, 300n
  true 194
  see also fitness
anal glands
  dog 259n
  functions 68
  wolves 68
androgens 154–155, 289n
androstenedione 154–155, 289n
anestrus 180, 182
anosmia 71, 72–73
appeasement sounds 75–76
aromatic compounds, vomeronasal organ 254n
assault, aggression 51
attachment
  definitions 306n
  infantile 220, 229

bark-mobbing, dogs 262–263n
barking
  acoustical features 77–78
  acoustical range 80

co-adapted signaling hypothesis 82–83
  dogs 82–83, 261n, 262
    frequency 261n
    hypertrophied trait 263n
  frequency 261n
  function 81
  isolation 263n
  mammals 262n
  pitch 78
  pups 208–209, 210
  receivers 263n
  silver foxes 82
  wolves 74, *76*, *77*
basal metabolic rate (BMR) 119–120
  canids *120*, 275–240n
bear, brown
  attack by wolves 280n
  competitors of wolves 131
beggar harassment 189
behavior
  agonistic 40–42n, 52, 252n
    haptic 45
  conflicted 52
  definition 33
  learning 39–40
  ritual 255
  signals 39–40
black wolves 15–17
  melanism 245n
body postures, dominance/submission
    135, 227
body-sucking 207–208
body temperature, neonatal pups 206
bonding, socialization 212–221
bottle feeding 207–208
breed familiarity 300n
breeding
  waiting for opportunities 301n
  see also courtship; mating; pregnancy;
    reproductive cycles
breeding females, dominance 51–52
breeding success, wolves 188–189
brood parasites 203

caching of food
  dogs 137, 144
  wolves 136–137, 282n
Canidae family 1
canids 1
  admixing 5
  basal metabolic rate 119–120
  care-giving behavior 204
  society 205
Canis, groups 14–15
Canis aureus (golden jackal) 1
Canis himalayensis (Indian Himalayan wolf) 4
Canis indica (Indian plains wolf) 4

Canis latrans see western coyote (*Canis latrans*)
Canis lupus see gray wolf (*Canis lupus*)
Canis lupus lycaon (Algonquin wolf) *see*
  Algonquin wolf (*Canis lycaon*)
Canis lycaon (Algonquin wolf) *see* Algonquin
  wolf (*Canis lycaon*)
Canis simensis see Ethiopian wolf (*Canis simensis*)
cannibalism, wolves 136
captivity
  impact on behaviors 192
  see also owned dogs; wolves, captive
care-giving behavior 204
carnivores 1
  vomeronasal receptor function 65
cheating 199
  free-ranging dogs 234
chemosensory organs
  mouse *60*
  see also main olfactory bulb (MOB); main
    olfactory epithelium (MOE); vomeronasal
    organ
chimpanzee, theory of mind 260n
chorus-howls *85*, 87–88, 131–132, 265n
coefficient of relatedness 193, 300n
color of wolves 15–18
communication xiii, 33
  agonistic behavior 40–42
  channel 38–39
  definition 33
  global 230
  howling 304–305n
  local 230
  metaphors 33–38
  motivation–structural hypothesis 79, 80–81
    close-contact sounds *79*
    sound frequency 261
  physiological stress response 42–43
  semiotics 33–38
  tactile/visual signaling 43–58
  wolf howls 83–89
  see also olfactory communication; signals;
    vocalizations
competition
  leadership 310n
  male–male 162
  wolves 130–131
conception, dogs 180
conflicted behavior 52, *215*
contact-barks 82
cooperators, free-ranging dogs 234
corpora lutea 174, 176
  metestrus 293n
  monestrus 293–294n
  regression 180–181
corticosteroids 42–43
  dominant animals 43
cortisol *178*

courtship
  dingoes 165–167
  free-ranging dogs 163–167
  owned dogs 158–163
  wolves 167–173
  see also mating
coydogs 26–28
  admixtures 27, 249n
  haplotype 26
  paternal care 250n
  scarcity 26
coyote, red see red wolf (red coyote)
coyotes 2
  admixture
    with dogs 26, 29–30
    with gray wolf 6–7, 8–9
    with Great Lakes wolf 7, 11
  body size 14
  competitors of wolves 130–131
  dog haplotype 248n
  expansion 4
  genetic variation 2
  genetics 10, 11–12
  genome sequence 8
  gorging 275n
  hunting 309n
  inbreeding
    environmental barriers preventing
      10–11
    with Great Lakes wolf 7
  infanticide 270n
  mating
    with Great Lakes wolves 7, 10, 242n
    with red fox 292n
    with wolves 29
  mRNA 28
  mtDNA 11, 13
  paternal care 30
  pup socialization 208
  reverse pairings 11
  sex preference for humans 303n
  western 14–15
  see also eastern coyote
Cuon alpinus (dhole) see dhole (Cuon alpinus)
Cynomys ludovicianus (prairie dogs) 301n

dangerous prey hypothesis 137
decisions
  combined 230
  consensus 231
deer
  metatarsal glands 130
  tarsal glands 130
defecation
  pups 208
  scent marking 68–69
delayed reciprocity 199

dens
  dingoes 186–187
  free-ranging dogs 186–187
dens, wolf 182–185
  absence from 183
  captive females 307n
  digging 183, 295n
  entrance tunnels 184
  location 183–184
  migratory wolves 184–185
  occupancy 188
  pups 185
  range restriction in breeding season 187
  shape/size 183
  social meetings 304–305n
  terminology 296n
  usage 183, 184
dhole (Cuon alpinus) xii
  chorus-howls 265n
  whistle-call 77, 261, 264n
diestrus 174–175, 178, 293n
  cytological 293n
diet
  dingo-dogs 145
  dingoes 144–145, 146–147
  wolf 124–125, 138
    cannibalism 136
    garbage 136
    vegetable matter 135–136
dingo-dogs xin, 31–32, 251
  diet 145
  dispersal 114
  home range 114–115, 116
  philopatry 114
dingoes xi, xii, 1, 30–32, 236
  activity 109
  attack by camp dogs 238, 310n
  birth timing 166
  bite force 147
  body size 284–285n
  courtship 165–167
  dens 186–187
  diet 144–145, 146–147
  dispersal 114, 116–117
  distribution 31
  domestic livestock predation 148, 286n
  domestication 310n
  dominant/subordinate behaviours 57–58
  food requirement 145
  foraging 144–149
  gestation length 294n
  groups 285n, 286
    formation 111
    size 148
  home range 114–115n, 117–118n, 273–274n
  human food 236, 311n
  human relationships 235–236, 310, 311n

hunting 148–149, 286n
  with humans 236–237, 238
infanticide 105, *106*
interbreeding with dogs 31–32
mating 165–167
  with dogs 32
morphology 31–32, 250n
opportunist predators 147
origin 30n, 248n, 250n
pack formation 115–117n, 274n
philopatry 114, 117
predation 145–146
  group 285n
prey 144–145, 146–147, 285n
  availability 117–118
  injuries 147, 285–286n
  size 285n
rearing of pups 192
rendezvous sites 192
reproductive cycle 165–167
sexual maturity 167
social rank *57*
socialization 234–238
socializing with humans 235–236, 310n
territory 273–274n
trophic cascade 149
watering sites 117
see also pups, dingo
dispersal 2–3, 96, 98, 100–104
  across ice 102
  age 102
  altruism impact 197
  benefits 142
  delaying *96*, 201–202, 203
  dingo-dogs 114
  dingoes 114, 116–117
  distance 101–102, 269–270n
  ecological constraints 301n
  fitness 201
  genetic factors 138–139
  habitat-biased 3, 138–139
    prey-based 140
  inbreeding prevention 100
  inhibition 203
  limited 300n
  lions 197
  male-biased 282n
  models 302n
  offspring 204
  population dynamics 104
  from prey-carrying habitat 139
  prey density changes 100
  prey selection 138–141
  rate 93
  risks 201
  saturation impact 301n
  season 102–103, 104

sex bias 269n
siblings 101
socialization 213–214
temporary forays 104, 270n
wolves 96, 98, *101*
  delayed *96*, 201–202, 203
  immigration into other packs 103–104
  inability in captive animals 222
  integration with new pack 213–214
  migration following prey 140–141, 283n
  pack splitting 139–140
  from packs 98, *101*, 226–227
  rate 93
disturbance-barks 82
division of labor, wolf packs 231–232
dogs
  accessory olfactory system size 65–66
  admixing
    with coyotes 26, 29–30
    with wolves 29–30
  age categories 163, 290n
  aggression to strangers 196
  agonistic behavior 55–56
  anal glands 259n
  appearance of early animals 22
  arrival in North America 24, 248n
  Asian 248n
  attachment to humans 220
  bark distinction 83
  boxer genome 246n
  breeds
    modern 20, 21, 247n
    recent archaic 24, 247n
  coat variation 249n
  confinement 83
  early 21–26n, 247n
  food animal 247n
  fossil bone DNA 22
  fossil record 22–23, 247n
  gene flow 20
  genetic bottleneck 21, 22
  genetic diversity 20, 25
    loss 22
  genetic lines 25–26
  genome sequence *8*
  hairless 25, 247n
  haplogroups 21
  haplotypes 25
    diversity 21
  helping behavior 204
  human relationships 229, 308
  IGF-1 22
  interbreeding with dingoes 31–32
  interdigital glands 259n
  isolation 83
  jackal cross 239n
  lifespan 298n

dogs (cont.)
  macrosomatism 65
  main olfactory system 65–66
  Mesolithic *23*
  mRNA 28
  mtDNA 23–24, 29
  nuclear microsatellite markers 21
  odor reception 65
  origins *24*, 25–26n, 246, 248n
  Palaeolithic 22
  paternal care 30
  pet role 245n
  pheromone receptor genes 257–258n
  pheromones 261n
  reproductive phase shifting 29–30
  scent discrimination 65
  scent glands 259n
  selective breeding 55–56, 256n
  sex preference for humans 303n
  SNP studies 21–22
  social patterns 19
  socialization 205–212
  survival in Alaskan winter 250n
  tails 55, 56–57
  tameness 82
  tracking of human odor 258n
  use by man 29
  vomeronasal organ function 65
  wolf crosses 23–24
  wolfish morphology 55–56
  see also feral dogs; free-ranging dogs; *named*
    topics; owned dogs; pups, dog
domestic livestock *see* livestock, domestic,
    predation of
domestication
  dogs 19–21, 248n
    hypertrophied trait 263
    morphology changes 27–28
    timing 21
  silver foxes 82
  tameness selection in red fox 310n
  wolves 25
dominance 40
  aggression relationship 252n
  agonistic behavior 41, 52, 309n
  body postures 227
  breeding females 51–52
  competitive 161
  dingoes 57–58
  food 51
  formal 255, 309n
  free-ranging dogs 227–228
  mate choice 161
  mating dogs 161, 162–163, 164–165
  mating wolves 169, 188, 221, 292n
  situational 51–52
  social hierarchy 41, 255n

  stress levels 43
  submission association 42
  wolves 45, 225–226
    captive 221–222n, 223–225,
      306n, 307
    feeding 135
    mating 169, 188, 221, 292n
    in the wild 227
dominance hierarchies 41n, 54, 252, 255n
  captive animals 55, 222, 223–225
  free-ranging dogs 227
  leadership 229–230
  wolves 225–226

eastern coyote 12–15
  body size 14
  genetics 15
  jaws 13–14
  origins 244n
  sweat glands 13–14
effective population size, wolves 173
embryo implantation, dogs 176
estradiol 153–154, 289n
  diestrus 178
  LH surge *156*
estrogen 153
  dogs 175–176
estrus 155, 157, 289n
  behavioral/cytological 157
estrus groups, dogs 164, 165, 171–172
  attacks 291n
Ethiopian wolf (*Canis simensis*)
    1, 239n
Eurasian wolves 21
evolutionarily stable strategy (ESS) 204
excitement, vocalizations 215
experience 35
eye opening, pups 207

feeding
  pups 210
  socialization 210, 217
  wolves 121–122, 135–137, 281n, 298n
    caching of food 136–137, 282n
  see also food regurgitation
feral dogs 107–108n, 108–109, 271n
feralization 108–109, 271n
fertilization 290n
fitness 188
  direct 194, 196, 201
  dispersal 201
  helping behavior 204, 301–302n
  inclusive 194, 196
    enhancement 197
  indirect 194–195, 196, 201
flavor 66
flehmen response 63, 254n

follicle-stimulating hormone (FSH) 153–155, 175, 181, *182*
  pseudopregnancy 295n
food caches
  scent marking 67
  see also caching of food
food consumption, wolves 121
food regurgitation 204
  free-ranging dogs 191
  wolves 189, 190, 297n
    energy deficit 196
    at rendezvous sites 301n
food sharing 189
foraging 119
  competitors of wolves 130–131
  dingoes 144–149
  energy costs 119–121
  facultative by wolves 274n
  free-ranging dogs 142–149
  human societies 301n
  travel distance 122
  see also predation
formants 81
fossil record, dogs 22–23
fox, red
  coyote mating with 292n
  socialization 310n
  tameness selection 310n
fox, silver 263n
  barking 82
  domestication 82
free-ranging dogs
  acting together 227–228
  activity 109, 272n
    crepuscular 109
  affiliative relationships 310n
  attacks on cattle 284n
  behavior patterns 109
  cooperators 234
  definition xi
  owned 272n
  packs 273n
  parental care 228
  promiscuity 190
  resource availability 109
  rural 228
  scavenging 142–143, 144
  space use 107–118
  survivorship 191
  urban street dogs *110*, 112–115, *186*, 228
  see also dingoes; *named topics*
friendship
  free-ranging dogs 234
  wolves 234n, 305n, 309
fruit, foraging by wolves 135–136
functional reference 34

functional summation 77
fur farms, fox domestication 82, 310n

game theory
  cooperative hunting 141
  evolutionarily stable strategy 204
garbage scavenging
  free-ranging dogs *107*, 144
  wolves 136
genes, introgression 7
genetic bottleneck 21, 22
genetic drift 3
genetic relatedness *8*
  kin recognition 198
genetics xii
gestation
  body mass 180
  length 178–180, 294n
gonadal recrudescence 151, 157
gonadotropin 295n
  placental 293
gonadotropin-releasing hormone (GnRH) 181, 295n
Goyet Cave canid skull 22
gray wolf (*Canis lupus*) xi, xii, 14–15
  admixture with coyotes 6–7, 8–9
  ancestor of domestic dog 1
  arrival in North America 239–240n
  dispersal 2–3
    habitat-biased 3
  distribution 1
  dominant 43
  environmental barriers preventing inbreeding 10–11
  genetic variation 2, 3, 239–240n
  litter size 104
  modern 2–4
  mtDNA 241n
  origins 1, 239n
  persecution 2, 3
  population decline 2
  prey species 2
  races 4–5
  range 240n
  regional clusters 3
  relatives 1
  reverse pairings 11
  skull morphology 4–5
  treatment by man 2
  types 4–5
  variation in appearance 7
Great Lakes wolf xi, 4–7, 14–15, *16*
  admixture with coyotes 6–7, 11
  appearance 5–6
  foreign gene introgression 7
  genetic distinction from red wolf 9
  genetics 241n

Great Lakes wolf (cont.)
    genome 6, 7
    inbreeding with coyotes 7
    mating with coyotes 7, 10, 242n
    mtDNA 241n
    size 6–7, 241n
    species recognition barrier disintegration 7
greetings, harmonic sounds 75–76
ground-scratching 70, 260n
group augmentation 199, 200
group-ceremony 49–50, 131–132, 220–221
groups
    free-ranging dog 110–111
    leadership 230
    self-organizing 230

habitat-biased dispersal 138–139
habitats
    multiple-prey 282n
    prey-based bias 140
    saturation by wolves 96
Hamilton's rule 193, 300n
hamstringing 280–281n
    dingoes attacked by camp dogs
        238, 310n
haplogroups, dog 21
haplotypes, dog 25
    diversity 21
haptic agonistic behaviors 45
hearing, pups 207
helping behavior
    dogs 204
    fitness component 203–204
    obligate 203–204
    reproduction deferral 299n
helping behavior, wolves 193–204
    benefits to adolescents 202
    cross-fostering experiments 202–203
    delayed dispersal 201–202, 203
    energy deficit 196
    fitness 301–302n
    kinship theory 202
    reproductive success 204
homage, paying/receiving 52–53
home range 90, 265n
    dingo-dogs 114–115, 116
    dingoes 114–115n, 117–118n, 273–274n
    dogs 109
    free-ranging dogs 112–115n, 186, 273n
        urban street dogs 228
    size 265n
homesites 296n
hormones
    pregnancy 174
    scent marking 69–70
howling
    chorus-howls 85, 87–88, 131–132, 265n

communication 304–305n
    dogs 83
howls, wolf 83–89, 264–265n
    amplitude modulation 84
    attenuation 85–86
    captive animals 89, 263–264n
    chorus-howls 87–88
    degradation of sound 264n
    frequency modulation 84
    frequency range 76, 264n
    function 84
    induction by humans 87, 89
    recipients 84
    signals 84–89
    sound scattering 86
humans
    dingo relationships 235–236, 310,
        311n
        eating 236, 311n
        hunting with 236–237, 238
    dog relationships 229, 308n
        attachment 220
    sex preference by animals 303n
    wolf relationships 229, 305n
        following 305n
        lack of aggression to 219–220
        socialization 215–217, 220–221
        training 305n
hunting
    African wild dog 133–134
        technique 281n
    chase strategy 133–134
    cooperative 141–142
    coyotes 309n
    dingoes 148–149, 286n
        with humans 236–237, 238
    dogs 248n
    excitement 280n
    wolves 119, 131–137
        chase strategy 133–134
        cooperative 141–142, 281n
        group 132–134, 141–142
        lone 121
        preparation for 131–132, 280n
        risks 134–135
        scrounging 141n, 283n
        snow-covered ground 133, 276n
        stalking 132
        techniques 133–134, 280–281n
hyaenas 279n

inbreeding 19, 268n
    avoidance in wolves 170–173, 292n
    depression 172, 292n
    hazards in wolves 292n
    limiting mechanisms 101
    prevention by dispersal 100

Indian Himalayan wolf (*Canis himalayensis*)
    4, 240n
Indian plains wolf (*Canis indica*) 4
Indian wolf populations 4
indigenous wolf 241n
infanticide 99–100, 104–105n, 270n
    dingoes *106*
    lions 270n
infantile attachment 220, 229
information 37–38
    exchange 34–35
    transmission 34
        coding for 35
injuries, wolves during hunting 134–135
insulin-like growth factor 1 (IGF-1) 22
intentionality 34
interdigital glands 259n, 260n, 279n
interdigital pockets 129–130
interprant 36
    message processing 37
Isle Royal population of wolves 93–95
    colonization 93–95, 267n
    decline 142
    density 267n
    immigration 292–293n
    inbreeding 173
    population isolation 292–293n
    social behavior 142, 267n
    spatial organization 267n
isolation-barking 263n

jackal, domestic dog cross 239n
jackal, golden (*Canis aureus*) 1
jaw-snapping 209
jaws, eastern coyote 13–14

kin discrimination 193
kin recognition 193, 196, 197, 198–199
kin selection 193, 197
kinship, affiliative relationships 310n
kinship theory 199, 202–203
    helping behavior 202
    natural selection 197

lactation
    cortisol *178*
    progesterone *178*
    prolactin *178*
    pseudopregnancy 299
language 34
leadership 229–234
    aggression 234
    combined display 234
    competitive 310n
    consistent 309n
    definition 229, 230
    development 233

distributed 231, 233
dominance hierarchy 229–230
followers 233–234
free-ranging dogs 232–233, 309n
    competition 310n
    measurement 308n, 309–310
    personal 230
    teaching 232
    variable 309n
    wolves 231–232
        packs 231–232
leadership groups 230
learning 35, 232
    behavioral 39–40
    dominance submission continuum 42
    observational 232
licking-up *48*
    human caregivers 229
lions
    dispersal 197
    infanticide 270n
    territory 197
        defence 270n
litters, dingo 190
litters, dog 190–192
    communal rearing 190
    free-ranging 190–192
    size 190
litters, wolf 187–190
    aggression over food 189
    multiple 188
    number in pack 307n
    size 104, 187–188
livestock, domestic, predation of
    dingoes 148, 286n
    free-ranging dogs 143, 144
    wolves 126–127
loafing spots 296n
luteinizing hormone (LH) 153–155, 175
    baseline levels 181–182
    estrus *156*
    pregnancy *181*, 293
    proestrus *156*
        induction 182
    pseudopregnancy 176, 293, 295n
    reproductive cycle *181*
    surge *156*, 180n, 289n, 295
luteolysis 174
Lycaon pictus (African wild dog) *see* African wild
    dog (*Lycaon pictus*)

macrosomatism 65
main olfactory bulb (MOB) 60
    evolution 67–68
    mouse *60*
    oscillation frequency 67
    size 67–68

main olfactory epithelium (MOE) 60
  chemical signal detection 171–172, 292n
  mouse *60*
main olfactory system (MOS) 60, 61–62
  chemical signal detection 171–172
  dogs 65–66
major histocompatibility complex (MHC) genes 171
mallards 192, 299n
mating
  coyotes
    with Great Lakes wolves 7, 10, 242n
    with red fox 292n
    with wolves 29
  dingoes 165–167
  dogs 158–163
    age 157
    aggression 162
    with dingoes 32
    dominance 161, 162–163, 164–165
    estrus groups 164, 165, 171–172, 291n
    female choice 158–163, 164, 171–172
    free-ranging 163–167
    indiscriminate 290n
    male choice 163
    male–male competition 162
    monogamy 164
    owned 158–163
    promiscuous 290n
    with wolves 28–29
  wolves 150–151, 167–173
    age 157
    breeding pairs 168–169
    captive 169–170, 173, 221, 291n
    with coyotes 29
    with dogs 28–29
    dominance 169, 188, 221, 292n
    inbreeding avoidance 170–173, 292n
    monogamy 168–169
    submission 169, 188
melanism 245n
mental state concept 251n
messages 34–35
  meaning 35, 38
  processing 37
metaphors 33–38
  ambiguity 251n
  conduit 33, 35
metestrus 293n
Mexican gray wolf 7, 10, 11–12
Middle Eastern wolf 22
migration
  den use by wolves 184–185
  inability in captive wolves 222
  wolves following prey 140–141, 283n
mitochondrial DNA (mtDNA) 5, 6, 11
  dogs 23–24
  male-biased dispersal 282n

monestrus 287n, 293–294
monogamy
  dogs 164
  wolves 168–169, 201
motivation–structural hypothesis 79, 80–81
  close-contact sounds *79*
  sound frequency 262n
movement
  neonatal pups 207
  transitional pups 208
musk ox, attack by wolves 280n

natural selection 197
  altruism 299n
New Guinea singing dog xii
New World wolves 14–15
noise, signals 38–39
nonaggression, sounds 75–76

odor reception 59–66
  dogs 65
odorant receptors (ORs) 60, 61–62, 256n
  genes 60
    pseudogenization 63
odorants 59
  aromatic compounds 254n
  reproductive 151–153, 288n
  ungulate 129–130, 279n
Old World wolves 14–15
olfaction
  definition 256n
  neonates 303n
  see also accessory olfactory system (AOS);
    main olfactory bulb (MOB); main
    olfactory epithelium (MOE); main
    olfactory system (MOS); vomeronasal
    organ; vomeronasal receptors (V1Rs
    and V2Rs)
olfactory communication 59–73
  anal glands 68
  genes 60, *61*, 256n
  ground-scratching 70
  odor reception 59–66
  pheromones 59, 62–65
  pups 196
  rolling 70–71
  rubbing 70–71
  scent marking 66–73
    over-marking 72
  sniffing 71–73
  urination 69–70
    over-marking 72
olfactory receptors 256n
olfactory signals, behavioral response 62–63
olfactory system 60
  MHC genes 171
  primates 63

oocyte maturation 156–157, 290n
operant conditioning 251–252n
outbreeding 20
ovarian follicles 153–154
ovulation
  dogs 156–157n, 288n, 289n, 290
  wolves 155
owned dogs 111–112
  courtship 158–163
  rearing of pups 192
  scrounging 144
  socialization 211
  wolf predation 125–126

packs
  African wild dog
    size 276n, 277n
    structure 277n
  dingoes 115–117n, 274n
  free-ranging dogs 273n
packs, wolf 116
  behavior 226–227
  breeding unit 173
  budding 98, 197–198
  definition 96–97
  disintegration 97
  dispersal from 98, *101*, 226–227
    delayed *96*
    splitting 97–98, 139–140
  division of labor 231–232
  dynamics 96–99
  forms 98
  leadership 231–232
  leadership groups 230
  membership 97
  new 172
  number of litters 307n
  pups 185
    introduced 307n
  range restriction in breeding season 187
  relatedness 198
  rendezvous sites 185
  size 97–98n, 142, 266, 276n
    kill rate 123
  splitting 97–99, 139–140
  structure 120, 226–227
paedomorphism 19, 55, 229
  selection *20*
  signaling *56*
parental care, free-ranging dogs 228
parenting 174
pariah dogs 107
parturition
  cortisol *178*
  dogs 175–176, 178, 180
  progesterone *178*
  prolactin *178*

peck order 307n
pekin ducks 192, 299n
pets
  dogs 245n
  wolves/wolfdogs 304n
pheromones 59, 62–65
  behavioral response to signals 62–63
  definition 62
  detection 61–62
    absence from humans 257n
  dog 261n
  flehmen response 63, 254n
  functions 62
  gene repertoires *61*, 257–258n
  neonatal rats 302n
  vomeronasal organ 59, 64–65
philopatry 90
  dingoes/dingo-dogs 114, 117
photoperiod, reproductive cycles 176–177
physiological stress response 42–43
play
  functions 212–213, 304n
  object *210*
  socialization 212–221
    pups 208–209
  species differences 213
  wolves 212–217
    precocial 219
play-barks 82
play fighting, pups 208
play-solicitation 209
  conflicted behavior *215*
  dogs *214*, *215*
  wolves *214*
population limitation/regulation 276n
population size, wolf 92, 93
  crash 94–95
  effective 173
  infanticide 99–100, 104–105
  mechanisms of control
    extrinsic 100
    intrinsic 99
  natural controls 99–105
  non-admixed *3*
  prey availability 100, 267
  prey regulation 268–269n
  rate of increase 93
  reproductive suppression 104, 270n
  self-regulation 99
  spatial organization 267
prairie dogs (*Cynomys ludovicianus*) 301n
precocial offspring 99, 268n
predation, dingoes 145–146
  alternation *146*
  capture success 147–148
  domestic livestock 148
  groups 285n, 286

predation, dingoes (cont.)
  formation 111
  size 148
  hunting 148–149
  killing of surplus prey 148–149
  opportunist 147
  technique 286n
  see also hunting, dingoes
predation, free-ranging dogs 143
  domestic livestock 143, 144
predation, wolf 119–130
  air temperature 127
  caching of food 136–137, 282n
  diel activity 127–128
  dogs 278n
  domestic livestock 126–127
  encountering prey 141
  facultative foraging 274n
  functional response 276n
  futile chase 132–133
  kill rate 122–123, 276n
  lone wolves 109–110, 121, 125
  migration following prey 140–141, 283n
  movements 123–124, 127–128
  musk ox 280n
  on owned dogs 125–126
  prey diversity 124–125
  prey selection 134–135, 137–141
  rest time 122
  scavenging 131–137
  scrounging 141n, 283n
  search distance 123–124
  small game 277n
  in snow 133, 276n
  surplus killing 126
  travel distance 122
  ungulates 125, 126
    age/physical condition 124
    odorants 129–130
  see also hunting, wolves
predators, prey population effects 268–269n
pregnancy
  dogs 175–180
    body mass 180
    nutritional requirements 180
  hormones 174
  luteinizing hormone 181, 293
  prolactin 177, 179
  relaxin 177
prey
  abundance 137–138
  age 124
  availability 94
    dingoes 117–118
    pack size 266n
    population size 100, 267n
  dangerous 137

density and kill rate 122–123
dingoes 144–145, 146–147, 285n
  availability 117–118
  injuries 147, 285–286n
  size 285n
  surplus 148–149
diversity 124–125
ease of capture 282n
encountering by wolves 141
escaping 132–133
migration following 140–141, 283n
physical condition 124
predator population 268–269n
resource distribution 308n
selection 134–135, 137–141
size 120
vulnerable 276n
wounded 132
prey-based habitat bias 140
prey–predator relationships 276n
primates
  olfactory system 63
  theory of mind 260n
  trichromatic vision 257n
proestrus
  dingoes 291n
  dogs 151, 287–288, 290n
  wolves 287–288
progesterone 153–154, 175–176, 293
  lactation 178
  LH surge 295n
  peripartum 178
  proestrus/estrus 156
prolactin 176–177
  lactation 178
  peripartum 178
  pregnancy 177, 179
  wolves 179
pseudopregnancy 174–175, 176, 299
  follicle-stimulating hormone 295n
  lactation 299
  luteinizing hormone 176, 293, 295n
  progesterone 293
  wolves 195–196
punishment, socialization impact 217
pups
  agonistic behavior 53
  allelomimetic behavior 210
  barking 208–209, 210
  coyotes 208
  defecation 208
  eye opening 207
  feeding 210
  hearing 207
  jaw-snapping 209
  movement 207, 208
  play 208–209

play fighting 208
scent trail following 210
socialization 205–212
   coyotes 208
   isolated pups 211
urination 208
vocalizations 206–207
weaning 210
pups, dingo
   growth of litters *106*
   litter size 190
   rearing 192
   recognition of removed pups 195
pups, dog
   agonistic behavior 53
   behavioral development 303n
   bottle feeding 207–208
   communal rearing 190
   litters 190–192
      communal rearing 190
      size 190
   neonatal behavior 303n
   rearing 191
      male involvement 191–192
   recognition
      of mother/littermates 196
      of removed pups 195
   regurgitation of food by adults 191
   socialization 205–212
      adolescent 212
      critical stage 208–212
      neonatal stage 206–207
      transitional stage 207–208
   survivorship 191, 298n
   urination 208, 304n
pups, free-ranging dog
   communal rearing 190
   litters 190–192
   mortality 228
   parental care 228
   rearing 191
   regurgitation of food by adults 191
   survivorship 191, 298n
pups, wolf 185–186, 187–190
   agonistic behavior 53
   bond with adults 217–219
   growth 296n
   litters 187–190
      aggression over food 189
      multiple 188
      size 104, 187–188
   mobbing of adult 189–190
   play 212–217, 219
   rearing 188–190, 301n
   recognition of removed pups 195
   regurgitation of food by adult
      189, 190

removal from mother 217–218
rendezvous sites 185–186, 189
scent-trail following 210, 303n
socialization 205–212
   adolescent 212
   critical stage 208–212
   neonatal stage 206–207
   transitional stage 207–208

radial olfactory gradient field 72
ravens, competitors of wolves 130
recognition, individual 195
red wolf (red coyote) xin, 8–12, 242
   diet 9
   distribution 243n
   genetic distinction from Great Lakes wolf 9
   genome 8
   genotype 9–10
   origins 9–10, 15, 243n
   skull 243n
   status 9–10
   vocalization 9
referent 36, 37
relatedness 300n
   altruism 195, 300n
   coefficient 193, 300n
relaxin *177*
rendezvous sites
   dingoes 192
   terminology 296n
   wolves 185–186, 301n
      occupancy 185
      pups 185–186, 189
reproductive cycles 150–158
   dingoes 165–167
      birth timing *166*
      proestrus 291n
   dogs 156–158, 174–182
      anestrus 180, 182
      conception 180
      courtship 158–167
      dens 186–187
      diestrus 174–175, 178
      duration 157–158
      embryo implantation 176
      estrogen 175–176
      gestation 180
      gestation length 178–180
      LH surge 180n, 289n
      luteal phase 174–175
      luteolysis 174
      monestrous 287n
      ovarian quiescence 180–181
      ovulation 156–157n, 288n, 289n, 290
      photoperiod 176–177
      proestrus 151, 182, 287–288n
      progesterone 175–176

reproductive cycles (cont.)
  prolactin 176–177
  testosterone *154*
fertilization 290n
monestrus 287n, 293–294
odorants 151–153
wolves 150–155
  breeding success 188–189
  courtship 167–173
  dens 182–185, 188
  effective population size 173
  estrus 155
  female 151, 153
  gestation length 178–180
  gonadal recrudescence 151, 157
  litter size 104, 187–188
  litters 187–190
  ovulation 155
  photoperiod 176–177
  proestrus 287–288
  prolactin 178
  puberty 151, 287n
  rendezvous sites 185–186
  reproductive life 187
  sexual maturity 169
  spermatogenesis 151
  timing 177
  visible signs 153
  see also lactation; mating; parturition;
      pregnancy; pseudopregnancy
reproductive phase shifting, dogs 29–30
reproductive success 188–189
  cost/benefits 301–302n
  helping behavior 204
reproductive suppression 104, 270n
reptiles, vomeronasal organ 257n, 258
ritual behavior 255
rodents
  accessory olfactory system size 65–66
  mouse chemosensory organs *60*
  vomeronasal organ 64–65
runways 266n
  urine-marking 271n

scats, wolf 68–69
scavenging 119
  free-ranging dogs 142–143, 144
  wolves 136–137, 279n
    marine mammals 140
scent discrimination, dogs 65
scent glands
  dogs 259n
  ground-scratching 260n
  see also anal glands
scent marking 66–73
  anal glands 68
  conspecifics 258n

counterproductivity 66
defecation 68–69
definition 258n
food caches 67
functions 66–67
ground-scratching 70
hormone-driven 69–70
territorial boundaries 67
urination 69–70
scent-posts, response to 72
scent trails, following by pups 210, 303n
scrounging 199–200
  owned dogs 144
  wolves 141n, 283n
self-organizing groups 230
semiotic triangle *47*
semiotics 33–38
  definition 35
separation anxiety 220
signaling *56*
  co-adapted signaling hypothesis 82–83
  quantum 251n
  tactile 43–58
  tails 55, 56–57, 256n
  visual 43–58
  vocal 84–89
signals 37, 38
  behavior 39–40
  definition 33, 251n
  degrading 264n
  encoding 35
  information value 38, 251, 260n
  interpretation 35, 38
  noise 38–39
  primary 39–40
  reinforcement 35
  representational symmetry 34
  response 38–40, 251–252n
  secondary 39–40
  vocalization 78–79
signs, semiotic 35–36, 37
single nucleotide polymorphisms (SNPs) 3
  dog origins 21–22, *24*
skull 241n
  morphology of gray wolf 4–5
  red wolf 243n
sniffing 71–73, 256n
social behavior xiii
  defensive 303n
  inclusive fitness enhancement 197
social familiarity 195
social hierarchy 54, 252n
  captive animals 55, 222, 223–225
  wolves 221–227
  see also dominance; submission; subordinate
      animals
social mammals 193–194

social repression, wolves 200–201
social stress 252n
socialization 205
    bonding 212–221
    dingoes 234–238
    dispersal 213–214
    dogs 205–212
        attachment to humans 220
        isolated pups 211
        owned 211
        pups 205–212
    feeding 210, 217
    foxes 310n
    infantile attachment 220, 229
    leadership 229–234
    mutual reinforcement 217–219
    pair bonds 218–219
    play 212–221
    punishment impact 217
    sequence 205–212
    wolves 205–212
        captive 211, 221–227
        deprivation 304n
        with humans 215–217, 220–221
        pups 205–212
sound
    attenuation of signal 85–86
    close-contact 79
    degrading of signal 264n
    frequency 262n
    generation 81
    scattering 86
    see also motivation–structural
        hypothesis
sounds, wolf 76, 80, 86
    bark 74, 76, 77
    categories 75–76, 262
    chorus-howls 85, 87–88, 131–132, 265n
    low-frequency 79–80
    squeaking 79–80
    whines 75–76, 79–80, 262n
space
    use of 90–95
        free-ranging dogs 107–118
    see also territorial boundaries; territory;
        territory, wolves
species 242
species-identification 303n
spermatogenesis, wolves 151
stalking
    African wild dog 280n
    hunting wolves 132
startle response 209
starvation 121
stray dogs 108, 271n
stress, social 252n
stress response, physiological 42–43

submission 40
    active 46–48, 52–53
        pups 209
    agonistic behavior 41
    body postures 135, 227
    captive wolves 223–225
    definition 252
    dingoes 57–58
    dominance association 42
    formal 255
    mating wolves 169, 188
    passive 46–48, 50–51
    sounds 75–76, 262n
    wolves 45, 225–226
subordinate animals
    behaviors 229
    breeding 252n
    feeding wolves 135
    stress levels 43
    suppression of females 104
sucking frustration 207–208
sweat glands, eastern coyote 13–14
sympatry 6

tactile signaling 43–58
tail-wagging, wolves 215
tails, signaling 55, 56–57, 256n
tameness 205
tastants 66
taste 59, 66
    neonates 303n
taste papillae 66
taste receptors (TRs) 66
teaching, leadership 232
territorial boundaries
    monitoring 91, 92
    olfactory map 72
    scent marking 67
    self-regulation of population 99
    social fence 98
    urine-marking 73
territoriality 265n
    free-ranging dogs 109–110, 111, 272n
    resources 308n
territory 90, 265n
    defense by females 99
        lions 270n
    defense by free-ranging dogs 227–228
    dingoes n, 273–274n
    females 99–100
    runways 266n
        urine-marking 271n
    size 99
territory, wolves 90–95
    aggression
        conspecific 95
        intraspecific 95

territory, wolves (cont.)
 defence 95
 disputes 95–96
 habitat saturation 96
 monitoring of periphery 91, 92
 overlapping 92, 95
  pack splitting 98
 population size 93
 size 91–92
 social fence 104, 105–107
 travel routes 92–93
 see also dispersal; population size, wolf
testosterone 154–155, 289, 292n
theory of mind 33–34
 chimpanzee 260n
thermotaxis 206
thigmotaxis 206
threat, aggression 51
touch, neonatal pups 206
trace amino-associated receptors (TAARs) 60
Tweed wolf 4

ungulates
 interdigital pockets 129–130
 odorants 129–130, 279n
 organization 309n
 predation by free-ranging dogs 143
 predation by wolves 124, 125, 126,
  129–130
  selection of prey 134–135, 137–138
  stalking 132
urination, pups 208, 304n
urination/urine-marking
 courtship 288n, 152–153
 effectiveness 106–107
 flexed-leg 69–70
 model *73*
 odorants 288n
  courtship 152–153, 288n
 over-marking 72, 271n
 postures 69–70n, 259n
 raised-leg 69, 106, 259n
 random walk modeling 106–107, 271n
 runways 271n
 social fence marking 105–107
 squat 69
 standing 69
 volume 259n

vegetation, foraging by wolves 135–136
vision
 trichromatic 257n
 wolves 128–129
visual behaviors 45
visual signaling 43–58
 ground-scratching 70
 vocalization association 77

vocal tract 81
vocalizations 35, 37, 73–89
 acoustic continuum 78
 affective 75, *76*
 categories 75–76
 context-specific 263n
 emotional range 81, 260–261n
 evaluation by conspecifics 80
 excitement 215
 formants 81
 frequency *76*, 77–78
 functional summation 77
 functions 74–75
 groans as distress signal 303n
 harmonic 80–81
 information value 38, 251, 260n
 motivation-structural hypothesis 79
 neonatal pups 206–207
 onomatopoeic 261n
 ontogeny 81
 receivers 74, 84, 263n
 referential 75, 82
 signals 78–79, 84–89
 sound complexity 81
 sound generation 81
 species-specific 263n
 stereotypical 78
 visual signal association 77
 see also barking; chorus-howls; dogs, barking;
  howling; howls, wolf; sounds, wolf;
  whines, wolf
vomeronasal organ 61
 animal groups 63
 aromatic compounds 254n
 chemical signal detection 171–172
 function 63, 257, 289n
  dogs 65, 257n
 pheromone uptake 59, 64–65
 reptiles 257n, 258
 rodents 64–65
 snakes 258n
 types 257n
vomeronasal receptors (V1Rs and V2Rs) 62,
  63–65, *64*, 289n,
 function in carnivores 65
 pseudogenes 65

watering sites, dingoes 117
weaning, pups 210
western coyote (*Canis latrans*) 14–15
whines, wolf 75–76, 79–80, 262n
whistle-call, dhole 77, 261, 264n
white wolves 17
wolfdog xi
 pet 304n
 predation on ungulates 143
wolverines, competitors of wolves 130

wolves
  activity 127, *128*
  admixing with dogs 29–30
  adolescent 202
    socialization 212
  anal glands 68
  basal metabolic rate 119–120, 275–240n
  bond with pups 217–219
  captive 89, 259n
    aggression 222–223
    agonistic behavior 225
    artifacts 221
    dominance 221–222n, 223–225, 306n, 307
    hierarchy 222, 223–225
    inability to emigrate 222
    inbreeding 173
    socialization 211
    submission 223–225
  conflicted behavior *50*
  distance travelled *128*
  dog crosses 23–24
  fitness 188
  food consumption 121
  friendship 234n, 305n, 309
  genome sequence *8*
  group augmentation 200
  in harness 249n
  helping behavior 193–204
  hierarchies 225–226
  indigenous 241n
  interactions 45
  lack of aggression to humans
      219–220
  leadership 231–232

  lifespan 187
  lone 109–110, 121, 125
    Arabia 277n
    attacking dogs 278n
    dispersal 142
    pairing 167, 307n
  migratory 91
  mRNA 28
  mtDNA 247n
  pair bonds 218–219
  paternal care 30
  pet 304n
  rest time 122
  scats 68–69
  sex preference for humans 303n
  societies 45
  starvation 121
  tail-wagging 215
  tails 55, 256n
  training by humans 305n
  travel distance 122
  urban areas 279n
  vision 128–129
  wounded 282n
  zoo animals 222–225
  see also named topics

xoloitzcuintle (hairless dog) 25, 247n

Y chromosome markers 242n

zoo animals 221
  wolves 222–225
    aggression 307n